a CORE Curriculum for Diabetes Education

Fifth Edition

Diabetes in the Life Cycle and Research

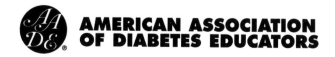

AMERICAN ASSOCIATION OF DIABETES EDUCATORS

a **CORE**
Curriculum
for Diabetes
Education
Fifth Edition

Diabetes in the Life Cycle and Research

Editor
Marion J. Franz, MS, RD, LD, CDE

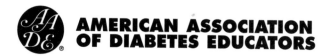

AMERICAN ASSOCIATION
OF DIABETES EDUCATORS

a CORE Curriculum for Diabetes Education, 5th Edition
Diabetes in the Life Cycle and Research
Published by the American Association of Diabetes Educators

©2003, American Association of Diabetes Educators, Chicago, Illinois.
ISBN 1-881876-14-4 (Volume Four)
ISBN 1-881876-15-2(Four-Volume Set)

Library of Congress Control Number: 2003108781

Printed and bound in the United States of America.

The information contained in a CORE Curriculum for Diabetes Education, 5th Edition is based on the collective experience of the diabetes educators who assisted in its production. Reasonable steps have been taken to make it as accurate as possible based on published evidence as of June 2003. But the Association cannot warrant the safety or efficacy of any product or procedure described in a CORE Curriculum for Diabetes Education, 5th Edition for application in specific cases. Individuals are advised to consult an appropriate healthcare professional before undertaking any diet or exercise program or taking any medication referred to in a CORE Curriculum for Diabetes Education, 5th Edition. Healthcare professionals must use their own professional judgment, experience, and training in applying the information contained herein. The American Association of Diabetes Educators and its officers, directors, employees, agents, and members assume no liability whatsoever for any personal or other injury, loss, or damages that may result from use of a CORE Curriculum for Diabetes Education, 5th Edition.

COPYRIGHT ADDENDUM
If you would like to make a request for permission to reproduce information from a CORE Curriculum for Diabetes Education, 5th Edition for non-commercial, not-for-profit, educational purposes meeting the requirements listed above, please call 1-800-338-3633 or e-mail products@aadenet.org.

a CORE Curriculum for Diabetes Education

Diabetes in the Life Cycle and Research

In this Volume:

Table of Contents

Diabetes in the Life Cycle and Research

Introduction/Acknowledgements

It is an exciting and challenging time for diabetes education. Exciting because of the many advances that help people better manage their diabetes—new medications, technologies, research that makes lifestyle recommendations easier to understand and apply, the empowerment approach to education, to name just a few. The challenges and frustrations are the difficulties of sharing this information with individuals with diabetes, the lack of opportunities to individualize care, and the lack of time to assist in facilitating behavior changes. Resources—personnel, payment for services, maintaining education centers—are other challenges. The CORE Curriculum cannot solve all the challenges, but it can update healthcare providers' knowledge and skills and provide suggestions for facilitating behavior changes in persons with diabetes.

The CORE Curriculum was originally planned to help educators prepare for the Certified Diabetes Educator (CDE) exam. This has continued to be a goal for subsequent editions; however, the use and the scope of the CORE Curriculum has expanded. It is a key reference for the Advanced Diabetes Management credential exam. The CORE Curriculum has also evolved into being an authoritative source of information for diabetes education, training, and management. Just as all medicine is moving toward evidence-based practice, this must also be a goal for education. Chapters must have appropriate and adequate references, and as a reader you have the right to question statements in the CORE Curriculum that do not have adequate documentation. Continuing this focus will result in the CORE Curriculum becoming more evidence-based. Another goal is to have the CORE Curriculum reflect a team approach to education and management. It is exciting to see the number of management chapters written by a team of healthcare providers.

As with all projects of this size, there are many individuals to whom we are indebted. It begins with the chapter authors, who are willing to share their expertise and provide up-to-date information and management skills for the reader. It continues to the chapter reviewers, who provide suggestions to make the chapters stronger. The authors and reviewers are listed in each volume of the CORE Curriculum. When you see these individuals, please extend your thanks to them for the valuable service they provide. The Editorial Board—Janine Freeman, Barbara McCloskey, Charlotte Nath, and William Polonsky—provide suggestions to improve the CORE Curriculum and valuable reviewer assistance. Dr. Lois Book, RN, Director of Professional Relations, at the AADE National Office provides valuable suggestions for CORE content and support for the process of writing and editing of the CORE Curriculum. We are fortunate to work with very competent editorial and publishing professionals. Mary Beach at Stenson Bauer Communications keeps the process moving efficiently. Nancy Williams uses her copyreader and editing skills to make sure small details and mistakes are not missed. Karen Lloyd provides editorial assistance for the new chapters, and Michele Montour at Montronics makes sure text is accurately typeset. To all these important professionals, the AADE owes a great deal of gratitude.

The CORE Curriculum would not be possible without the contributions of previous editors—Diana Guthrie, Julie Meyer, Kathryn Godley, Virginia Peragallo-Dittko, and Martha Funnell. Each edition moved the professionalism of the CORE Curriculum forward, and those who worked on this edition sincerely hope to have continued that tradition. As authors, reviewers, and editors, we have done our best to make this edition a valuable resource for all diabetes educators and healthcare providers. We welcome suggestions from you as you read and use the CORE Curriculum as to how it can become a better and more useful resource. Please use the CORE Curriculum to improve the education and care that you provide for people with diabetes. That ultimately is the final goal, to enrich the lives of persons with diabetes who have been, for all of us, our best educators!

Marion J. Franz, MS, RD, LD, CDE
Editor, CORE Curriculum, 5th Edition

Authors

Susan A. Biastre,
RD, LDN, CDE
Women & Infants Hospital
Providence, Rhode Island

Angela D'Antonio, RD
University of South Carolina
Norman J. Arnold School
of Public Health
Columbia, South Carolina

James A. Fain,
PhD, RN, BC-ADM, FAAN
University of Massachusetts
Worcester
Graduate School of Nursing
Worcester, Massachusetts

Stephanie H. Gerken,
RD, LD, CDE
International Diabetes Center
Minneapolis, Minnesota

Carol Homko,
RN, PhD, CDE
Temple University Hospital
Philadelphia, Pennsylvania

Elizabeth J. Mayer-Davis,
PhD, RD
University of South Carolina
Norman J. Arnold School of
Public Health
Columbia, South Carolina

Terri McGee, MS, RD, CDE
Children's Hospital of
Pittsburgh
Pittsburgh, Pennsylvania

Anne T. Nettles,
RN, MS, CDE
Diabetes CareWorks
Minneapolis, Minnesota

Jean Betschart Roemer,
MSN, MN, CPNP, CDE
Children's Hospital of
Pittsburgh
Pittsburgh, Pennsylvania

Karin R. Sargrad,
MS, RD, CDE
Temple University Hospital
Philadelphia, Pennsylvania

Laura Shane-McWhorter,
PharmD, BCPS, FASCP,
BC-ADM, CDE
College of Pharmacy
University of Utah
Salt Lake City, Utah

Julie Slocum, RN, MS, CDE
Women & Infants Hospital
Providence, Rhode Island

Susan L. Sullivan,
RN, BSN, CDE
Driscoll Children's Hospital
Corpus Christi, Texas

Catrine Tudor-Locke, PhD
University of South Carolina
Norman J. Arnold School of
Public Health
Columbia, South Carolina

Reviewers

Jo Ann Ahern,
APRN, MSN, CDE
Yale–New Haven Hospital
Yale University/Pediatric
Endocrinology
New Haven, Connecticut

Mary Jo Dudley,
RN, BSN, CDE
Diabetes Education Center
Lamprey Health Care
Dover, New Hampshire

Alison B. Evert, RD, CDE
Joslin Diabetes Center and
Woodinville Pediatrics
Seattle and Woodinville,
Washington

Janine Freeman,
RD, LD, CDE
Diabetes Nutrition Specialist
Atlanta, Georgia

Barbara A. McCloskey,
PharmD, BCPS, CDE
Diabetes Services
Baylor Medical Center
Irving, Texas

Susan McLaughlin, RD, CDE
On-Site Health and
Wellness, LLC
Omaha, Nebraska

Charlotte R. Nath,
MSN, RN, EdD, CDE
West Virginia University
Department of Family
Medicine
Robert C. Byrd Health
Sciences Center
Morgantown, West Virginia

Carol Henderson Nelson,
RN, BSN, CDE
Cottage Health
System/Education
Santa Barbara Cottage
Hospital
Santa Barbara, California

Belinda O'Connell,
MS, RD, CDE
Diabetes Nutrition Specialist
Hudson, Wisconsin

William H. Polonsky,
PhD, CDE
Department of Psychiatry
University of California
San Diego, California

Barbara Schreiner,
RN, MN, BC-ADM, CDE
Texas Children's Hospital
Diabetes Care Center
Houston, Texas

Madelyn L. Wheeler,
MS, RD, CD, FADA, CDE
Department of Medicine,
Division of Endocrinology
Indiana University School
of Medicine
Indianapolis, Indiana

Judy Wylie-Rosett, EdD, RD
Epidemiology and
Population Health
Albert Einstein College of
Medicine
Bronx, New York

A Core Curriculum for Diabetes Education
Diabetes in the Life Cycle and Program Management

Lifestyle for Diabetes Prevention

1

Elizabeth J. Mayer-Davis, PhD, RD
Angela D'Antonio, BS, RD
Catrine Tudor-Locke, PhD
University of South Carolina, Norman J. Arnold School of Public Health
Columbia, South Carolina

Introduction

1 The prevalence of type 2 diabetes, pre-diabetes, and the metabolic syndrome is increasing rapidly.[1-4] In 1991, the prevalence of diabetes was 4.9%. By 1999, the prevalence had increased to 6.9% and by 2001, the prevalence further increased to 7.9%, a 61% increase from 1990.[2] The prevalence of pre-diabetes, the stage between normal glucose regulation and diabetes, among adults ages 40 to 74 is approximately 15.8% with the highest rates in the 60 to 74 age range.[3] It is also estimated that approximately 22% of US adults have the metabolic syndrome.[4]

2 The increase in occurrence of type 2 diabetes is associated with an increasing prevalence of overweight and obesity, physical inactivity, and pre-diabetes.[1] In 1991, the prevalence of obesity (BMI >30 kg/m^2) was 12.0%. By 2001, the prevalence increased to 20.9%.[2] Similar trends have been observed for diagnosed diabetes.

3 Scientific evidence is accumulating that lifestyle modifications for sustained, moderate weight loss through a low-fat, hypocaloric diet, regular physical activity, and programs that provide regular participant contact and education can markedly reduce the incidence of type 2 diabetes.[5-8]

4 Although conclusive evidence is lacking, reducing the intake of total fat (particularly saturated fat), increasing the intake of whole grains and dietary fiber, and increasing physical activity may improve insulin sensitivity and reduce the risk of diabetes, independent of obesity.

5 The American Association of Diabetes Educators[9] (AADE) and the American Diabetes Association[10] (ADA) have issued statements supporting the role of lifestyle strategies and education in prevention of type 2 diabetes.

A The AADE white paper[9] states that those at risk for diabetes can individually benefit from working with a diabetes educator to heighten their knowledge, to assess their risk, and to mutually establish goals and strategies to reduce their risk and maintain good health practices.

B The ADA[10] concluded that individuals at high risk of developing diabetes can be identified early. Diabetes prevention policies that focus on lifestyle modifications, specifically modest weight loss and increased physical activity, are very likely to have additional health benefits. Public health messages, healthcare providers, and healthcare systems should all encourage behavior changes to achieve a healthy lifestyle.

6 The Executive Summary of the Clinical Guidelines on the Identification, Evaluation, and Treatment of Overweight and Obesity in Adults,[11] prepared by the National Institutes of Health (NIH) and based on extensive review of the literature to date, indicates that a combined intervention of behavior therapy with a low-calorie diet and increased physical activity constitutes the most successful therapy for weight loss and maintenance.

7 Both the Centers for Disease Control (CDC) and the NIH have initiated studies to determine the prevalence, incidence, and risk factors for type 2 diabetes in youth and its complications. Evidence for effective lifestyle approaches for preventing type 2 diabetes in youth is insufficient at this time to justify specific recommendations.

8 Evidence for preventing type 1 diabetes is insufficient at this time to justify specific recommendations. Therefore, this chapter focuses on weight management through a hypocaloric, low-fat diet and regular physical activity for preventing type 2 diabetes in adult populations.

Objectives

Upon completion of this chapter, the learner will be able to

1 Identify individuals likely to be at increased risk for type 2 diabetes.

2 Discuss observational and intervention studies supporting lifestyle strategies for diabetes prevention.

3 Identify community and healthcare facility issues that may impact the potential success of weight-management strategies (either individual or community based) for preventing type 2 diabetes.

4 Explain how lifestyle interventions to reduce type 2 diabetes risk need to address cultural and familial influences that affect food and physical activity choices.

5 Collaborate with the individual to determine appropriate weight-management goals, considering both short-term and long-term goals, and emphasizing the potential benefit of sustained moderate weight loss.

6 Collaborate with the individual to develop an appropriate nutrition/food plan to meet weight-management goals and nutritional adequacy for overall health.

7 Collaborate with the individual to develop an appropriate physical activity plan to meet weight-management goals.

8 Respond appropriately to questions regarding the use of weight-loss medications and surgery for weight loss, considering both safety and efficacy.

9 Respond appropriately to questions regarding popular diets and nutritional supplements, considering both safety and efficacy.

Identifying Individuals at High Risk

1 Individuals with a positive family history of type 2 diabetes have an increased risk of type 2 diabetes. The occurrence of multiple cases of diabetes within a family can be the result of genetic susceptibility, shared environment or lifestyles that increase the risk of diabetes, or, most likely, a combination of genetic and behavioral influences.

2 Individuals who are overweight or obese may be at high risk for type 2 diabetes.

A Based on body mass index (BMI, kg/m^2), the current classification of overweight and obesity in adults from the NIH is as follows[11]:

Classification	BMI (kg/m^2)
Underweight	<18.5
Normal	18.5 to 24.9
Overweight	25.0 to 29.9
Obese	>30.0

B Asian Americans with a BMI >22 kg/m^2 can be considered at high risk for type 2 diabetes.[12] Intraabdominal fat deposition is associated with insulin resistance and risk of cardiovascular disease, independent of total adiposity. Although Asian Americans' BMI may not place them in a high risk category for type 2 diabetes, intraabdominal fat distribution may (see next paragraph).

3 Individuals who have increased central (ie, visceral) obesity, which is deposited around abdominal organs, appear to have a greater risk for type 2 diabetes than those with subcutaneous fat. Intraabdominal obesity has a greater supply of capillaries, making it more metabolically active than subcutaneous fat or fat in the hips and thighs. As a result, there is a greater flux or turnover of free fatty acids (FFA). In the liver, these FFA contribute to insulin resistance (lipotoxicity). Furthermore, FFA may be used as a fuel source instead of glucose, thus contributing to hyperglycemia.

A Based on waist circumference, the current classification of central obesity in men and women from the NIH is as follows[11]:

Waist circumference

Men >102 cm (>40 in)

Women >88 cm (>35 in)

B The vast majority of individuals who meet the current criteria for central obesity are also overweight or obese and, thus, would be candidates for diabetes prevention strategies focused on weight management.

C There is insufficient evidence for interventions that uniquely address central obesity, independent of overall obesity. Thus, the focus for diabetes prevention in centrally obese individuals would be reduction in overall fat mass (including visceral fat deposits) through healthy eating and physical activity.

4 Native Americans, Hispanics/Latinos, African Americans, Asian Americans, and Pacific Islanders are all at higher risk for type 2 diabetes than Caucasians.[3]

A Native Americans have a fivefold increase in risk for the development of type 2 diabetes. In American Indians and Alaska Natives the prevalence varies among tribes, bands, pueblos and villages and ranges from 5% to 50% for diagnosed diabetes.

B The risk in Hispanic Americans, particularly individuals of either Puerto Rican or Mexican origin, is approximately 2.5 times higher than in Caucasians.

C The risk for US African Americans is increased twofold.

D Diabetes is an emerging problem among Asian Americans and Pacific Islanders, who are more likely to have diabetes than Asians in their countries of origin.

5 Individuals with either impaired fasting glucose (IFG) or impaired glucose tolerance (IGT) are at high risk for type 2 diabetes. The recommended terminology for this group is pre-diabetes.

A Current American Diabetes Association (ADA) guidelines define IFG as a fasting glucose level between 110 mg/dL and 125 mg/dL (6.1 and 6.9 mmol/L).[13]

B Current ADA guidelines define IGT as a 2-hour post-75-g glucose load glucose concentration of between 140 mg/dL and 199 mg/dL (7.8 and 11.0 mmol/L).

C Over a 5-year period, approximately 30% to 40% of individuals with IGT or IFG develop type 2 diabetes.

6 The incidence of diabetes also increases rapidly with age. Factors that predispose the older adult to diabetes include age-related decreases in insulin and insulin sensitivity, adiposity, decreased physical activity, multiple prescription medications, and coexisting illnesses.

7 Women with a diagnosis of gestational diabetes have a 40% to 60% chance of developing type 2 diabetes as they age.[14] This prevalence rate can be reduced to 25% with appropriate weight loss and physical activity.

  A The prevalence of gestational diabetes varies based on both the population of interest and the diagnostic criteria utilized.[15]

  B Prevalence estimates range between 1% to 14% of all pregnancies.[15]

Evidence for Type 2 Diabetes Prevention

1 Given the importance of lifestyle factors in the development of diabetes, type 2 diabetes would appear to be a largely preventable disease. Evidence to support this comes from both observational studies and clinical trials.

2 Observational studies addressing physical activity, weight loss, and dietary intake have provided evidence for factors that can delay or prevent type 2 diabetes.

  A An active lifestyle prevents or delays the development of type 2 diabetes and has been demonstrated in a number of prospective studies.[16-20] The effect persists after adjusting for BMI. Based on observational studies, it appears that a 30% to 50% reduction in risk would be associated with regular or vigorous exercise versus a sedentary lifestyle.[21]

  - Protection from diabetes occurs from moderate-intensity activities, such as brisk walking, as well as from vigorous physical activity.
  - Benefits of physical activity are particularly apparent in overweight individuals and in those at greatest risk for diabetes.
  - The goal is to accumulate at least 30 minutes of physical activity nearly every day.

  B Moderate, sustained weight loss has the potential to reduce risk of type 2 diabetes.[22-24] Obesity and weight gain are associated with an increased risk of diabetes and despite the difficulty maintaining weight loss, intentional moderate and sustained weight loss has the potential to reduce risk.

  - Besides the observational studies, there are 2 other small intervention trials using lifestyle and orlistat[25] and bariatric surgery[26] reporting decreased risk of type 2 diabetes with weight loss.
  - Short-term studies lasting 6 months or less have demonstrated that weight loss is associated with decreased insulin resistance. Long-term data assessing the extent to which these improvements can be maintained are not available.[27]
  - The reason long-term weight loss is difficult for most people to accomplish is because energy intake and energy expenditure and, thereby, body weight are controlled and regulated by the central nervous system.

  C An inverse relationship between total and whole-grain intake and fiber and risk of type 2 diabetes has been observed.[28-30] In a small study, insulin sensitivity improved in overweight and obese subjects consuming a whole grain diet compared to a diet of processed carbohydrates.[31]

D Increased intake of dietary fat, independent of total caloric intake, has been associated with an increased incidence of type 2 diabetes.[32,33] Dietary fat has been identified as a contributor to insulin resistance, independent of obesity.[34-36] All types of dietary fat, except n-3 fatty acids, may have an adverse effect on insulin sensitivity, with saturated fat having the greatest effect.[37] However, other studies have not detected an effect of dietary fat on diabetes incidence or insulin resistance. These effects may be greater in individuals with either obesity or low levels of physical activity.

E Observational studies in nondiabetic individuals suggests that light-to-moderate alcohol ingestion in adults is associated with decreased risk of type 2 diabetes and increased insulin sensitivity.[38-42] The type of beverage consumed does not appear to make a difference.[43] Data is insufficient to support making recommendations for the use of alcohol in diabetes prevention, especially as potential adverse effects of heavy drinking are of concern.

3 Several intervention studies have provided support for the benefits of lifestyle intervention, however, early studies had methodological limitations.[5,6] The greatest behavior change occurred initially between 3 and 12 months, with a gradual return to baseline. By the end of the studies, the behavior changes were minimal. Despite this, decreases in the incidence of diabetes were seen, suggesting that even modest behavior changes may have an impact on risk reduction.

   A The Finnish Diabetes Prevention Study[7] and the Diabetes Prevention Program (DPP)[8] were designed to investigate the effects of lifestyle interventions on prevention in those at high risk for diabetes. They provide strong support for the role of lifestyle interventions in the prevention of type 2 diabetes and will be discussed in more detail.

   B Three diabetes prevention trials used pharmacological therapy and also demonstrated a significant lowering of the incidence of diabetes:

   • The DPP used metformin, which reduced risk of developing diabetes by 31%[8]; STOP-NIDDM used the alpha-glucosidase inhibitor, acarbose, which reduced risk by 32%[44]; and TRIPOD used the thiazolidinedione, troglitazone, in women with a history of gestational diabetes, which reduced risk by 56%.[45]

   • The American Diabetes Association concluded that when all factors are considered, the use of drug therapy as a substitute for, or for routine use in addition to, lifestyle modification is not recommended.[11]

4 In the Finnish Diabetes Prevention Study, 522 middle-aged, overweight subjects with pre-diabetes, were randomly assigned to an intensive lifestyle or control group.[7] Each subject in the control group was given general information about diet and exercise. Each subject in the intervention group received detailed counseling by nutritionists. Lifestyle goals were to reduce weight, reduce total intake of fat and saturated fat, and increase intake of fiber and physical activity.

   A The mean duration of follow-up was 3.2 years. Mean weight loss by the end of year 2 was 3.5 kg in the intervention group and 0.8 kg in the control group.

   B The risk of developing diabetes was reduced by 58% in the intervention group. The reduction in the incidence of diabetes was directly associated with changes in lifestyle. Thirteen subjects in the intervention group and 48 in the control group did not achieve any of the lifestyle goals; diabetes developed in 38% and 31% of these subjects, respectively. Diabetes did not develop in any of the 49 subjects in the intervention group and 15 subjects in the control group who achieved 4 or 5 of the lifestyle goals.

5 The Diabetes Prevention Program (DPP) was designed to compare a lifestyle intervention and a pharmacologic intervention (metformin) with a placebo to determine the safest and most effective approaches to preventing or delaying development of type 2 diabetes among an ethnically diverse group of individuals with impaired glucose tolerance.[8] The DPP enrolled 3234 subjects; approximately 45% of the participants were from ethnic groups (eg, African Americans, Hispanic) and 20% were 60 years of age or older.

A Subjects in the placebo and metformin arms received written information regarding lifestyle recommendations and an annual 20- to 30-minute individual session.

B Participants in the lifestyle arm met with a case manager 16 times over the first 6 months (a 16-lesson curriculum was used[46]) and then monthly thereafter. Group courses on exercise and weight loss lasting 4 to 6 weeks were offered every 3 months and telephone contact was at least monthly.

C The lifestyle intervention focused on achieving a weight loss of 7% of initial body weight by decreasing daily caloric intake by 500 to 1,000 calories, eating less than 25% of total calories from fat, and increasing physical activity to at least 150 minutes per week. Over the entire DPP, the average weight loss in the lifestyle intervention group was 5.6 kg.
  - At week 24, 50% of the participants in the lifestyle arm achieved the weight loss goal of >7% of body weight; at study end, 38% achieved this goal.
  - At week 24, 74% of the participants in the lifestyle arm exercised 150 minutes a week; at study end, 58% did.

D Due to the tremendous success of both intervention groups, the study ended one year early; average follow-up was 2.8 years. Results showed that among individuals randomized to the lifestyle intervention group, there was a 58% reduction in risk of developing type 2 diabetes over a three-year period of time. Among individuals randomized to the pharmacologic intervention, risk was reduced by 31%.
  - Treatment effects did not differ according either to sex, race, or ethnic group. The lifestyle intervention was highly effective in all groups.
  - Metformin was nearly ineffective in older individuals (>60 years of age) or in those with lower BMI (BMI <30). Metformin was as effective as lifestyle in individuals ages 24 to 44 or in those with a BMI >35.
  - To delay or prevent diabetes, 14 persons would need to be treated with metformin to prevent 1 case; whereas, only 7 persons would need to be treated with lifestyle to prevent 1 case.

Lifestyle Modifications for Weight Loss for Delay or Prevention of Type 2 Diabetes

1 The remainder of this chapter covers topics related to lifestyle modifications aimed at eliciting weight loss for purposes of preventing or delaying the development of type 2 diabetes. Consideration is given to broader issues related to the community and healthcare facility within which strategies are utilized as well as to cultural and familial influences affecting individuals.

2 Setting appropriate weight management goals and nutrition and physical activity recommendations are discussed. Information regarding weight loss medications, popular diets, and nutritional supplements related to diabetes prevention is also presented.

The Community and Healthcare Facility

1 Before implementing weight-management strategies on an individual basis, it is important to have an understanding of the community and healthcare facility with which the individuals are associated. Many diabetes educators have contact with individuals in a traditional clinical setting. However, the term "healthcare facility" could include any setting in which an individual receives support for lifestyle changes aimed at preventing type 2 diabetes. Having a broad perspective of factors that shape lifestyle behaviors provides better preparation for dealing with barriers on an individual level.

2 Understanding the community and healthcare facility allows better implementation of risk-reduction activities on a community level. Community-based screening programs are not recommended, however, due to cost-ineffectiveness, low turnout, and lack of follow-up. Screening in high-risk populations may prove effective, if used as part of routine medical care, but at this time the evidence is not complete.[47]

3 At the community level, it is important to understand the factors that impact those living in the area, including regional food preferences; available resources such as grocery stores, locally available foods, restaurants, and monetary resources; and opportunities for physical activity. Local establishments such as businesses, churches, hospitals, schools, health departments, and parks/recreation departments are examples of resources for such information. Once the information is gathered, it then becomes important to use it when discussing barriers to behavior change, building support systems, and dealing with issues of availability and accessibility.

4 At the facility level, it is important to consider the healthcare providers' perspective on weight loss/maintenance and the information they provide to their patients. Communicating with the other healthcare providers is paramount to assure that there is continuity in the care being provided to the individual. Providers who are made aware of patients' efforts toward weight loss can provide additional support and encouragement when seeing the patient for a routine medical visit.

5 At the individual level, it is important to evaluate how a program delivered at the facility could be tailored to target specific needs. This can be achieved through the use of focus groups made up of small groups of individuals who are representative of those seen at the facility. The use of focus groups provides an opportunity to do the following:
  A Explore topics related to weight management (physical activity, nutrition/food, behavioral strategies, motivational factors, common barriers) that are important to the group.
  B Explore types of services that the group sees as helpful in achieving weight loss/maintenance. Examples may include phone support and transportation.
  C Test comprehension and usability of a sample of intervention materials.

Cultural and Familial Influences

1 It is important to make use of the community and facility information that has been gathered while recognizing that not all group information will apply to each individual.

2 The information can be used to have ongoing discussions with these individuals to achieve a better understanding of the factors that shape their individual lifestyle behaviors. These discussions should not be structured interviews but rather a time for the individual to speak openly, guided by probing questions. The following topics should be included in this discussion:

A What are the individual's feelings about weight loss? Encourage the individual to share any past experiences, positive or negative.

B Does the patient want to lose weight? If so, why? This question is important because not all patients see themselves as needing to lose weight, regardless of the medical benefits. This topic requires sensitivity in dealing with a variety of people whose cultures vary in their body image perceptions. It is important to share with those individuals, spouses, and/or families who feel they do not want to be "too skinny" that the goal for them will be to achieve a moderate weight loss that is important for their health. Goals should be realistic and sensitive to the individual's preferences, not those of the healthcare provider.

C What are the individual's food preferences? What types of foods do they commonly eat? A 24-hour food recall in combination with a regionally and ethnically appropriate food frequency questionnaire is often helpful in providing information about the patient's current eating habits, including food choices and food preparation methods.

D Does the individual have access to regular transportation? What are the individual's available monetary resources? Are there important time constraints to consider? These factors affect the individual's ability to access opportunities for physical activity, ability to purchase healthy food, and ability to participate in a weight-loss program that includes frequent visits for ongoing instruction and support.

E How often is food purchased? Recommendations that involve eating fresh fruits and vegetables may not be realistic for those who only shop for groceries once a month. Their diet is likely to be focused on nonperishable foods, so any recommendation given should take this into account. Similarly, recommendations for preparing low-fat foods at home may not be realistic for a person who eats out on a regular basis.

F What is the individual's role in family situations? Do they prepare the food or do they eat food prepared by another person? Who does the food shopping? Do they work outside the home? What types of social support are available to the individual (eg, family, friends, community group)? Be aware of any mention of foods or physical activities that may be constrained by the health or preferences of family members. All of these questions are important to consider when making recommendations for physical activity and healthy eating.

G Throughout the conversation and when counseling the individual, take notice of the individual's comprehension level and literary skills when new concepts are presented. This information will help to better tailor the way in which information is presented to suit the individual's needs.

Determining Appropriate Weight-Management Goals

1 It is essential to engage the individual in goal setting. If the plan that is developed is not collaboratively negotiated, it is likely to fail. The role of the healthcare provider in goal setting is twofold: (1) to provide information related to what is medically appropriate for the individual and (2) to facilitate development of weight-loss goals and behavioral goals that are realistic and desirable, both in the short term and long term. The role of the individual is to provide information related to what is feasible at this time, barriers likely to be faced, and meaningful supports and reinforcements for behavior change.

2 Review of the literature provides strong evidence that sustained, moderate weight loss in persons who are overweight or obese reduces the risk of diabetes and cardiovascular disease.

A Moderate weight loss refers to a 5% to 10% reduction in baseline weight. For example, the range of weight loss for a person who weighs 200 lb (90.9 kg) would be 10 to 20 lb (4.5 to 9.0 kg).

B A weight-loss rate of 1 to 2 lb (0.5 to 0.9 kg) per week is recommended. Weight loss at a more rapid rate, in most cases, results in later weight regain.[48] For individuals with a BMI between 27 and 35, a net decrease of 300 to 500 kcal/day (either through increased physical activity and/or decreased food intake) would yield ½ to 1 lb (0.2 to 0.5 kg) weight loss per week. For more severely obese individuals with a BMI >35, a 500 to 1000 kcal/day decrease would yield a 1 to 2 lb (0.5 to 0.9 kg) weight loss per week. In both cases, this rate of sustained weight loss would yield a 10% weight reduction in 6 months.

• On average, individuals lose approximately 10% of their starting weight within a relatively short period of time after starting a weight loss program. At this point, weight plateaus because of compensatory mechanisms that prevent excessive weight loss. Appetite is controlled by the central nervous system and is likely programmed to prevent "starvation."

• If treatment stops during this time, weight gain occurs. Therefore, continued treatment including follow-up and support is essential to maintain weight loss.

C Moderate weight loss achieved through lifestyle change (eg, changes in eating habits and physical activity) produces improvements in a wide range of risk factors for the development of chronic diseases. Among overweight and obese individuals, weight loss has been shown to lower blood glucose, blood pressure, serum/plasma lipid levels (total cholesterol, LDL cholesterol, and triglycerides) and to increase levels of HDL cholesterol.[49-53]

3 There are important considerations for individuals who smoke. Overweight or obese individuals who are trying to quit smoking should be encouraged to do so because of the marked reduction in risk for a number of chronic diseases. However, weight gain occurs in approximately 80% of quitters and the average weight gain is 4.5 to 7 lb (2.0 to 3.2 kg).[54] In 13% of women and 10% of men, weight gain is more than 28 lb (12.7 kg). Weight gain associated with smoking cessation is generally very resistant to typical behavioral approaches for weight management. Individuals should be realistic in their expectations about weight loss during a smoking cessation effort. It is generally most appropriate to simply provide support to minimize excess weight gain and to encourage weight loss at a later time.

4 It is critical to involve the individual in specific goal setting, both long-term and short-term.

    A The long-term goal should specify an agreed-upon target weight (5% to 10% weight loss) and a target date by which to reach the goal.

- If the individual wants to lose more weight, encourage him/her to focus on the initial goal first before progressing beyond. Once the initial goal has been met, a decision can be made regarding further weight loss.
- If the individual wants to lose weight more quickly, inform the patient that an extended period of weight loss at a rate that markedly exceeds the more prudent rate of 1 to 2 lb (0.5 to 0.9 kg) per week tends to promote excess loss of muscle mass and water rather than optimizing loss of fat mass.
- If the individual wants to lose less weight, try to reach a compromise on a weight that the person feels comfortable with that is still within the 5% to 10% range to elicit health benefits. It is important to be sensitive to the patient's body image perception, especially if the patient is concerned with losing too much weight.
- If the individual does not want to lose weight, stress the importance of taking steps to prevent further weight gain. The strategies used to lose weight and the strategies used to prevent weight gain involve the same subject matter, the difference being that more calories are needed for maintenance of weight than for weight loss. Therefore, success in preventing weight gain may lead to interest in weight loss.

    B Short-term goal setting is a means for achieving the long-term goal. Short-term goals allow the individual and the provider to focus on goals (both for weight and behaviors) that are manageable and to experience success within a reasonably short time.

- Short-term goals provide focus for the individual and the provider in small blocks of time; however, simply setting the goal is not enough. At each visit, the progress toward the goal should be reviewed, including a discussion of what the individual learned and what barriers were encountered. This information should be used in subsequent goal setting along with problem-solving strategies to determine ways to handle the barriers in the future.
- Short-term goals should be simply stated and targeted toward specific behaviors, such as "This week I will pull the skin off the chicken before cooking it" instead of "I will cook low-fat foods this week." Or "I will walk for 30 minutes each morning this week" instead of "I will exercise more this week." The participant should be involved in deciding which behaviors to change and what actions to take to improve the behavior. The provider should keep the individual focused on goals that are feasible, manageable, and specific, and not more than a few goals should be set at a time.
- It is important to take into account the time between visits so that the short-term goals are realistic to achieve in the time allotted. If the time between visits is long, tools such as weekly logs for monitoring food/eating or activity behaviors or reminder postcards or phone calls from the healthcare provider can be used effectively. Behavior therapy that elicits successful weight loss requires frequent sustained contact with the individual. When the patient is actively making attempts to lose weight, it is recommended that, at a minimum, monthly visits occur. These visits provide support and encouragement to the patient and opportunities to problem-solve and review/reinforce concepts related to short-term goals for the behavior change needed to achieve sustained weight loss.

Determining and Implementing Appropriate Nutrition and Eating Recommendations

1 Negative energy balance is the essential factor in weight loss. As evidenced by the plethora of weight-loss programs marketed to the public, there are a variety of ways to achieve negative energy balance that relate to increased physical activity or some type of reduction in food consumption. Some intervention programs begin by teaching participants to count fat grams as a means of achieving negative energy balance, which has been shown to elicit weight loss.[55] After mastering this technique, participants are often given a calorie goal and taught to keep track of daily calories consumed as a means of achieving further weight loss.

2 The role of the healthcare provider is to teach and counsel the individual in healthy approaches to achieve negative energy balance that will maximize health benefits and optimize nutritional status. Participants will have different needs and expectations for instruction and support to achieve behavior change. Be aware of and sensitive to the individual's needs to achieve the most effective balance of specific direction, encouragement, and support.

A Interventions that include culturally appropriate, reduced-energy meal plans (with reduced intake of total and saturated fat), increased physical activity, and behavior therapy have provided the strongest evidence for reducing the risk of diabetes through sustained, moderate weight loss. Common elements of successful behavior therapy are frequent and sustained contact with the interventionist and use of self-monitoring tools (see Chapter 3, Cultural Competence in Diabetes Education and Care, in Diabetes Education and Program Management, for more information)

B Very-low-calorie diets (VLCDs), those containing <800 kcal/day, initially produce a large weight loss.[48] However, comparison of VLCDs to a reduced-calorie, low-fat diet showed that both resulted in similar weight loss at 1 year. A VLCD provides little opportunity for acclimation to the new behavior strategies that are necessary for maintaining weight loss over time. When used under proper medical supervision, however, VLCDs may prove effective with obese patients who are highly motivated and for whom conventional weight-loss approaches have not been successful.

C Meal replacements can be used to help a patient achieve weight loss, provided that the product is used as part of the meal plan followed by the individual. The product should be assessed for nutritional adequacy prior to incorporating it into the diet. Meal replacement products should be used in combination with regular food and can provide a viable alternative for dealing with temptations at meal times.[56]

3 The following are healthy nutrition recommendations for weight loss and reducing risk factors for diabetes and cardiovascular disease:

A Total dietary fat should be limited to 25% to 30% of total calories, and saturated fat should be limited to 8% to 10% of total calories. General strategies to reduce dietary fat include eating smaller amounts of high-fat foods, eating high-fat/high-calorie foods less often, and/or substituting with low-calorie/low-fat foods. Food substitutions can include use of fat-modified food products (amount eaten still must be monitored), alternative cooking methods (eg, broiling instead of frying), or alternative food choices (eg, fruit for dessert instead of ice cream).

■ Individual modifications in macronutrient composition may be necessary on a case-by-case basis. For example, persistently elevated triglyceride levels may necessitate moderation in carbohydrate intake if carbohydrate intake has been >55% of total energy intake. This is usually a concern in a small number of individuals. Individuals with markedly high triglycerides (over 1000 mg/dL) should severely restrict fat intake. (See Chapter 1, Medical Nutrition Therapy for Diabetes, in Diabetes Management Therapies, for more information.)

■ The Food Guide Pyramid, based on the Dietary Guidelines for Americans, 2000,[57] provides a basic outline to follow on a daily basis for healthful eating (Figure 1.1[58]). These recommendations translate to a reduced-energy, low-fat diet focused on carbohydrate-rich foods (preferably whole grains), fruits, and vegetables and supplemented with servings from the dairy and meat groups. Fats, sweets, and oils are to be used in limited quantities and frequencies. Using the Food Guide Pyramid to select foods from each food group on a daily basis also encourages a varied diet.

Figure 1.1. Food Guide Pyramid

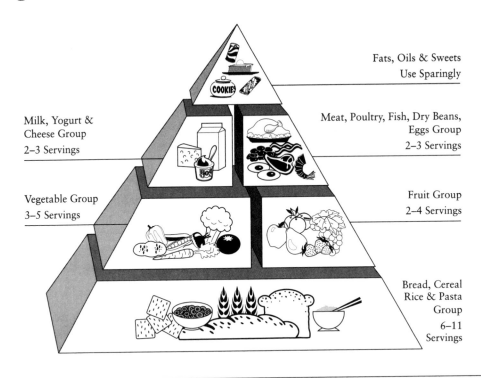

Source: US Department of Agriculture/US Department of Health and Human Services.[58]

4 There are key steps to implementing a healthy weight-loss/weight-maintenance program.

■ After gaining an understanding of the community and healthcare facility, have a discussion with the individual, being sure to cover topics that influence lifestyle behavior.

B Determine with the individual a mutually agreeable long-term weight-loss goal and target date for reaching the goal. Discussions should include health implications and behavioral changes that will be necessary to accomplish the goal.

C Conduct a 24-hour food recall, and a regionally and ethnically appropriate food frequency interview, to learn about foods commonly eaten, typical food preparation methods, frequency of eating out, and general patterns of meals and snacks.

D Based on the Dietary Guidelines for Americans, 2000, discuss key aspects of a healthy low-fat and low-energy diet, stressing the importance of eating whole grains, fruits, and vegetables.

E Introduce the principles of self-monitoring. Explain that this is an important tool that provides continuous feedback to patients about their progress in making behavior changes. It also helps identify patterns of behavior that should be encouraged or need to be improved. Patients should be taught how to record the type of food eaten, portion size, fat grams, and calories. The level of detail of these records will vary based on patients' comprehension level, literacy skills, and commitment. Patients should be encouraged to write down and keep track of as much as possible.

F Determine with the individual a mutually agreeable short-term goal to achieve by the next visit. The goal should apply new information to a lifestyle behavior that can be improved.

G Encourage patients to weigh themselves weekly and to record their weight.

H Subsequent contacts can be used to review and revise goals as needed, to identify barriers to success and problem-solve, to introduce new information related to ways to reduce fat and calories in the diet, and to provide support for ongoing success.

Determining and Implementing Appropriate Physical Activity Recommendations

1 Physical activity may contribute to a decreased risk of type 2 diabetes either as an adjunct to healthy eating for weight-loss maintenance or by directly improving insulin sensitivity.[59-61]

2 At the first session with the individual, determine what moderate physical activities he/she regularly engages in, for how long, and for how many days during the week. As with weight loss, set realistic, manageable, and specific goals for physical activity. At subsequent visits, check progress toward these goals.

3 Compare the individual's current activity habits with public health recommendations; the ADA clinical guidelines[62] include the US Surgeon General's recommendations to accumulate 30 minutes or more of moderate activity on most, preferably all, days of the week.

A Moderate physical activity is any activity performed at an intensity of 3 to 6 METs (work metabolic equivalent/resting metabolic rate). Brisk walking at 3 to 4 miles per hour is considered moderate physical activity whereas a slow stroll is not.

B Cultural and family influences as well as time and money factors shape the type of physical activity preferred. Examples of moderate physical activities include walking, swimming, cycling, mowing the lawn with a power mower, general house cleaning, and home repair. Walking is the most frequently reported physical activity choice. Walking throughout the day is convenient, inexpensive, and accessible for most people.

C The lifestyle recommendation emphasizes that moderate physical activity can be accumulated throughout the day in relatively short bouts, such as engaging in 10 minutes of activity 3 times during the day.[63] Strategies for accumulating moderate physical activity throughout the day include taking the stairs, walking for short-distance transportation and errands, pedaling a stationary cycle while watching TV, and raking leaves. While the recommendation to accumulate 30 minutes or more of moderate activity on most, preferably all, days of the week will help with weight maintenance, achieving a duration of 60 minutes of moderate physical activity is recommended to achieve weight loss and weight maintenance.[64]

D The recommendation for physical activity emphasizes the importance of frequency. Daily activity is recommended for weight loss and management. Self-monitoring using a calendar and/or pedometer is an excellent way to keep track of progress toward a goal.

4 Identify individualized and realistic opportunities for improvement, such as counseling on types of moderate physical activities, strategies to accumulate activity on a daily basis, and strategies to increase frequency during the week, especially when weight loss or weight management is a desired goal.

A Individuals who prefer more structured exercise may choose to take dance or fitness classes, walk, jog, swim, or do sports. Individuals planning to begin a program of vigorous exercise should consult their physician, especially if they have a history of heart disease.[62]

B Individuals who do not regularly engage in any of these activities should slowly incorporate a few minutes of physical activity each day and gradually build up to at least 30 minutes daily of accumulated moderate physical activity. Additional benefits accrue when the individual progresses by adding more time (eg, up to 60 minutes) and/or increasing the pace.

Responding to Questions About Weight-Loss Medications

1 Extensive review of the literature to date indicates that a combined intervention of behavior therapy with a low-calorie diet and increased physical activity constitutes the most successful therapy for weight loss and weight maintenance. It is recommended that such therapy be maintained for at least 6 months prior to considering pharmacotherapy.[9]

A Pharmacotherapy is not a replacement for behavioral approaches to weight loss; rather, it should be considered an adjunct to ongoing behavioral strategies.

B Individuals for whom use of FDA-approved pharmacologic agents for weight loss may be useful include those with a BMI >30 with no concomitant risk factors or obesity-related diseases or those with a BMI >27 with concomitant risk factors or obesity-related diseases.[65] Such conditions (other than diabetes) include hypertension, dyslipidemia, coronary heart disease, and sleep apnea.

C Careful initial and ongoing assessment by the individual's physician for safety and efficacy of the specific drug therapy is required.[66-68] Major side effects can include increases in blood pressure and heart rate for sibutramine and inadequate absorption of fat-soluble vitamins for orlistat.

D Although the FDA-approved agents demonstrated efficacy in clinical trials, the current agents appear, on average, to increase weight loss and to facilitate sustained weight loss by only a modest amount, typically well under 11 lb (5 kg) compared with lifestyle modification alone. However, limited clinical trial data suggest a reduced risk of type 2 diabetes with such therapy.[25]

E Further information about the safety and efficacy of the available pharmacologic agents for weight loss should be obtained from a healthcare provider knowledgeable in this field.

Responding to Questions About Weight-Loss Surgery

1 Weight-loss surgery may be an option in a limited number of individuals with severe obesity (BMI >40 or BMI >35 with comorbid conditions).[9] Such surgery should be considered only for motivated individuals with acceptable operative risks in whom medical therapy has failed and who are suffering from complications of extreme obesity.

A One long-term clinical trial showed a reduced risk of type 2 diabetes in severely obese individuals who underwent weight loss surgery.[26]

B Further information about the available options for weight-loss surgery, and the behavioral and social support strategies required preoperatively and postoperatively, should be obtained from a healthcare provider knowledgeable and actively working in this field.

Responding to Questions About Popular Diets and Nutritional Supplements for Diabetes Prevention

1 Several basic concepts should be kept in mind when dealing with questions about popular diets for weight loss.

A Weight management is a long-term process. Therefore, diets should promote good health, and as such, should conform to the Dietary Guidelines for Americans, 2000.

B Diets that promote rapid weight loss through extremes of food and/or nutrient sources (ie, very high-protein, low-carbohydrate diets) result in weight loss simply because the total caloric intake is less than the individual's usual diet.

C The general composition of lost weight is a combination of water, fat, and protein. A healthy weight-loss program (hypocaloric with moderate-to-low fat intake, consistent with Dietary Guidelines for Americans, 2000) with regular physical activity can optimize the composition of the weight that is lost (ie, maximize the loss of fat mass). Many rapid weight-loss programs can result in excess loss of muscle mass and body water, with a smaller proportion of lost fat.

D Because many popular diets are expensive and socially difficult to maintain, they are unlikely to lead to sustained weight loss.

E If a patient is interested in a particular diet, review the diet relative to the guidelines for healthy weight-loss diets described in this chapter and discuss the information with the patient. Consider the safety of the diet as well as the patient's ability and likelihood of sustaining the diet.[69,70]

2 To date, no nutritional supplements have been proven to be safe and effective in preventing diabetes and for weight loss. (For more information, see Chapter 7, Biological Complementary Therapies in Diabetes, in Diabetes in the Life Cycle and Research.)

  A The National Academy of Sciences' Food and Nutrition Board recently updated recommendations regarding micronutrients commonly taken as supplements, including vitamin E.[71] Intakes exceeding those recommendations have not been demonstrated to have specific health benefits for the generally healthy population.

  B The position of the American Dietetic Association on nutritional supplements[72] is that "the best nutritional strategy for promoting optimal health and reducing the risk of chronic disease is to wisely choose a wide variety of foods. Additional vitamins and minerals from fortified foods and/or supplements can help some people meet their nutritional needs as specified by science-based nutrition standards such as the Dietary Reference Intakes (DRI)."

  C The healthcare professional should be aware that use of nutritional supplements is widespread, with sales in 1998 estimated at nearly $14 billion.[72]

  • It is estimated that during 1996 through 1998, 17.2 million Americans used nonprescription weight loss products, 5.0 million used phenylpropanolamine, and 2.5 million used products containing ephedra.[73]

  • Of great concern is the use of ephedra-containing products. The Food and Drug Administration in 1997 proposed that these products must (1) be labeled with all possible adverse effects, including death, (2) contain no more than 8 mg of ephedrine per serving, (3) be labeled to include maximum daily dose of 24 mg, (4) be used for no more than 7 days, and (5) not be allowed to be marketed when combined with caffeine.[74] However, this regulation was never put into effect.

  D The marketing and sales of nutritional supplements (broadly defined to include herbs and botanicals) is largely unregulated; thus, information provided by the manufacturer to the consumer may be inaccurate.

  E There is considerable interest in the scientific community in the careful study of nutritional supplements, including herbal and botanical products and other aspects of complementary and alternative medicine. In the future, new approaches may be identified for use in conjunction with weight management for preventing type 2 diabetes. At this time, however, individuals should be informed that (1) no supplements have been shown to reduce the risk of type 2 diabetes and (2) the safety of many supplements is uncertain (see Chapter 7, Biological Complementary Therapies in Diabetes, in Diabetes in the Life Cycle and Research, for more information).

Key Educational Considerations

1 Individuals at high risk for developing type 2 diabetes include those with a family history of diabetes; overweight or obese individuals (including central obesity); individuals of Native American, Hispanic/Latino, African American, Asian American, or Pacific Islander race/ethnicity; and individuals with either impaired fasting glucose or impaired glucose tolerance.

2 The lifestyle approach to preventing type 2 diabetes, which is supported by scientific evidence, consists of sustained moderate weight loss through hypocaloric, low-fat diets; regular physical activity; and behavioral strategies that identify and reinforce appropriate patterns for healthy eating and physical activity and programs that provide ongoing support and education.

3 Prior to providing individual counseling, it is important to take time to learn about the patient's community, healthcare facility, familial influences, and culture, all of which have an impact on an individual's lifestyle behaviors. These factors can be used to tailor the behavior change strategies to the individual. Furthermore, understanding why the patient wants to avoid diabetes assists in developing behavioral change strategies as well. The patient also must believe his or her actions can delay or prevent the onset of diabetes.

4 Goal setting should be used to help the patient achieve the desired health benefits. A long-term goal for moderate weight loss (5% to 10% of baseline weight) should be established with an average rate of weight loss of 1 to 2 lb (0.5 to 0.9 kg) per week. Short-term goals related both to weight and specific food/eating and activity behaviors should be used to help achieve the long-term goal in a stepwise fashion.

5 Determine which moderate physical activities the individual regularly engages in, for how long, and for how many days per week.

6 Explain the US Surgeon General's recommendation[75] of 30 minutes accumulated physical activity per day endorsed by the American Diabetes Association. Compare the individual's reported activity level with these recommendations.

7 Identify individualized and realistic opportunities for improvement such as counseling on types of moderate physical activities, strategies to accumulate activity on a daily basis, and strategies to increase frequency during the week, especially when weight loss or weight management is a desired goal.

8 Assist the individual in committing to this lifestyle change, taking into consideration real-world obligations and barriers.

9 Lifestyle approaches to weight management should be maintained for at least 6 months prior to considering pharmacotherapy for weight loss. Pharmacologic agents for weight loss should be used as an adjunct to ongoing behavioral strategies, never in place of such strategies.

10 Weight-loss surgery may be considered as an option only for a limited number of individuals with severe obesity. Such surgery should be considered only for motivated individuals with acceptable operative risks in whom medical therapy has failed and who are suffering from complications of extreme obesity.

11 To date, no nutritional supplements (including micronutrients, herbals, and botanicals) have been proven to be safe and effective in preventing diabetes.

Self-Review Questions

1 Identify 5 groups of individuals who may be at high risk for developing type 2 diabetes.

2 Describe the essential elements of a lifestyle approach to preventing diabetes that is supported by scientific evidence.

3 What are 3 sources of information that are important in understanding community and facility issues that may impact weight-management success?

4 What information can be used to incorporate sensitivity to cultural and familial influences into recommended strategies for achieving weight loss for an individual?

5 Explain what moderate weight loss is and identify the recommended rate of weight loss.

6 How does quitting smoking affect attempts to lose weight? How should you handle an overweight or obese patient who is attempting to quit smoking and would like to also lose weight?

7 Why are short-term goals important?

8 What are the recommended healthy eating recommendations for weight loss?

9 What are the steps for implementing nutrition recommendations?

10 State the US Surgeon General's recommendations for physical activity.

11 State 5 examples of moderate physical activity.

12 Describe 3 strategies for accumulating moderate physical activity throughout the day.

13 What is the recommended frequency of moderate physical activity if weight loss or weight maintenance is the desired goal?

14 Describe how a sedentary individual should begin a lifestyle physical activity change.

15 What is the role, if any, of pharmacologic treatment of obesity or weight-loss surgery in preventing type 2 diabetes?

Learning Assessment: Case Study 1

GH is a 40-year-old African-American female with a family history of diabetes. She is 5 ft 4 in (162 cm) and weighs 175 lb (79.5 kg) (BMI = 30.1 kg/m²). Recently her doctor recommended that she lose weight and referred her for weight-loss counseling. She says that she is worried about becoming too skinny because her husband is happy with the way she looks. She explains that she has tried losing weight in the past but became frustrated when she was unsuccessful. She has tried preparing healthier foods at home, but her husband and 3 teenage boys refused to eat these foods.

Questions for Discussion

1 What cultural and familial influences seem to be affecting GH's feelings about weight loss?

2 How should you deal with her apprehensions about losing weight?

3 What long-term goal would be appropriate for GH?

4 What weight-loss topics should you initially begin to discuss with her?

5 What initial short-term goal(s) could be recommended to help GH?

Discussion

1 Begin the session by assessing GH's desire to lose weight at this time and what she hopes to gain from this counseling session.

2 GH's apprehension with weight loss is probably also affected by her failed attempt at weight loss and the negative feedback she received from her family regarding the healthy food she prepared. Probing techniques should be used to find out more details about these experiences to tailor strategies to her specific needs.

3 Explain to GH the benefits of weight loss, especially as they relate to possibly reducing the risk factors for type 2 diabetes, and why this is important given her family history of diabetes. Describe how GH can reduce her risk with moderate weight loss. The apprehension she has about weight loss associated with her husband's preferences is a real concern and should be addressed early in the discussion.

4 After getting feedback from GH during discussions about weight loss, determine a weight-loss goal to recommend to her that is between the 5% to 10% range. Make sure that GH views this goal as feasible and agree on a target date for reaching the goal. If this approach seems undesirable or unfeasible, focus on short-term goals such as a 5-lb (2.2-kg) weight loss in the next 3 to 4 weeks.

5 Initial topics to discuss about weight loss include aspects of healthy eating and becoming more physically active. GH may also appreciate learning strategies related to food preparation. This discussion should also take into account other cultural and familial aspects of her lifestyle relating both to nutrition and physical activity that would affect her attempts at weight loss.

6 A short-term goal should be mutually agreed upon before GH leaves her initial visit. The goal should be reasonable to accomplish in the time before her next visit and targeted toward a specific behavior change. For example, if GH is returning for a follow-up visit in one week, help her identify a particularly high-fat food that she eats often (perhaps a food she prepares for her husband and sons on a regular basis). Her goal could be one of the following: eat the food less often (1 to 2 times per week versus 4 to 5 times per week), eat a smaller portion of the food (measure her food before eating it), or try using low-fat preparation techniques (perhaps work with her to generate low-fat flavorful alternatives).

Learning Assessment: Case Study 2

DL is a 38-year-old man who is married and has 3 children. At a routine physical his fasting plasma glucose was 115 mg/dL (6.4 mmol/L), which was confirmed with a second test later that week. His job requires a great deal of out-of-town travel and commuting by car. Evenings and weekends he stays close to home and watches sports on TV. He goes to the gym 1 or 2 days a week at lunchtime to walk on the treadmill for 20 to 25 minutes. He would like to spend more time with his children. He has been referred to you for lifestyle counseling with regard to weight loss.

Questions for Discussion

1 DL's glucose tests place him in what category of glucose tolerance?

2 How do DL's current activity habits compare with the US Surgeon General's recommendations for physical activity?

3 How might DL go about achieving weight-loss goals through increased lifestyle activity while also meeting his personal goal of spending more time with his children?

Discussion

1 DL is diagnosed as having pre-diabetes. Modest weight loss and increased physical activity are recommended.

2 Although DL has an apparent interest in physical activity, the frequency of his exercise habit falls short of current recommendations. If he is realistically not able to increase his attendance at the gym, he needs help in identifying strategies to meet his weight-loss goals through increased daily lifestyle activity. It would be a good idea to help DL plan activities that also engage his children.

3 Assist DL in identifying types of preferred moderate physical activities. For example, he already likes to walk and therefore may enjoy incorporating more walking into his day (eg, walking for errands, walking the children to school, going for walks in the evening or on weekends). Since he enjoys sports, there may be some sports or games that he would like to participate in (eg, tossing a frisbee with the children).

Learning Assessment: Case Study 3

ND, the daughter of one of your patients with newly diagnosed type 2 diabetes, has a BMI of 27. She has a history of losing and then regaining weight. ND has expressed a strong motivation to avoid diabetes. She tells you that she has recently purchased a chromium supplement and a weight-loss product containing ephedra.

Questions for Discussion

1 ND asks you for advice about her diet, but does not ask for specific information about the chromium supplement or the ephedra-containing product. What do you do?

2 Without the perceived support of the chromium supplement and the ephedra-containing product, ND is discouraged, especially given her history of regaining lost weight. How can you encourage her to try to lose weight on her own?

Discussion

1 Since ND volunteered the information that she purchased these products, you should advise her that neither has been shown to prevent diabetes or promote lasting weight loss. It may be helpful to do some research on the products in question so you can have a more detailed discussion with ND. There is some evidence that chromium may improve insulin sensitivity, but the overall scientific evidence for a lasting, clinically significant effect that would prevent diabetes is lacking. Thus, chromium sup-

plementation is not recommended. The efficacy of ephedra-containing products for sustained weight loss is not certain, and serious questions regarding safety of ephedra have arisen. Thus, it is not recommended. ND should be advised of the risks of using ephedra-containing products.

2 For individuals with a history of weight-loss recidivism (ie, weight cycling), supplements of any sort can be seen as the answer to the problem. Unfortunately, they are not. Counseling should focus on determining what specific approaches were most effective in the past and what determinants of weight regain could be avoided in the future. In general, it has been shown that adherence to low-fat diets in conjunction with increased physical activity, along with some form of social support, have the greatest likelihood of contributing to successful weight-loss maintenance.

References

1 King H, Aubert RE, Herman WH. Global burden of diabetes, 1995–2025: prevalence, numerical estimates, and projections. Diabetes Care. 1998;21:1414-1431.

2 Mokdad AH, Ford ES, Bowman BA, et al. Prevalence of obesity, diabetes, and obesity-related health risk factors, 2001. JAMA. 2003;289:76-79.

3 Harris MI, Flegal KM, Cowie CC, et al. Prevalence of diabetes, impaired fasting glucose, and impaired glucose tolerance in US adults. The Third National Health and Nutrition Examination Survey, 1988-1994. Diabetes Care. 1998;21:518-524.

4 Ford ES, Giles WH, Dietz WH. Prevalence of the metabolic syndrome among US adults. Findings from the Third National Health and Nutrition Survey. JAMA. 2002; 287;356-359.

5 Eriksson KF, Lindgärde F. Prevention of type 2 (non-insulin-dependent) diabetes mellitus by diet and exercise: the 6-year Malmo feasibility study. Diabetologia. 1991;34:891-898.

6 Pan XR, Li GW, Hu YH, et al. Effects of diet and exercise in preventing NIDDM in people with impaired glucose tolerance: the DaQing IGT and Diabetes Study. Diabetes Care. 1997;20:537-544.

7 Tuomilehto J, Lindstrom J, Eriksson JG, et al. Prevention of type 2 diabetes mellitus by changes in lifestyle among subjects with impaired glucose tolerance. N Engl J Med. 2001;344:1342-1350.

8 Knowler WC, Barrett-Connor E, Fowler SE, et al. for the Diabetes Prevention Research Group. Reduction in the evidence of type 2 diabetes with lifestyle intervention or metformin. N Engl J Med. 2001; 346:393-403.

9 American Association of Diabetes Educators. White paper on the prevention of type 2 diabetes and the role of the diabetes educator. The Diabetes Educator. 2002;28:964-971.

10 American Diabetes Association and National Institute of Diabetes, Digestive and Kidney Diseases. The prevention or delay of type 2 diabetes (position statement). Diabetes Care. 2003;26(suppl 1):S62-S69.

11 National Heart, Lung, and Blood Institute. Clinical Guidelines on the Identification, Evaluation, and Treatment of Overweight and Obesity in Adults. Bethesda, Md: National Heart, Lung, and Blood Institute; 1998.

12 Yamashita S, Nakamura T, Shimomura I, et al. Insulin resistance and body fat distribution. Diabetes Care. 1996;19:287-291.

13 The Expert Committee on the Diagnosis and Classification of Diabetes Mellitus. Report of the expert committee on the diagnosis and classification of diabetes mellitus. Diabetes Care. 2003;26(suppl 1):S5-S20.

14 Kim C, Newton KM, Knopp RH. Gestational diabetes and the incidence of type 2 diabetes. A systematic review. Diabetes Care. 2002;25:1862-1868.

15 American Diabetes Association. Gestational diabetes mellitus (position statement). Diabetes Care. 2003;26(suppl 1):S103-S105.

16 Helmrich SP, Ragland DR, Leung RW, Paffenbarger RS Jr. Physical activity and reduced occurrence of non-insulin dependent diabetes mellitus. N Engl J Med. 1991;325:147-152.

17 Manson JE, Rimm EB, Stampfer MJ, et al. Physical activity and incidence of non-insulin-dependent diabetes in women. Lancet. 1991;338:774-778.

18 Manson JE, Nathan DM, Krolewski AS, Stampfer MJ, Willett WC, Hennekens CH. A prospective study of exercise and incidence of diabetes among US male physicians. JAMA. 1992;268:63-67.

19 Perry IJ, Wannamethee M, Walker MK, Thomson AG, Whincup PH, Shaper AG. Prospective study of risk factors for development of non-insulin-dependent diabetes in middle aged British men. BMJ. 1995;310:560-564.

20 Wei M, Gibbons LW, Mitchell TL, Kampert JB, Lee CD, Blair SN. The association between cardiorespiratory fitness and impaired fasting glucose in type 2 diabetes in men. Ann Intern Med. 1999;130:89-96.

21 Wing RR. Lifestyle and the prevention of diabetes. In: Franz MJ, Bantle JP, eds. American Diabetes Association Guide to Medical Nutrition Therapy for Diabetes. Alexandria, Va: American Diabetes Association; 1999:351-368.

22 Moore LL, Visioni AJ, Wilson PW, et al. Can sustained weight loss in overweight individuals reduce the risk of diabetes mellitus? Epidemiology. 2000;3:269-273.

23 Wannamethee SG, Shaper AG. Weight change and duration of overweight and obesity in the incidence of type 2 diabetes. Diabetes Care. 1999;22:1266-1272.

24 Will JC, Williamson DF, Ford ES, Calle EE, Thun MJ. Intentional weight loss and 13-year diabetes incidence in overweight adults. Am J Public Health. 2002;92:1245-1248.

25 Heymsfield SB, Segarl KR, Hauptman J, et al. Effects of weight loss with orlistat on glucose tolerance and progression to type 2 diabetes in older adults. Arch Intern Med. 2000;160:1321-1326.

26 Sjostrom CS, Lissner L, Wedel H, Sjostrom L. Reduction in incidence of diabetes, hypertension and lipid disturbances after intentional weight loss induced by bariatric surgery. Obes Res. 1999;5:477-484.

27 American Diabetes Association. Evidence-based nutrition principles and recommendations for the treatment and prevention of diabetes and related complications (position statement). Diabetes Care. 2003;26(suppl 1):S51-S61.

28 Meyer KA, Kushi LH, Jacobs DR, Slavin J, Sellers TA, Folsom AR. Carbohydrates, dietary fiber, and incident type 2 diabetes in older women. Am J Clin Nutr. 2000;71:921-930.

29 Liu S, Manson JE, Stampfer MJ, et al. A prospective study of whole-grain intake and risk of type 2 diabetes mellitus in US women. Am J Public Health. 2000;90:1409-1415.

30 Fung TT, Hu FB, Pereira MA, et al. Whole-grain intake and risk of type 2 diabetes: a prospective study in men. Am J Clin Nutr. 2002;76:535-540.

31 Pereira MA, Jacobs DR, Pins JJ, Raatz SK, Gross MD, Slavin JL, Seaquist ER. Effect of whole grains on insulin sensitivity in overweight hyperinsulinemic adults. Am J Clin Nutr. 2002;75:848-855.

32 Tsunehara CH, Leonetti DL, Fujimoto WY. Diet of second-generation Japanese American men with and without non-insulin-dependent diabetes. J Am Clin Nutr. 1990;52:731-738.

33 Lovejoy JC, Windhauser MM, Rood JC, de la Bretonne JA. Effect of a controlled high-fat versus low-fat diet on insulin sensitivity and leptin levels in African-American and Caucasian women. Metabolism. 1998;47:1520-1524.

34 Marshall JA, Bessesen DH, Hamman RF. High saturated fat and low starch and fiber are associated with hyperinsulinemia in a non-diabetic population: the San Luis Valley Diabetes Study. Diabetologia. 1997;40:430-438.

35 Mayer-Davis EJ, Monaco JH, Hoen HM, et al. Dietary fat and insulin sensitivity in a triethnic population: the role of obesity. The Insulin Resistance Atherosclerosis Study. Am J Clin Nutr. 1997;65:79-87.

36 Mayer EJ, Newman B, Quesenberry CP Jr, Selby JV. Usual dietary fat intake and insulin concentrations in healthy women twins. Diabetes Care. 1993;16:1459-1469.

37 Maron DJ, Fair JM, Haskell WL. Saturated fat intake and insulin resistance in men with coronary artery disease. Circulation. 1991;84:2070-2074.

38 Ajani UA, Hennekens CH, Spelsberg A, Manson JE. Alcohol consumption and risk of type 2 diabetes mellitus among US male physicians. Circulation. 2000;102:500-505.

39 Tsumura K, Hayashi T, Suematsu C, Endo G, Fuji S, Okada K. Daily alcohol consumption and the risk of type 2 diabetes in Japanese men: the Osaka Health Study. Diabetes Care. 1999;22:1432-1437.

40 Wei M, Gibbon LW, Mitchell TL, Kampert JB, Blair SN. Alcohol intake and incidence of type 2 diabetes in men. Diabetes Care. 2000;23:18-22.

41 Facchini F, Chen Y-D, Reaven GM. Light-to-moderate alcohol intake is associated with enhanced insulin sensitivity. Diabetes Care. 1994;17:115-119.

42 Davies MJ, Baer DJ, Judd JT, Brown ED, Campbell WS, Taylor PR. Effects of moderate alcohol intake on fasting insulin and glucose concentrations and insulin sensitivity in postmenopausal women. JAMA. 2002;287:2559-2562.

43 Mukamal KJ, Conigrave KM, Mittleman MA, Camargo CA, Stampfer MJ, Willett WC, Rimm EB. Roles of drinking pattern and type of alcohol consumed in coronary heart disease in men. N Engl J Med. 2003;348:109-118.

44 Chiasson J-L, Josse RG, Gomis R, Hanefeld M, Karasik A, Laaski M; the STOP-NIDDM Trial Research Group. Acarbose for prevention of type 2 diabetes mellitus: the STOP-NIDDM randomised trial. Lancet. 2002;359:2072-2077.

45 Buchanan TA, Xiang AH, Peters RK, et al. Preservation of pancreatic beta-cell function and the prevention of type 2 diabetes by pharmacological treatment of insulin resistance in high-risk Hispanic women. Diabetes. 2002;51:2796-2803.

46 The Diabetes Prevention Program (DPP) Research Group. The diabetes prevention program (DPP). Description of lifestyle intervention. Diabetes Care. 2002;25:2165-2171.

47 American Diabetes Association. Screening for diabetes (position statement). Diabetes Care. 2003;26(suppl 1):S21-S24.

48 Wadden TA, Foster GD, Letizia KA. One-year behavioral treatment of obesity: comparison of moderate and severe caloric restriction and the effects of weight maintenance therapy. J Consult Clin Psychol. 1994;62:165-171.

49 Bourn DM, Mann JI, McSwimming BJ, Waldron MA, Wishart JD. Impaired glucose tolerance and NIDDM: does a lifestyle intervention program have an effect? Diabetes Care. 1994;17:1311-1319.

50 Elmer PJ, Grimm R, Laing B, et al. Lifestyle intervention: results of the treatment of mild hypertension study (TOMHS). Preventive Med. 1995;24:378-388.

51 Wing RR, Koeske R, Epstein LH, Nowalk MP, Gooding W, Becker D. Long-term effects of modest weight loss in type II diabetic patients. Arch Intern Med. 1987;147:1749-1753.

52 Wood PD, Stefanick ML, Williams PT, Haskell WL. The effects on plasma lipoproteins of a prudent weight-reducing diet, without exercise, in overweight men and women. N Engl J Med. 1991;325:461-466.

53 Brown SA, Upchurch S, Anding R, Winter M, Ramirez G. Promoting weight loss in type 2 diabetes. Diabetes Care. 1996; 19:613-624.

54 Varner LM. Impact of combined weight-control and smoking-cessation interventions on body weight: review of the literature. J Am Diet Assoc. 1999;99:1272-1275.

55 Astrup A, Grunwald GK, Melanson EL, Saris WHM, Hill JO. The role of low-fat diets in body weight control: a meta-analysis of ad libitum dietary intervention studies. Int J Obes. 2000;24:1545-1552.

56 Rothacker DQ, Staniszewki BA, Ellis PK. Liquid meal replacement vs traditional food: a potential model for women who cannot maintain eating habit change. J Am Diet Assoc. 2001;101:345-347.

57 US Department of Agriculture and US Department of Health and Human Services. Nutrition and Your Health: Dietary Guidelines for Americans, 2000. 5th ed. Hyattsville, Md: USDA/DHHS; 2000. Home and Garden Bulletin 232.

58 US Department of Agriculture. The Food Guide Pyramid. Hyattsville, Md: USDA Human Nutrition Information Service; 1992. Home and Garden Bulletin 252.

59 Mayer-Davis EJ, D'Agostino R, Karter AJ, et al. Intensity and amount of physical activity in relation to insulin sensitivity: the Insulin Resistance Atherosclerosis Study. JAMA. 1998;279:669-674.

60 Hu FB, Sigal RJ, Rich-Edwards JW, et al. Walking compared with vigorous physical activity and risk of type 2 diabetes in women: a prospective study. JAMA. 1999;282:1433-1439.

61 Duncan GE, Perri MG, Theriaque DW, Hutson AD, Eckel RH, Stacpoole PW. Exercise training, without weight loss, increases insulin sensitivity and postheparin plasma lipase activity in previously sedentary adults. Diabetes Care. 2003;26:557-562.

62 American Diabetes Association. Physical activity/exercise and diabetes mellitus (position statement). Diabetes Care. 2003; 26:S73-S77.

63 Pate RR, Pratt M, Blair SN, et al. Physical activity and public health: a recommendation from the Centers for Disease Control and Prevention and the American College of Sports Medicine. JAMA. 1995;273:402-407.

64 Institute of Medicine of the National Academies. Dietary Reference Intakes. Energy, Carbohydrate, Fiber, Fat, Fatty Acids, Cholesterol, Protein, and Amino Acids. Washington, DC: The National Academies Press; 2002.

65 US Food and Drug Administration. Draft Guidance Clinical Evaluation of Weight Control Drug. Rockville, Md: US Food and Drug Administration;1996.

66 Apfelbaum M, Vague P, Ziegler O, Hanotin C, Thomas F, Leutenegger E. Long-term maintenance of weight loss after a very-low-calorie diet: a randomized blinded trial of the efficacy and tolerability of sibutramine. Am J Med. 1999;106:179-184.

67 Hauptman J, Lucas C, Boldrin MN, Collins H, Segal KR. Orlistat in the long-term treatment of obesity in primary care settings. Arch Fam Med. 2000;9:160-167.

68 Rossner S, Sjostrom L, Noack R, Meinders AE, Noseda G, European Orlistat Obesity Study Group. Weight loss, weight maintenance, and improved cardiovascular risk factors after 2 years treatment with orlistat for obesity. Obes Res. 2000;8:49-61.

69 Kennedy ET, Bowman SA, Spence JT, Freedman M, King J. Popular diets: correlation to health, nutrition, and obesity. J Am Diet Assoc. 2001;101:411-420.

70 Freedman MR, King J, Kennedy E. Popular diets: a scientific review. Obesity Research. 2001;9(suppl 1):1S-40S.

71 Institute of Medicine, Food and Nutrition Board. Dietary Reference Intakes for Vitamin C, Vitamin E, Selenium, and Carotenoids: A Report of the Panel on Dietary Antioxidants and Related Compounds. Subcommittees on Upper Reference Levels of Nutrients and Interpretation and Uses of Dietary Reference Intakes, and the Standing Committee on the Scientific Evaluation of Dietary Reference Intakes. Washington, DC: National Academy Press; 2000.

72 American Dietetic Association. Position statement. Food fortification and dietary supplements. J Am Diet Assoc. 2001; 101:115-125.

73 Blanck HM, Khan LK, Serdula MK. Use of nonprescription weight loss products. Results from a multistate survey. JAMA. 2001;286:930-935.

74 Kemper KJ. Ephedra monograph. Boston, Longwood Herbal Task Force; May 2000. Available from: www.mcp.edu/herbal/ephedra.pdf.

75 US Surgeon General. Surgeon General's report on physical activity and health. From the Centers for Disease Control and Prevention. JAMA. 1996;276:522.

Suggested Readings

American College of Sports Medicine position stand. Exercise and type 2 diabetes. Med Sci Sports Exerc. 2000;32:1345-1360.

Diabetes Prevention Program Research Group. The Diabetes Prevention Program. Design and methods for a clinical trial in the prevention of type 2 diabetes. Diabetes Care. 1999;22:623-634.

Edelstein SL, Knowler WC, Bain RP, et al. Predictors of progression from impaired glucose tolerance to NIDDM. An analysis of six prospective studies. Diabetes. 1997; 46:701-710.

Eriksson J, Lindstrom J, Valle T, et al. Prevention of type II diabetes in subjects with impaired glucose tolerance: the Diabetes Prevention Study (DPS) in Finland. Study design and 1-year interim report on the feasibility of the lifestyle intervention program. Diabetologia. 1999;42:793-801.

Freedman MR, King J, Kennedy E. Popular diets: a scientific review. Obesity Research. 2001;9(suppl 1):1S-40S.

Klem ML, Wing RR, McGuire MT, Seagle HM, Hill JO. A descriptive study of individuals successful at long-term maintenance of substantial weight loss. Am J Clin Nutr. 1997;66:239-246.

Kumanyika SK, Ewart CK. Theoretical and baseline considerations for diet and weight control of diabetes among blacks. Diabetes Care. 1990;13(suppl 4):1154-1162.

Maggio CA, Pi-Sunyer FX. The prevention and treatment of obesity. Diabetes Care. 1997;20:1744-1746.

Norris JM, Scott FW. A meta-analysis of infant diet and insulin-dependent diabetes mellitus: do biases play a role? Epidemiology. 1996;7:87-92.

Prochaska JO, Velicer WF. The transtheoretical model of health behavior change. Am J Health Promotion. 1997;12:38-48.

Shick SM, Wing RR, Klem ML, McGuire MT, Hill JO, Seagle H. Persons successful at long-term weight loss and maintenance continue to consume a low-energy, low-fat diet. J Am Diet Assoc. 1998;98:408-413.

Williams KV, Mullen ML, Kelley DE, Wing RR. The effect of short periods of caloric restriction on weight loss and glycemic control in type 2 diabetes. Diabetes Care. 1998;21:2-15.

Wing RR. Use of very-low-calorie diets in the treatment of obese persons with non-insulin dependent diabetes mellitus. J Am Diet Assoc. 1995;95:569-672.

Wing RR. Physical activity in the treatment of the adulthood overweight and obesity: current evidence and research issues. Med Sci Sports Exerc. 1999;31(suppl 11):S547-S552.

For further information regarding the Diabetes Prevention Program lifestyle session, materials, and learning objectives, see: http://www.bsc.gwu.edu/dpp/manuals.htmlvdoc.

Learning Assessment: Post-Test Questions

Lifestyle for Diabetes Prevention

1

1 Based on the scientific literature, which of the following can be recommended for preventing type 2 diabetes?
A Increased vitamin E intake
B Increased chromium intake
C Reduced fat intake
D All of the above
E None of the above

2 Factors that are useful in better understanding cultural and familial influences on lifestyle behaviors include:
A Medical history of the individual
B The individual's feelings about weight loss, access to transportation, and available monetary resources
C Notes about the patient's compliance written in the clinic medical chart by the primary care provider
D Experiences of other similar patients

3 What type of intervention provides the best evidence of sustained, moderate weight loss?
A A very-low-calorie diet sustained for an extended period
B The use of meal replacements
C A reduced-calorie, low-fat diet along with increased physical activity
D Weight-loss medications

4 The recommended rate of weight loss is:
A 2 lb or more per week
B Variable depending on the individual
C No more than ½ lb per week
D 1 to 2 lb per week

5 Behavioral techniques that enhance an individual's success with weight loss include:
A Self-monitoring of foods that are eaten
B Self-monitoring of physical activity
C Frequent sustained contact with the healthcare provider
D All of the above

6 Which of the following is not an example of moderate physical activity?
A Vacuuming
B Shuffleboard
C Walking to work
D Reading while riding a stationary bicycle

7 How frequently should you engage in moderate physical activity for weight loss?
A Three times per week
B Every other day
C Daily
D Five times per week

8 Moderate physical activity is equivalent to:
A Walking at 3 to 4 miles per hour
B Walking a mile in 15 to 20 minutes
C Brisk walking
D All of the above

9 Pharmacologic agents to support weight-loss efforts can be considered after:
A 6 weeks of behavioral therapy
B 6 months of behavioral therapy
C Never (none have been shown to be effective)
D None of the above

See next page for answer key.

Post-Test Answer Key

Lifestyle for Diabetes Prevention 1

1 C

2 B

3 C

4 D

5 D

6 B

7 C

8 D

9 B

A Core Curriculum for Diabetes Education
Diabetes in the Life Cycle and Research

Type 1 Diabetes in Youth
2

Jean Betschart Roemer, MSN, MN, CPNP, CDE
Children's Hospital of Pittsburgh
Pittsburgh, Pennsylvania

Terri McGee, MS, RD, CDE
Children's Hospital of Pittsburgh
Pittsburgh, Pennsylvania

Introduction

1 The impact of type 1 diabetes is unique for each developmental stage of childhood and adolescence.

2 Diabetes can profoundly affect the normal physical, cognitive, and emotional developmental stages of childhood and adolescence. Likewise, each developmental stage has implications for diabetes management and care.

3 The unrelenting demands of type 1 diabetes management are difficult for families, affect their social network, and may disrupt the child's developmental tasks within the family.

4 Diabetes management for children and adolescents involves the education and training of the child and caregivers. Management issues include medical nutrition therapy, insulin administration and adjustment, monitoring, and exercise.

5 Understanding the unique considerations of diabetes management in children and adolescents with type 1 diabetes, the impact of diabetes on normal development, the effect of the diagnosis on parents, and the dynamic nature of managing diabetes in youth can help health professionals provide appropriate support, flexible care, and age-specific education.

Objectives

Upon completion of this chapter, the learner will be able to

1 State the major developmental concerns about type 1 diabetes in infants and toddlers, preschool/school-age children, and preadolescents/adolescents.

2 Explain how diabetes self-management training (DSMT) in children and adolescents with diabetes and their parents is different from that of adults.

3 Describe the concepts of medical nutrition therapy for children and adolescents so that there is provision for normal growth and development and optimal glycemic control.

4 Describe the parental burden of managing a child's diabetes and the benefit of social networks and support.

5 Describe the acute and chronic complications of type 1 diabetes in childhood.

6 Identify age-appropriate educational materials and considerations for each age group.

Incidence of Type 1 Diabetes in Youth

1 Type 1 diabetes occurs in children and adolescents at a rate of 13.8 to 16.9 per 100 000 for Caucasian-American children and from 3.3 to 11.8 per 100 000 for African-American children.[1] Approximately 151 000 children and adolescents under the age of 20 years have type 1 diabetes.[2] The worldwide prevalence and incidence of type 1 diabetes varies from one geographic location to another, with the highest incidence being in the Scandinavian countries of Sweden, Finland, and Norway, and lowest incidence in Japan. Evidence suggests that the incidence of type 1 diabetes is increasing globally.[3]

2 Type 1 diabetes occurs in approximately 55% to 98% of new onset diabetes in children and adolescents.[3]

    A The incidence of type 1 diabetes increases with age and peaks at puberty.

    B Seasonal variations have also been reported, with diabetes being diagnosed more frequently in the winter than in the summer months.[3]

    C Beta cell destruction is immune-mediated and usually leads to absolute insulin deficiency. It results from a cellular-mediated autoimmune destruction of the beta cells of the pancreas. Markers of immune destruction include islet cell autoantibodies (ICAs), autoantibodies to glutamic acid decarboxylase (GAD) and autoantibodies to the tyrosine phosphatases (IA-2 and IA-2ß). The rate of beta cell destruction can happen slowly or rapidly, explaining the wide variability in the severity of onset of symptoms from one child to another.[4]

Diagnostic Criteria

1 Criteria for type 1 diabetes in children and adolescents are the same as those for adults (see Chapter 1, Pathophysiology of the Diabetes Disease State, in Diabetes and Complications).

2 Classification can be reliably made on the basis of clinical presentation and course of the disease. Other tests may be required to clarify the diagnosis (islet cell, GAD, IA-2, IA-2ß, or insulin autoantibodies).[4]

3 General goals of therapy for children or adolescents with diabetes include the following:

    A Normal growth and development

    B Optimal glycemic control

    C Minimal acute or chronic complications (Table 2.1)

    D Positive psychosocial adjustment to diabetes

Growth, Weight Gain, and Developmental Issues

1 Growth, weight gain, and developmental milestones should be normal. The following are considerations when growth is poor.

    A Diminished height gain after diagnosis has been reported.[5]

    B Poor growth or weight gain and developmental lags must be evaluated to be sure that they are not a result of other medical or psychosocial problems.

    C Height and weight need to be carefully plotted at 3- to 4-month intervals on a standard growth chart. (See Figures 3.1 to 3.5 in Chapter 3, Type 2 Diabetes in Youth, in Diabetes in the Life Cycle and Research.)

    D If height and weight fall below the child's normal growth percentile, the child should be evaluated for glycemic control, insulin sufficiency, nutritional adequacy, celiac disease, or the presence of other endocrine disorders or other disease.

2 Adequate growth and appropriate pubertal development are important indices of insulin sufficiency.

    A With insulin sufficiency, children with type 1 diabetes have normal onset of puberty and normal sexual maturation.

    B Impaired growth and delayed pubertal development might occur when metabolic control is poor.[6]

Table 2.1. Possible Complications of Diabetes in Childhood and Adolescence

Acute Complications	• Hypoglycemia (often unrecognized in young children) • Ketoacidosis • Vaginal yeast infections/thrush • Cellulitis due to infection/injury (rare)
Chronic Complications*	• Hypertension • Nephropathy • Neuropathy • Retinopathy • Eating disorders • Depression • Cognitive deficits
Other Complications	• Lipohypertrophy and lipoatrophy at injection sites • Mauriac syndrome (rare; characterized by insulin insufficiency, growth, and pubertal delay) • Necrobiosis lipoidica diabeticorum (rare)

*Not usually seen before puberty.

C Mauriac syndrome, a diabetes-related growth disorder, is characterized by delayed linear growth, delayed sexual maturation, hepatomegaly, and joint contractures among other findings. Although rarely seen today in its severe form, mild variations are seen in children and adolescents with poorly controlled diabetes.

Insulin Therapy Considerations Unique to Children and Adolescents

1 Determinants of insulin type, method of delivery, and dosage are the following:

A Therapy takes into account fluctuating food intake, insulin requirements, and physical activity levels of the growing and developing child.

B The type of insulin, number of injections, and insulin delivery method are based on the individual needs of the child and family. This may include meal schedules, supervision issues, and glycemic patterns.

C Most children require approximately 0.7 to 1 unit of insulin per kilogram of body weight per day (other than during remission).[6] A range of 0.5 to 1.5 units/kg/day is acceptable and allows for individual differences based on age, activity, eating habits, and metabolic requirements.

• Approximately 50% to 65% of the total dose (given as glargine, NPH, or Ultralente) will cover basal insulin needs. The remainder (given as rapid-acting insulins such as insulin lispro, insulin aspart, or short-acting insulin such as regular insulin) prevents postprandial hyperglycemia.

D Multiple daily injections (such as an insulin glargine and rapid-acting insulin regimen) or an insulin pump will provide the flexibility necessary for most children and adolescents. Three injection regimens might work in children who have very structured schedules and consistent eating habits. A child or teen with psychosocial limitations may do best on a simplified regimen such as mixed insulins, fixed doses.

E Frequent adjustments of insulin dosages are necessary to balance food and exercise excursions. Young children may require dose adjustments in half-unit increments or less when on a pump. Commercially prepared premixed insulins do not allow for the flexibility of daily dosage adjustment based on blood glucose values and exercise levels, which are especially variable in children. They may be useful for those who are unable or unwilling to regularly adjust insulin doses.

F Approximately 70% of children and adolescents with diabetes move into a remission phase (or "honeymoon" phase), requiring decreased insulin dosages.[7] This period can be highly variable in duration, ranging from approximately 2 weeks to 2 years after diagnosis.

- Evidence suggests that beta cell preservation may be enhanced by provision of basal insulin. Therefore, providing round-the-clock basal insulin to maintain tight glycemic control without frequent or severe hypoglycemia during remission may be desirable.[7-10]

2 Developmental expectations of self-care include the following:

A School-age children are frequently capable of giving their own insulin injections with supervision although broad differences have been identified in their ability to master and share responsibility for self-care tasks.

B When determining the ability of a child to perform self-care skills, it is important to identify readiness and individual considerations (locus of control, maturity, and family factors) rather than define specific age ranges for task performance.

- Parental involvement and/or supervision appears to enhance self-care behaviors and glycemic control.[11,12]
- Diabetes self-management education programs for children can be effective for facilitating greater responsibility for self-care.[13]

3 Considerations for insulin injections in children and teens are the following:

A Usual injection sites for young children are the legs, arms, and the upper/outer quadrant of the buttocks.

B School-age children and adolescents can be encouraged to use the abdomen on a regular basis. Abdominal injections may not be advisable in children with little subcutaneous abdominal fat or in very young children. For these children, the abdomen is usually the least favored site.

C Rotating sites in a consistent manner (eg, arms in the morning, legs in the evening) might help provide a consistent rate of absorption.

D It is not clear whether the findings from adult studies about insulin absorption are applicable to children.[14]

E Using 30-gauge (short) or "mini" pen needles might provide more comfortable injections for the very young or the very lean.

F Half-unit increments can now be measured on certain insulin syringes.

G Avoiding injections into even mildly hypertrophied sites is recommended so that insulin absorption problems can be avoided.

4 Insulin pump therapy, also known as continuous subcutaneous insulin infusion (CSII), is a popular and viable alternative to multiple daily injection (MDI) insulin therapy for children and teens of all ages.[15,16]

   A The use of an insulin pump requires a solid educational foundation in the child (as appropriate for age), parent or caregiver, and school personnel.

   B An insulin pump provides a greater ability to have a flexible lifestyle and can but does not necessarily provide improved glycemic control. The need to balance insulin with the special characteristics of childhood, such as eating variability and activity can be managed more easily with insulin pump therapy.

   C Children and parents who choose pump therapy must be willing to monitor blood glucose levels at least 4 times daily and during the night weekly as needed.

   D Young children and others with little subcutaneous abdominal fat can successfully use the upper/outer quadrant of the hip as the pump site. (See Chapter 7, Insulin Pump Therapy, in Diabetes Management Therapies, for more information on insulin pumps.)

Management of Physical Activity in Youth

1 There are benefits from physical activity in children. In youth with diabetes, physical activity is strongly encouraged even though it may not result in better glycemic control.

   A Benefits include cardiovascular fitness, long-term weight control, and improved well-being.[17]

   B It is important to balance play and activity with insulin adjustments to provide glycemic control and prevent hypoglycemia.[18]

   C Physically fit adolescents with diabetes have greater insulin sensitivity.[19] In youths with type 1, as well as type 2 diabetes, physical activity is encouraged to increase insulin sensitivity, lower blood glucose levels, and improve long-term maintenance of weight loss.

   D Physical training in young children with a short duration of diabetes may improve glycemic control when their A1C is high. However, changes in A1C appear to be independent of changes in fitness.[20]

2 There is both an immediate and delayed effect of hypoglycemia with exercise. Additionally there is a possibility of hypoglycemia during the night.

   A To replenish glycogen stores depleted during high-intensity exercise, additional food at bedtime or later may be required.

   B Bedtime monitoring may help identify children who are at risk for nocturnal hypoglycemia.[21] (See Chapter 2, Physical Activity/Exercise, in Diabetes Management Therapies, for additional information about physical activity and hypoglycemia.)

   C Children and teens must wear a medical ID during exercise. Wearing a nylon bracelet or anklet identification is safe and practical during strenuous or contact sports.

Monitoring of Blood Glucose and Blood or Urine Ketone Levels

1 Blood glucose monitoring must be done regularly to enable parents and children to make management decisions and adjustments in food, scheduling, and/or insulin.

　A In general, the recommended frequency for blood glucose monitoring for children is before each meal and bedtime snack, with additional tests performed if the child has symptoms of hypoglycemia, hyperglycemia, ketosis, or illness.

　　• For children in optimal glycemic control, on multiple daily injections, or pump therapy, a 3 or 4 AM monitoring is often recommended on a weekly basis. Night-time monitoring is important after unusual exercise, hypoglycemia, or poor appetite.

　　• Testing blood glucose levels before lunch is necessary for children and adolescents. The child, parent, medical team, and school personnel will need to find a safe and comfortable way for the child to perform these required self-management tasks.

　B There has been no consensus on adapting glycemic goals for pediatric use.

　　• Goals must be individualized with each family based on age, ability to recognize hypoglycemia, self-management capabilities, and history of severe hypoglycemic episodes or seizures.

　　• Target ranges for blood glucose levels of children and adolescents vary depending on the judgment of the provider or healthcare team and the individual goals set with the child and his/her parents.[17]

　　• Target goals must be individualized, with the overall goal being to achieve the lowest achievable A1C possible without frequent or severe hypoglycemia.[22] For example, most children may have a target goal range of 80 to 140 mg/dL (4.4 to 7.8 mmol/L) during the day.

　　• Children under 6 years of age may have a target that is higher (such as 90 to 200 mg/dL (4.9 to 11.1 mmol/L) in order to prevent frequent or severe hypoglycemia in a child too young to recognize and report symptoms.[6,22] Still, most children should have the same goal of 80 to 140 mg/dL (4.4 to 7.8 mmol/L) in order to grow properly and delay or avoid complications.

　　• Blood glucose monitoring results help caregivers make decisions in order to balance activities and type and quantity of food to provide.

2 The general recommendation regarding ketone testing for children and adolescents is to test when blood glucose levels exceed 240 mg/dL (13.3 mmol/L) and when illness occurs.

　A Some centers advise regular ketone testing before breakfast and as an indicator of antecedent insulin deficiency (the dawn phenomenon).[6]

　B When significant levels of ketones are present, it is important for caregivers to report such to their healthcare provider. Additional fluids and/or insulin might be required. Continued ketone monitoring is essential.

Provision of Family Education and Support

1 All family members of the child or adolescent with diabetes (including grandparents, babysitters, and other caregivers when possible) should receive diabetes management training. (See Key Educational Considerations, later in this chapter.)

A The educational process needs to be an open-ended, ongoing experience between the child, family, friends, and the diabetes team.[23]

B Developing effective stress management/coping skills and problem-solving skills is considered as important to successful therapy as insulin administration, nutrition therapy, monitoring, and exercise.[24] (See Chapter 3, Behavior Change, in Diabetes Education and Program Management, for information about coping skills.)

C It is important for the medical team to recognize and encourage those who problem-solve diabetes management problems by making changes in food, insulin doses, schedules, or physical activity.[22]

2 Intervention strategies must be culturally appropriate, sensitive to family resources, and provided for all caregivers.

3 The diagnosis of diabetes, as in other chronic illnesses, often causes parents to grieve the loss of their healthy child. Anger, sadness, and depression can ensue.

A The role of the parent in diabetes management tasks varies greatly depending on the child's age and ability to perform self-care activities.

- The tasks of adjustment of insulin, food, monitoring, and physical activity are either assumed by or supervised by a parent or caregiver. Responsibility is shared among the child or teen, family, caregivers, school personnel, and medical team.
- The demands of daily diabetes management are stressful to most parents and cause worry, anxiety, and family disruption.

B In some instances, both the child and the family respond by developing dysfunctional methods of coping.[25,26]

- Healthcare providers must make every effort to support adaptive coping strategies.
- The educator can help provide parents with the guidance and support needed by teaching extended family members, encouraging counseling, closely reviewing blood glucose monitoring results, and enhancing family support networks.

4 Children with diabetes who come from families with minimal support, lower socio-economic status, or a chaotic home environment may be at greater risk for acute and chronic complications.[24]

A Even families who have health insurance still incur a larger out-of-pocket healthcare expense than those who do not have a child with diabetes. Families coping with diabetes have additional financial burdens.[27]

B The burden of responsibility for constant care can be quite difficult for caregivers. Supportive extended family, friends, or babysitters are important to offer respite.

Developmental Issues of Infants and Toddlers (Birth to 2 Years) With Diabetes

1 Characteristics normal in the development of young children must be taken into account when diabetes management regimens are determined. Normal growth and development for infants and toddlers progresses rapidly and predictably.

A Infants may require significant amounts of sleep, and toddlers usually need daily naps. This can influence the timing of snacks and will need to be considered when determining insulin types. Naps should fit into the schedules at a time that does not interfere with meals or snacks. Understandably, the child does not always cooperate!

B Regularly scheduled nighttime feedings are important for avoiding hypoglycemia in infants and the very young.

2 An understanding of normal developmental tasks of very young children is essential when developing the diabetes management plan.
  A In normal development, differentiation begins at around 4 to 5 months of age; tentative experimentation with separation-individuation begins at around 6 months; and early practicing of crawling begins at around 9 months.
  B Infants 10 to 12 months of age practice walking and manual skills and have been described by Mahler as having "a love affair with the world."[28]
  C As toddlers approach 2 years of age, they begin to separate and individuate, testing their separateness by saying no and behaving in an oppositional manner. Most parents know this stage as the "terrible twos." Providing choices at this age can give the toddler with diabetes some control, but the choices need to be framed in such a way that the child is not allowed to make important decisions. For example, asking, "Which finger shall we choose?" works better than asking "Do you want to do your blood test now?"
  D Infants usually nurse or eat predictably.
  E Appetite may become erratic in toddlers when rapid growth begins to subside. Food and feedings can become problematic for parents and caretakers of a selective eater.
  F Toddlers usually eat 3 meals and 3 snacks daily, but additional snacks may be required.
  G Normal activity in toddlers is sporadic and spontaneous, interspersed with sudden bursts of whole body movement.
  H The younger the child, the greater the likelihood that behavioral or neuroglycopenic, rather than autonomic symptoms, will be reported.

3 There are food considerations in the infant and toddler with diabetes.
  A Balancing food with insulin and activity to prevent hypoglycemia can be challenging, particularly because of the sporadic and spontaneous nature of physical activity in infants.
    • 3- to 4-hour flexible feeding schedule is effective for maintaining a steady blood glucose level.
    • In order to prevent hypoglycemia, infants older than 4 months of age may be given additional cereal by spoon along with milk at feedings prior to the peak effect of insulin.
    • To prevent hypoglycemia, activity needs to be balanced with intake of extra food or beverages such as milk or juice.
  B The normal sporadic eating habits of toddlers can be worrisome for parents who try to balance food with insulin and activity. Insulin lispro or insulin aspart can be given after the caregiver observes what and how much the child has eaten. This must be done with caution due to the poor matching of the rapid-acting insulin with the glucose peak from food. This can cause high postprandial glucose levels and hypoglycemia later as the insulin peak does not always match the food peak.
  C If a toddler will not eat, offer favorite foods and substitute alternative choices of carbohydrate-containing beverages (eg, milk, juice). However, parents should avoid becoming a short-order cook for a demanding toddler.

D Infancy is a time when feedings not only provide nutrition to maintain life and physiologic well being, but also build a relationship. A positive feeding interaction between the infant and caregiver fosters the ingestion of an appropriate amount of food.

E A feeding pattern that imitates family meal times should evolve by the end of the first year of life to incoporate the infant into the family's normal meal schedule.

F Young children require small portions of food and need to eat more frequently than adults. Snacks and regularly scheduled meals are necessary.

4 Parents of infants and toddlers must rely on frequent blood glucose monitoring to distinguish normal infant and toddler behaviors from symptoms of hypoglycemia. Infants and toddlers are often defiant, demanding, sleepy, or cranky as part of their normal development.

A Blood for glucose monitoring can be obtained from the child's fingers, big toes, and external, lateral aspect of the heel. Meters which take measurements from the arm, thigh, or buttock are useful for children with limited testing sites. However, children do not tolerate fingers or feet as testing sites very well.

B Blood glucose readings in young children most often are erratic, at best, and the number of injections is not necessarily related to the tightness of glycemic control.

C Onset of diabetes early in life is associated with impaired cognitive functions (eg, abstract and visual reasoning) or attention deficits.[29,30] The reason for cognitive differences in those with diabetes is not yet clear, and it is not conclusive that an association exists between impaired cognitive function and hypoglycemia.[31] Differences may be due to undetected hypoglycemia or a seizure resulting from hypoglycemia which causes varying levels of cognitive dysfunction. However, not all children with an early onset of diabetes show neuropsychological effects.

D Treatment guidelines for mild or moderate hypoglycemia are to test blood glucose, provide 5 to 15 g of carbohydrate, wait 10 to 15 minutes and if symptoms persist, repeat the process. Treatment should be followed by the ingestion of additional carbohydrate or the next meal or snack. Treatment for severe hypoglycemia is urgent and consists of glucagon or IV glucose.[17]

E Hypoglycemia in children is much more difficult to predict and therefore prevent. Even mild hypoglycemia should be considered as having potentially dangerous consequences.[32]

5 Illnesses in the very young child are another concern.

A Infants and young children may become dehydrated quickly because they have a large percentage of body surface area and are unable to consume large volumes of fluids taken by mouth.

- Dehydration can take place rapidly in any child when illness occurs; this effect is enhanced in the infant or toddler with diabetes.
- The potential for rapid dehydration makes infants and young children with diabetes especially vulnerable when illness, vomiting, or diarrhea occurs. Parents must be taught to notify their diabetes care provider whenever a young child is ill and carefully monitor blood glucose and blood or urine ketone levels.

B Infants, toddlers, and preschool-age children are especially vulnerable to elevated blood glucose values and ketonuria when acute infections of childhood occur (eg, otitis media, vomiting illnesses, or the common cold). Conversely, hypoglycemia can also result.

- Wide excursions in blood glucose levels are common and can be frustrating and frightening for parents.
- Dehydration and diabetic ketoacidosis (DKA) can develop rapidly, especially in children with poor glycemic control.
- Intravenous therapy may be necessary either to prevent further dehydration and to treat ketoacidosis or to acutely provide glucose to treat hypoglycemia if the child is unable to eat or drink.
- Intravenous hydration may be necessary if vomiting does not subside and/or the child shows signs of dehydration, urinary or blood ketones, ketoacidosis, or hypoglycemia. (See Chapter 9, Illness and Surgery, in Diabetes Management Therapies, for information about diabetes management during illness.)

Developmental Issues in the Preschool-Age Child (3 to 5 Years)

1 Physical growth slows after the toddler stage but is still relatively rapid. Development of fine motor skills continues and cognitive language is rapid.

2 Children engage in magical thinking, believing that if they think or wish something they can cause it to happen.[33]
   A Separation-individuation continues as children learn to distinguish themselves as being separate from their parents.
   B Body integrity, or the intactness of the body, is important.
   C Fear of intrusive procedures is characteristic of this age, and children may act out their anxieties at the times when insulin injections and blood testing are done.

3 Preschoolers have difficulty understanding the need for insulin injections and blood tests, particularly if they are feeling well. Describing the need in terms of "keeping you healthy" fosters a positive outlook.
   A The use of adhesive bandages is helpful to the preschool child, as they help to address concerns about body integrity.
   B Allowing the child to have some control by providing limited choices can be helpful. ("Do you want mashed potatoes or macaroni for dinner?")

4 The advantages and use of play therapy as a coping strategy have been well recognized.[34-36] Children establish a balance between their inner life and reality by continually exploring and testing through their play.
   A Guided play, or play therapy, provides a forum and vehicle for children to express their concerns and provides a mechanism for emotional release by helping the child learn to deal with these issues through creative expression.
   B Giving a child a "safe" syringe, family and health professional dolls, meter supplies, and other diabetes paraphernalia will provide an opportunity for supervised play.
   C Children may choose one of the dolls to have diabetes and will play out their personal life issues and concerns about having diabetes through doll or puppet play.
   D Forms of artwork also help young children express themselves.

5 Illness concerns are similar to the illness concerns for infants and toddlers (see point 5 in Developmental Issues of Infants and Toddlers With Diabetes).

6 Appetites may be very erratic and are often unpredictable in the preschool child. Variability in eating is not considered harmful but rather normal from a developmental point of view. (For example, children may want to eat only bananas and peanut butter for days at a time, and then they will switch to grilled cheese and apples.) Children may eat only a few foods or may want the same item meal after meal. These eating patterns typically last a few days or weeks. When treated casually, the behaviors are forgotten after a brief period.

  A Increased appetites tend to precede growth spurts, and food intake is usually balanced over a period of weeks.

  B This erratic eating makes glucose control difficult for this age group because parents worry about hypoglycemia when their child will not eat.

  C Parents can allow the child some control over eating by providing reasonable choices without allowing the child to control eating situations. By giving young children limited choices, parents may avoid a battle of wills.

  D Meats and vegetables are foods which are often rejected.

7 Undetected hypoglycemia is a risk in the preschool years.

  A Frequent blood glucose testing helps in making management decisions.

  B Many preschool-age children are able to identify symptoms of hypoglycemia and can alert adults.

  C Educating the staff in preschool or daycare centers is critical for the management of acute and chronic diabetes-related problems. Recognition, detection, and treatment of hypoglycemia are essential. The number of daycare centers able and willing to accommodate blood glucose monitoring and other procedures is increasing as a result of the Americans With Disabilities Act and other national efforts.

Developmental Issues in the School-Age Child (6 to 10 Years)

1 A school-age child is physically well-coordinated, has a vivid fantasy life, speaks fluently, has a conscience, and is able to share and cooperate. The child has concrete reasoning and likes repetition, which is played out in sports, games, and skills.

  A Although the school-age child has increasing need for independence, the power and protection of the parent are very important to the child's feeling of well-being.

  B One of the greatest drives of school-age children is to avoid failure. They acquire strategies to keep from feeling different from peers.

2 In terms of diabetes management, the parent's role is to perform diabetes care tasks while moving the child toward independence through supervision, encouragement, and support. At times the child may be willing and able to perform blood glucose monitoring, prepare his or her own snacks, and administer insulin. At other times, the parent will need to perform the test or administer insulin. Parent-child sharing of these responsibilities is essential during the school-age years and beyond.[11]

  A Parents of the school-age child with diabetes may be more understandably protective than other parents. This attitude can make it difficult for the child with diabetes to attain the same level of independence as a nondiabetic child of the same age.

  B Diabetes management planning for special events and activities is important to promote independence and minimize differences. By planning ahead, most children can safely participate in all childhood activities.

    C Monitoring, eating special snacks, taking injections, and fear of peers witnessing symptoms of hypoglycemia can alter diabetes self-care routines and ultimately affect self-esteem.

    D Helping the child to fit diabetes management into normal routines both at home and at school can minimize feelings of being different. For example, a snack break can be implemented for all children in the classroom. If children desire, they should be able to check glucose in the classroom to avoid losing classroom time.

    E All children should carry a source of carbohydrate with them at all times and need to be able to treat hypoglycemia in the classroom.

3 Children usually accept a greater variety of foods and develop increased autonomy regarding eating behaviors. Meal times and snacks are less frequent than preschoolers as children spend their time in school and other organized activities.

4 Because school-age children spend a large portion of their day in school, it is reasonable to expect school personnel to become informed about diabetes care. School districts and personnel are obligated to provide an individualized plan to accommodate a child's special healthcare needs.

    A Certain federal laws address these issues. The Education for All Handicapped Act of 1975, commonly referred to as Public Law No. 94-142, is a federal mandate that entitles all physically, developmentally, emotionally, and other health-impaired children to free, appropriate public education.[37] Any school that receives federal funding or facility considered open to the public must reasonably accommodate the special needs of children with diabetes.[38]

    B The other law, Section 504, is a more general civil rights law that makes it illegal for any agency or organization that receives federal funds to discriminate in any way against qualified people with disabilities.[37]

    C Beginning each school year with a conference involving the child with diabetes, parents, and school personnel is an effective way to establish a plan of care, communication, and a means of addressing important issues and concerns.

    D Knowledgeable trained personnel are essential if the student is to avoid the immediate health risks of low blood glucose and achieve the metabolic control required to decrease risks for complications.[38]

        • Parents need to provide basic information about diabetes, the causes of hypoglycemia, the specific requirements of their child's daily management plan, and their child's usual signs and symptoms. This information is used to develop a plan of care that satisfies the needs of the child, parents, and school policies. This written plan includes who will administer the care and the location of the treatment supplies. Children should be allowed to check glucose in the classroom and always be able to treat hypoglycemia in the classroom.

    E The administration of glucagon in schools must be provided if recommended by the student's treating physican.[38] Therefore, when a physician's order is provided, the school must designate a person to administer glucagon in the written plan of care.

    F When scheduling changes occur in the daily school routine (eg, field trips or parties), the school needs to notify parents prior to the event so that appropriate care can be administered. However, parents cannot be required to attend all field trips.

G A review of the food/meal plan basics provides school personnel with a general awareness of what the child eats. Providing a plan to enable the child to manage parties and snacks in school is also beneficial.

5 Children with diabetes can have feelings of sadness, anxiety, friendlessness, and isolation.[26]

    A Support groups, individual counseling, or diabetes camps can be useful for assisting the child in resolving these feelings.

    B Determining the child's individual coping skills, supporting adaptive strategies, and providing interventions should be initiated early.[22]

Issues of Adolescent Development

1 There are large differences between the 3 stages of adolescence. These stages are early adolescence or preadolescence (12 years), middle adolescence (13 to 15 years), and late adolescence (16 to 21 years).

2 At no other time of life do environment and heredity produce such a variance in individual development. Broad differences normally occur in emotional, social, and physical development.

    A In girls, the onset of breast budding and the growth of pubic hair occur at an average age of 10 to 11 years; in boys, the growth of pubic hair and the enlargement of testicles occur at an average age of 12 to 16 years.

    B Changes in size, weight, body proportions, muscular development, strength, coordination, and skill are seen at this age. These changes may occur slowly or rapidly.

    C The age of onset of pubescent growth is determined by genetic familial factors but can also be affected by economy, nutrition, health, and habitat.

    D Puberty is characterized by the onset of hormonal activity, which is under the influence of the central nervous system, especially the hypothalamus and pituitary gland. The major effects of puberty are the increased production of adrenocortical and gonadal hormones and the production of mature ova and spermatozoa.

3 Metabolic control, as represented by increasing A1C levels, deteriorates during adolescence despite significantly higher insulin doses.[39-41] This can be avoided by increasing insulin levels rapidly enough to meet the adolescent's needs.

    A Poor glycemic control can delay the onset of puberty.

    B It has been suggested that the hormonal changes of puberty cause a state of relative insulin resistance as a result of declining peripheral insulin action and changing counterregulatory hormonal responses.[39] However, the etiology of the insulin resistance associated with puberty is not fully understood and is likely multifactorial.

4 Characteristics of early adolescence are

    A The child becomes acutely aware of body image.

    B Dependent versus independent struggles begin between parent and child.

    C There may be great vacillation between childlike and adult behaviors.

    D There is less social involvement with family and more with peers.

    E Parental criticism becomes difficult to accept.

    F Turmoil and conflict within the parent-child relationship may begin.

5 Characteristics of middle adolescence are
  A Peer group allegiance develops.
  B Greater experimentation and risk taking occurs.
  C Physical and social activity increases.
  D Sexual relationships emerge and are important.
  E Formal operational thinking begins with the beginning of abstract reasoning.
  F Teens and parents often struggle and experience conflict in their relationship.

6 Characteristics of late adolescence are
  A Cognitive abilities and abstract morals develop.
  B The peer group loses its primary importance.
  C There is increasing separation from the family unit.
  D Teens become future oriented.
  E Conscience is able to stand without support or validity from others.

7 Diabetes affects normal adolescent development. Identity and self-image concerns can revolve around diabetes concerns such as the appearance of the injection site or self-identification as "a diabetic."
  A Normal independence issues may be thwarted as a result of parental protectiveness or the teen's failure to assume responsibility for self-care.
  B Physical growth and development have a strong impact on a teen's self-image.[42,43] Adolescents with diabetes can become particularly concerned about their growth and sexual maturation even though they usually display normal growth patterns and normal onset and progression of pubertal development.
  C Attitudes of experimentation and rebellion and risk-taking behaviors normally associated with adolescence can revolve around diabetes issues such as taking insulin regularly, monitoring, and the quality and quantity of food consumption.

8 Educators must be aware of and address issues of substance abuse (tobacco use, alcohol consumption, drug use) and sexual practices and attitudes in their assessment of adolescent diabetes management.
  A Risk taking and lack of health-promoting behaviors is widespread, especially among adolescents.
  B Family dynamics, family health beliefs, communication style, and support networks all affect adolescents' ability to do what is necessary to manage diabetes.

9 Food intake becomes less consistent due to issues such as participation in athletics, busier schedules, preoccupation with body weight and/or appearance, and the search for self-identity.
  A Proper eating habits are still important to ensure continued growth and development and to develop good patterns to be used for a lifetime.
  B Adolescents give low priority to their nutritional needs regarding recommended amounts and type of food.
  C Typical food-related behaviors include skipping meals, eating away from home, experimenting with fad diets, and attempting to change their weight.

10 Adolescent females with diabetes must be taught the importance of planning pregnancy and meticulously using contraception and the effects of diabetes on reproductive health, sexuality, and pregnancy. Their instruction should include a frank dialogue about the potential fetal/maternal health risks of an unplanned pregnancy in a woman with diabetes. Females might also have questions regarding diabetes and their menstrual cycle or yeast infections.

A Discuss sexual issues in a relaxed, comfortable manner. Comfort in discussing sexual topics comes with practice and a sense of control over the subject matter. The comfort level of the educator is communicated to the patient and sets the tone for the discussions.

B Begin sex education in the preteen ages so that it becomes a routine part of diabetes assessment and education.

C The use of unbiased, gender-neutral language is important when assessing sexual orientation, practice, frequency, use of contraceptives, and consistency of contraceptive practices.

D Remind teens that abstinence is the only 100% effective contraceptive method for preventing pregnancy, sexually transmitted diseases (STDs), and acquired immune deficiency syndrome (AIDS). Emphasize that use of a condom during sexual activity will help to prevent STDs and AIDS, but is not the most effective method of preventing pregnancy.

E Include the female's partner, whenever possible, as part of the contraception and other education process. It is important to ask for the date of last intercourse and whether the female or couple wants to have a baby.[44]

11 The privilege of driving is an adult responsibility. Health professionals and parents of teens who are approaching the age to drive should begin discussions with the teen about the responsibility of safety when driving. Guidelines for safety include responsible diabetes self-care, desire or motivation to consider the safety of self and others, monitoring before driving, testing blood glucose at 2-hour intervals while driving, carrying appropriate supplies, including carbohydrates, wearing a medical ID, and never driving if there are signs of hypoglycemia.

Conditions Associated With Poor Glycemic Control and/or Health Outcomes

1 Biologically, the adolescent's earlier and greater epinephrine responses to drops in blood glucose concentrations, combined with heightened insulin resistance, may contribute to some of the lability in metabolic control.

2 A chaotic home environment, chronic family stress, or parental over- or under-involvement can contribute to poorer metabolic control for children and adolescents as a result of increased epinephrine responses to physical or psychological neglect or abuse, or to the frank omission of insulin.

3 Knowledge and cognitive maturity levels are important elements of diabetes self-management. Occasionally, developmental delay or learning disabilities may hamper understanding of diabetes care.

4 Emotional disturbance can cause disequilibrium and precipitate frequent episodes of ketoacidosis.

A Insulin insufficiency may occur by insulin omission or in response to physical or emotional stress, resulting in overproduction of counterregulatory hormones.

B Early-adolescent girls who are extraordinarily sensitive to emotional stress are most likely to demonstrate recurrent DKA.[22]

C Repeated episodes of DKA warrant investigation, as DKA can be deliberately induced to displace family tensions. Family patterns of interaction may reveal family enmeshment, rigidity, poor communication, and overprotectiveness.[45] Treatment may include family counseling and aggressive insulin therapy when illness, stress, or ketones appear.

D Adolescents frequently develop DKA because they fail to take their insulin.

E Insulin doses can be missed when parents are not involved in an adolescent's diabetes management.[45,46]

5 Adolescent females may decide to skip injections for the purpose of weight control, which is a variant of an eating disorder.

A Diabetes and the regimen may provide the right conditions for those who are at risk of developing an eating disorder because of the focus on food and discipline required.

B Educators need to be aware of the possibility of pathologic eating behaviors, particularly among adolescent and young adult females. (See Chapter 6, Psychological Disorders, in Diabetes Education and Program Management, for more information about eating disorders in people with diabetes.)

Medical Nutrition Therapy (MNT) in Youth

1 The goal of MNT for children and adolescents with diabetes is to assist in achieving blood glucose goals and to provide for normal growth and development.[47] Specific goals of medical nutrition therapy for children are shown in Table 2.2.[48]

Table 2.2. Goals of Medical Nutrition Therapy (MNT) for Children and Adolescents With Diabetes

1 Maintenance of near-normal glucose levels by balancing food intake with insulin and activity levels
2 Achievement of optimal lipid levels
3 Provision of adequate calories for normal growth, weight, and development
4 Prevention, delay, or treatment of nutrition-related risk factors and complications
5 Improvement of overall health through optimal nutrition

Source: Adapted from Holzmeister.[48]

2 Nutritional recommendations for children and adolescents are based on a nutrition assessment.

A An assessment involves evaluating parameters such as age, weight, height, growth percentiles on a growth chart, gender, recommended daily allowances (RDAs) for caloric range, schedules, treatment modalities, and blood glucose patterns for each child.

B In general, children need sufficient calories for growth and pubertal development without excessive hypoglycemic episodes. Monitoring weight gains and growth patterns can reveal if energy intake is appropriate.[47]

C The child's height and weight are plotted on a growth chart to determine trends. If the growth parameters are deemed to be appropriate for age, the child's meal plan includes calories adequate for growth and development. Children and teens who are normal weight do not need to focus on weight control issues other than to follow prudent recommendations important for the general population.

D If the weight percentile is elevated, a body mass index (BMI) may also be calculated. BMI is used to estimate total body mass and is considered an indicator of body fatness.

- The calculation to determine BMI is as follows: BMI = weight (kg)/height (m²)
- The result is then plotted according to the child's age and gender to determine if it is in an acceptable range. BMI does not distinguish fat from muscle when determining if body weight is excessive.
- For children who are above an ideal weight range, encouraging alterations in food selection and physical activity levels can decrease possible insulin resistance and increase metabolic status. The success of MNT interventions as well as physical activity regimens can be based upon the child's cessation of excessive weight gain and the maintenance of blood glucose levels within the goal range.[47]

3 Meal plans must be individualized to meet each child's food preferences, cultural influences, family eating patterns and schedules, age, weight, activity level, and insulin action peaks. Insulin therapy can be integrated into usual eating and exercise habits. Therefore, it is important to determine the meal plan before determining an insulin regimen.

A The distribution of calories from fat and carbohydrate can vary and be individualized based on the nutrition assessment and treatment program.

B The child's appetite should be considered when determining the total caloric level provided in the meal plan.

- Withholding food or having the child overeat consistently without an appetite for food in an effort to control blood glucose should be discouraged. Withholding food can feel punitive to a child and eventually promote reluctance to honestly report extra food or high glucose values. Forcing children to eat when they are not hungry or when they are no longer hungry is not only difficult but also unnecessary.

C Children under the age of 6 years typically require 3 meals per day plus 3 snacks.

D Most children over the age of 6 require three meals per day plus snacks in mid-afternoon and at bedtime. Children should have a snack if meals are more than 4 hours apart.

E If older children and adolescents dislike having to eat during school time, insulin types or dosages can be adjusted to make snacks at school unnecessary.

F Meals and snacks are timed to correspond with the peak action of the injected insulin. For this reason, it is generally recommended that children and teens try to not deviate from their normal schedules by more than 1 hour. In the summer, for example, the daily schedule can be started later if the child wants to sleep later.

G Children and teens who sleep very late in the morning may awaken hypoglycemic because it has been a long time since they have eaten or hyperglycemic due to insulin insufficiency. A reasonable guide suggests that insulin be taken and breakfast eaten by 9:00 AM. A child who wants to sleep later can take the scheduled insulin, eat breakfast, and then go back to bed. However, if the patient is on an insulin pump, the basal dose can be set to accommodate sleeping in late. An insulin regimen of long-acting insulin (glargine) and rapid-acting insulin before meals can also be used to accommodate sleeping in late and can provide flexibility for meal times and food choices.

4 Carbohydrate counting principles are the same for children as adults and can allow greater flexibility and alternatives in a child's meal plan if an insulin pump or multiple daily injection therapy is utilized. (See Chapter 1, Medical Nutrition Therapy for Diabetes, in Diabetes Management Therapies, for more information on carbohydrate counting.)

A Children and their caregivers need to be carefully instructed when carbohydrate counting to not allow caloric consumption levels to drop significantly below caloric needs for growth and possibly delay development.

B Meat (and meat substitutes) and fat servings should not be viewed as free foods while children are counting carbohydrate grams as this could lead to unwanted weight gain from increased caloric intake.

5 Additional carbohydrate may be eaten before physical activity to decrease the risk of a hypoglycemic episode during or after exercise. Typical pre-activity snacks might be a sandwich or cheese and crackers. Adolescents may prefer to use various beverages such as sport drinks or fruit juice during or after sports because of the difficulty of exercising with a full stomach. If an insulin pump is used, the pump may be removed for up to 2 hours for exercise. This eliminates the need to eat before exercise. However, testing glucose after exercise is still important to prevent late-onset hypoglycemia.

6 School personnel, especially gym teachers and coaches, must know that children and adolescents with diabetes require a snack before and/or during strenuous exercise. They must also be prepared to identify and treat hypoglycemia with a form of readily available glucose.

Key Educational Considerations

1 Parents, friends, neighbors, caretakers, babysitters, and any other support persons can either help or hinder a child's adjustment to diabetes and self-care. For this reason, it is important to be consistent and provide the same information to all who are involved with the child.

2 All education must be developmentally appropriate to the child or adolescent. Learning materials, content, demonstration skills, and expectations must be adjusted to the age, abilities, and attention span of each child. See Table 2.3 for a summary of educational topics that are unique to children and adolescents with diabetes and their parents.

Table 2.3. Educational Topics Unique to Children and Adolescents and Their Parents

Children with diabetes have needs different from adults

Anticipatory guidance regarding the impact of diabetes on developmental issues
• Individuation
• Trust
• Independence

School issues: how to set up a conference and who should attend
• Developing a medical plan of care at school
• Training of personnel
• Observing for and treating hypoglycemia in school

Concerns for parents
• Seeking support for self and marriage
• Sharing the burden of responsibility
• Staying involved in your child's care, yet promoting independence

School-age and adolescent issues
• Addictive behaviors – alcohol, tobacco, drugs
• Athletics and diabetes
• Wearing a medical ID
• Feeling different
• Sexuality (menstrual periods, body maturation, sex, contraception and pregnancy)
• Safe driving
• Dating
• Special occasions management (prom, parties, sleep-overs, etc.)
• Preparing for college

3 Educating the preschool child is often limited to spontaneously occurring opportunities that revolve around diabetes management and questions asked by the child.

A Young children often do well when provided with simple choices such as "Do you want raisins or a banana?"

B The need for insulin injections and finger-sticks can be explained in terms of "keeping you healthy."

4 Parents and caregivers must treat for hypoglycemia if they are in doubt.

5 Diabetes management tasks should never be used as rewards or punishments. They are not negotiable.

6 Preschool and school-age children process what they have learned primarily through play. Doll play and puppet play are valuable teaching/learning methods for children of this age.

7 An essential topic for the young child is hypoglycemia: identifying the symptoms, knowing that treatment involves consuming juice or food, and recognizing the need to tell an adult about any symptom of hypoglycemia. Discussing how the child felt before each hypoglycemic episode can help a child recognize the symptoms the next time. Many young children are able to identify the symptoms of hypoglycemia and tell an adult about what they are experiencing.

A Parents often are concerned that they may not recognize an episode of hypoglycemia. They are likely to benefit from reading a detailed description of the symptoms of hypoglycemia and/or seeing a video about hypoglycemia. Parents can be assured that over a short time they will be able to identify very subtle changes in the child when they become hypoglycemic.

8 The school-age child needs to be assessed individually for learning readiness, which can be highly variable in this age group. School-age children are able to learn most effectively when the information about diabetes is presented in an interesting and fun way. They also have the ability to learn concrete survival skills quite well.

A Games, puzzles, and videos are effective educational tools.

B The school-age child also learns well through play.

9 Most health professionals agree that the most difficult task for the adolescent with diabetes is not learning educational content, but rather assuming responsibility for self-management.

A Adolescents learn best when the educational content is pertinent to adolescent issues. Topics of particular concern to adolescents are diabetes and sexuality (including contraception), alcohol and tobacco use, drugs, diabetes identification, driving issues, and special concerns such as party advice, managing diabetes and sports, prom-night management, career information, and travel.

B Educational materials can include books and videos, but discussion groups among peers are often most effective.

10 Educators can use a number of strategies for dealing with teens with diabetes.

A Enhance self-esteem by promoting feelings of normalcy. The behavior of teens frequently matches their self-image.

B Develop a primary relationship with teens and a collaborative one with parents.

C Provide honest communication and don't minimize feelings.

D Listen to what is being said as well as what is not being said. Negative feelings exist before negative acts.

E Solve problems together and negotiate treatment strategies.

F Enlist the assistance of a supportive person (boyfriend, girlfriend, sibling).

G Candidly discuss perceptions of barriers.

H Provide ongoing positive reinforcement.

I Convey enjoyment in working with adolescents.

11 Diabetes camps provide an excellent setting for facilitating formal and informal learning. Children and adolescents learn from each other in an environment where they share the common thread of having diabetes. They can relate to each other in terms of similar feelings, concerns, and experiences from living with diabetes; no one feels different because of the diabetes.

12 Support groups also promote learning and are most effective when structured around an activity that is fun.

13 Factors that contribute to impaired self-care are family dynamics (including the family's health belief model), communication style, emotional tone, and inappropriate expectations of children and adolescents.

14 It is important for both children and adolescents that blood glucose results be treated as information only and not as bad or good numbers. Less judgmental expressions for blood glucose readings should be used, such as "in range" or "out of range." The same is true for the commonly used word "cheating" to describe making food choices outside of the meal plan. This word is judgmental, meaning to defraud or deceive, and may create more anger, guilt, and acting-out behaviors.

Self-Review Questions

1 What are 3 characteristics for each of the following developmental stages: infancy and toddlerhood; preschool age; school age; and early, middle, and late adolescence?

2 What is the potential impact of diabetes on each developmental stage?

3 Describe the burden of care and potential stress that falls on parents and caretakers; what are 2 possible sources of support?

4 List 3 conditions that may be associated with poor glycemic control or health outcomes.

5 State 2 educational considerations regarding learning styles and abilities for each of the following age groups: preschool, school age, and adolescent.

Learning Assessment: Case Study 1

HP is a 21-year-old single mother whose 11-month-old son (BP) has just been hospitalized and diagnosed with type 1 diabetes. The mother is a high-school graduate currently employed part-time as a waitress and working a 4 PM to midnight shift. HP is having financial problems. Her sister, who has 4 children of her own, has agreed to watch BP on the nights his mother works.

BP's doctor has prescribed 2 injections of NPH insulin per day, which BP receives before breakfast and bedtime. Lispro insulin was tried and discontinued at this time because of hypoglycemia. BP is still being bottle-fed and receives a bottle before bedtime. The dietitian and HP have developed a 1200-calorie meal plan with 3 meals and 3 snacks per day.

Questions for Discussion

1 What are the primary management and social issues?

2 What are potential educational strategies?

3 What interventions could be implemented immediately and which can be planned for a later time?

Discussion

1 One of the main concerns for this single mother is finding the support and resources needed to adequately care for her child. One approach might be to ask if the mother needs additional support and who could provide it. Or the diabetes educator could explore relationships with other people besides the sister, such as neighbors and friends, and include them in the educational process.

2 Include all individuals in HP's support network in the diabetes education process from the beginning so they are fully aware of the seriousness of her needs.

3 Discuss with the sister her willingness and assess her ability to learn to give insulin injections, do monitoring, and so forth.

4 Social service workers might be able to assist with community resources and explore financial considerations such as expansion of Social Security benefits for this mother.

5 HP also will most likely need a great deal of support, close follow-up, and a positive relationship with her son's healthcare providers. Ongoing evaluation of her level of stress and coping should provide indications for the direction of follow-up care.

6 The infant should not be weaned from the bottle during the period of diagnosis and hospitalization, although this is an appropriate goal to work toward after BP is settled at home. Because hospitalization is a traumatic experience for a very young child, the stress should not be compounded by weaning him at this time from an obvious comfort.

7 Home healthcare nurses might be consulted to look in on and assist this young mother in her efforts to provide a regular schedule and care for her child.

Learning Assessment: Case Study 2

JJ is a 15-year-old male who was diagnosed with type 1 diabetes 8 years ago. As a child his blood glucose was reasonably well controlled, and he had no hospital admissions. Over the past year, JJ has been admitted to the hospital 3 times for DKA and once for severe hypoglycemia. His A1C concentration has risen over the past 2 years from 10.3% to 14.8% (normal = 5.5% to 7.4%). He has been frank about admitting to not testing his blood glucose level. JJ also states that he occasionally forgets to take his insulin, especially the second injection of the day. He lives at home with both parents and 2 younger siblings, does average work in school, and has a girlfriend. He has become very oppositional at home and argues frequently with his parents.

Questions for Discussion

1 What are the primary goals of therapy for this young man?

2 What educational approaches might be effective?

3 What concerns described above are typical adolescent behaviors from a developmental perspective?

Discussion

1 The main goals of therapy are to (1) prevent the recurrent DKA, (2) prevent severe hypoglycemia, and (3) decrease JJ's A1C concentration.

2 Critical to achieving these goals is JJ taking his prescribed doses of insulin and eating regularly.

3 Exploring JJ's goals and the reasons for not taking his insulin might reveal insights that can help JJ to address and problem-solve about his difficulties.

A JJ needs to understand the positive and negative consequences of his decisions and goals, focusing on the present.

B If JJ is out with friends and is either too embarrassed to take his insulin or has not had the foresight to bring it, these issues can be addressed. An insulin regimen that is easy for him to follow and provides for flexibility may be useful. He may like the idea of insulin glargine and a lispro pen. The more portable and convenient his regimen is, the greater the likelihood that he will take his second injection.

C If JJ agrees, his friends, including his girlfriend, can be asked to support these efforts and be invited to attend education classes.

D Asking parents to observe JJ taking his insulin can reinforce the importance of this request.

4 JJ also probably needs an updated educational review because he was at a developmentally younger age when he last received diabetes education.

5 JJ might contract with the educator for small behavior changes that are achievable and mutually agreeable and maintain frequent contact to monitor progress.

6 One motivating factor for JJ may be the potential inability to obtain a drivers license. He may be motivated by the understanding that the adult responsibility of driving is based on safety issues for himself and others on the road. Demonstrating responsibility and safety in his diabetes self-care is a sign that he is ready to take on the adult responsibility of driving.

7 JJ can be assisted in the problem-solving process using hypothetical adolescent situations. One strategy might be to remove the parents from the center of the conflict and communicate directly with JJ without eliminating parental involvement.

8 A referral for counseling, peer support groups, or camp might also be beneficial as JJ passes through a very difficult period of development.

9 Developmental concerns include declining glycemic control due to the insulin resistance of the hormones of puberty and the accompanying characteristics of middle adolescence. In particular, JJ is most likely striving for greater independence and is increasingly busy with his girlfriend and social agenda. He is showing experimentation and risk-taking behaviors. In addition, he is having increasing conflict with his parents. These are typical developmental characteristics of middle adolescence, all of which can affect glycemic control.

References

1 Tull ES, Roseman JM. Diabetes in African Americans. In: National Diabetes Data Group. Diabetes in America. 2nd ed. Bethesda, Md: National Institute of Diabetes and Digestive and Kidney Diseases; 1995:613-625.

2 1997-1999 National Health Interview Survey (NHIS), National Center for Health Statistics, Centers for Disease Control and Prevention.

3 LaPorte RE, Matsushima M, Chang YF. Prevalence and incidence of insulin-dependent diabetes. In: National Diabetes Data Group. Diabetes in America. 2nd ed. Bethesda, Md: National Institute of Diabetes and Digestive and Kidney Diseases; 1995:37-45.

4 Expert Committee on the Diagnosis and Classification of Diabetes Mellitus. Report of the Expert Committee on the Diagnosis and Classification of Diabetes Mellitus. Diabetes Care. 2003;26:S1-S5.

5 Salerno M, Argenziano A, Di Maio S, et al. Pubertal growth, sexual maturation and final height in children with IDDM. Diabetes Care. 1997;20:721-724.

6 International Society for Pediatric and Adolescent Diabetes. Consensus Guidelines 2000. ISPAD Consensus Guidelines for the Management of Type 1 Diabetes Mellitus in Children and Adolescents. Medical Forum International. 2000.

7 Drash A. Management of the child with diabetes mellitus: clinical course, therapeutic strategies, and monitoring techniques. In: Lifshitz F, ed. Pediatric Endocrinology, A Clinical Guide. 2nd ed. New York: Marcel Dekker; 1990:681-700.

8 Shah SC, Malone JI, Simpson NE. A randomized trial of intensive insulin therapy in newly diagnosed insulin-dependent diabetes mellitus. N Engl J Med. 1989;320:550-554.

9 Atkinson MA, Maclaren NK, Luchetta R. Insulitis and diabetes in NOD mice reduced by prophylactic insulin therapy. Diabetes. 1990;39:933-937.

10 Zhang ZJ, Davidson L, Eisenbarth G, Weiner HL. Suppression of diabetes in nonobese diabetic mice by oral administration of porcine insulin. Proc Natl Acad Sci USA. 1991;88:10252-10256.

11 Follansbee D. Assuming responsibility for diabetes management: what age? what price? Diabetes Educ. 1989;15:347-353.

12 Wysocki T, Meinhold PA, Abrams KC, et al. Parental and professional estimates of self-care independence of children and adolescents with IDDM. Diabetes Care. 1992; 15:43-52.

13 McNabb WL, Quinn MT, Murphy DM, Thorp FK, Cook S. Increasing children's responsibility for diabetes self-care: the In Control study. Diabetes Educ. 1994;20: 121-124.

14 Becker D. Management of insulin dependent diabetes mellitus in children and adolescents. Curr Opinion Pediatr. 1991;3:710-723.

15 Boland E. A flexible option for adolescents with diabetes: insulin pump therapy. Adv Nurse Pract. 1998;6:38-44.

16 Kaufman FR, Halvorson M, Fisher L, et al. Insulin pump therapy in type 1 pediatric patients. J Pediatr Endocrinol Metab. 1999;12:759-764.

17 American Diabetes Association. Standards of medical care for patients with diabetes mellitus (position statement). Diabetes Care. 2003;26(suppl 1):S33-S50.

18 American Diabetes Association. Physical activity/exercise and diabetes mellitus (position statement). Diabetes Care. 2003; 26(suppl 1):S73-S79.

19 Arslanian S, Nixon PA, Becker D, Drash AL. Impact of physical fitness and glycemic control on in vivo insulin action in adolescents with IDDM. Diabetes Care. 1990;13:9-15.

20 Campaign BN, Lampman RM. Exercise in the Clinical Management of Diabetes. Champaign, Il: Human Kinetics Publishing; 1994:62.

21 Porter PA, Keating B, Byrne G, Jones TW. Incidence and predictive criteria of nocturnal hypoglycemia in young children with insulin dependent diabetes mellitus. J Pediatr. 1997;130:366-372.

22 Drash A. Clinical Care of the Diabetic Child. Chicago: Year Book Medical Publishers; 1987.

23 Boland EA, Grey M. Coping strategies of school-age children with diabetes mellitus. Diabetes Educ. 1996;22:592-597.

24 Drash A, Becker DJ. Behavioral issues in patients with diabetes mellitus with special emphasis on the child and adolescent. In: Rifkin H, Porte D Jr, eds. Ellenberg and Rifkin's Diabetes Mellitus Theory and Practice. 4th ed. New York: Elsevier Publishing; 1990:922-933.

25 Kovacs M, Feinberg T. Coping with juvenile onset diabetes mellitus. In: Singer JE, Baum A, eds. Handbook of Medical Psychology. Vol 2. Hilldale, NJ: Lawrence Erlbaum Associates; 1982:165-212.

26 Almeida CM. Grief among parents of children with diabetes. Diabetes Educ. 1995;21:530-532.

27 Songer TJ, LaPorte R, Lave JR, Dorman JS, Becker DJ. Health insurance and the financial impact of IDDM in families with a child with IDDM. Diabetes Care. 1997;20:577-584.

28 Mahler M, Pine F, Bergman A. The Psychological Birth of the Human Infant. New York: Basic Books; 1975.

29 Ryan C, Vega A, Drash A. Cognitive deficits in adolescents who developed diabetes early in life. Pediatrics. 1985;75:921-927.

30 Rovet J, Alvarez M. Attentional functioning in children and adolescents with IDDM. Diabetes Care. 1997;20:803-810.

31 Becker D, Ryan C. Hypoglycemia: a complication of diabetes therapy in children. TEM 2000;11(5):198-201.

32 Nordfeldt S, Ludvigsson J. Severe hypoglycemia in children with IDDM. Diabetes Care. 1997;20:497-503.

33 Fraiberg S. The Magic Years. New York: Charles Scribner's Sons; 1959.

34 Rogerson C. Play Therapy in Childhood. New York: Oxford University Press; 1939.

35 Pothier P. Resolving conflict through play fantasy. J Psychiatr Nurs. 1967;5:141-147.

36 Marcus S. Therapeutic puppetry. In: Philpott AR. Puppets and Therapy. New York: Plays Inc; 1977:94-142 and 504.

37 Numbers that Add Up to Educational Rights for Children With Disabilities. Washington, DC: Children's Defense Fund; 1989.

38 American Diabetes Association. Care of children with diabetes in the school and day care setting (position statement). Diabetes Care. 2003;26(suppl 1):S131-135.

39 Daneman D, Wolfson D, Becker DH, Drash AL. Factors affecting glycosylated hemoglobin values in children with insulin-dependent diabetes mellitus. J Pediatr. 1981; 99:847-853.

40 Blethen S, Sargeant DT, Whitlow MG, Santiago JV. Effect of pubertal age and recent blood glucose control on plasma somatomedin C in children with insulin-dependent diabetes mellitus. Diabetes. 1981; 30:868-872.

41 Amiel SA, Sherwin RS, Simonson DC, Lauritano AA, Tamborlane WV. Impaired insulin action in puberty: a contributing factor to poor glycemic control in adolescents with diabetes. N Engl J Med. 1986; 315:215-219.

42 Committee on Adolescence/Group for the Advancement of Psychiatry. Normal Adolescence: Its Dynamics and Impact. New York: Charles Scribner's Sons; 1968.

43 Blos P. On Adolescence: A Psychoanalytic Interpretation. New York: Free Press of Blencoe; 1962.

44 Betschart J. Oral contraception and adolescent women with insulin-dependent diabetes mellitus: risks, benefits and implications for practice. Diabetes Educ. 1996;22:374-378.

45 Anderson BJ, Auslander WC. Research on diabetes management and the family: a critique. Diabetes Care. 1980;3:696-702.

46 Golden MP, Herrold AJ, Orr DP. An approach to prevention of recurrent diabetic ketoacidosis in the pediatric population. J Pediatr. 1985;107:195-200.

47 American Diabetes Association. Evidence-based nutrition principles and recommendations for the treatment and prevention of diabetes and related complications. Diabetes Care. 2003;26(suppl 1):S51-S61.

48 Holzmeister LA. Medical nutrition therapy for children and adolescents with diabetes. Diabetes Spectrum. 1997;10:268-274.

Child-Friendly Internet Resources

www.bam.gov. Bam! Body and Mind. Atlanta, Ga: US Dept of Health and Human Services, Centers for Disease Control and Prevention. Accessed June 11, 2003.

www.childrenwithdiabetes.com. Hamilton, Ohio: Diabetes123/Children with Diabetes/ Diabetes Monitor. Accessed June 11, 2003.

www.diabetes.org/wizdom. Alexandria, Va: American Diabetes Association. Accessed June 11, 2003.

www.VERBnow.com. Atlanta, Ga: US Dept of Health and Human Services, Centers for Disease Control and Prevention. Accessed June 11, 2003.

Educational Materials for Children, Adolescents, and Parents

Betschart J. A Magic Ride in Foozbah Land [Book and audiotape]. New York: John Wiley & Sons; 1995.

Betschart J. Diabetes Care for Babies, Toddlers and Preschoolers. New York: John Wiley & Sons; 1999.

Betschart J, Thom S. In-Control: A Guide for Teens With Diabetes. New York: John Wiley & Sons; 1995.

Betschart J. It's Time to Learn About Diabetes. New York: John Wiley & Sons; 1995.

Betschart J. It's Time to Learn About Diabetes [Video]. Available though the Internet at: www.diabetes.fyi.net. 1993. Accessed October 2000.

Brackenridge B, Rubin R. Sweet Kids: How to Balance Diabetes Control and Good Decision Making With Family Peace. Alexandria, Va: American Diabetes Association; 1996.

Chase PH. Understanding Insulin-Dependent Diabetes. The Pink Panther. 9th ed. Denver: The Guild of the Children's Diabetes Foundation; 2002.

Franz MJ. Exchanges for All Occasions. Now With Carbohydrate Counting. 4th ed. Minneapolis: IDC Publishing; 1997.

Franz MJ. Fast Food Facts. 5th ed. Minneapolis: IDC Publishing; 1997.

Hayes J. Necessary Toughness. Alexandria, Va: American Diabetes Association; 1990.

International Diabetes Center. My Food Plan for Kids & Teens. Minneapolis: IDC Publishing; 1998.

Mazur M. The Dinosaur Tamer. Alexandria, Va: American Diabetes Association; 1998.

Mitchell MK. Nutrition Across the Lifespan. Philadelphia: W.B. Saunders Company; 1997.

Monk A, Cooper N. Convenience Food Facts. 4th ed. Minneapolis: IDC Publishing; 1997.

Satter E. How to Get Your Kid to Eat...But Not Too Much. Palo Alto, Ca: Bull Publishing; 1987.

Siminerio L, Betschart J. Raising A Child With Diabetes: 2nd ed. Alexandria, Va: American Diabetes Association; 2000.

Wysocki T. The Ten Keys to Helping Your Child Grow Up With Diabetes. Alexandria, Va: American Diabetes Association; 1997.

Suggested Readings

American Diabetes Association. Care of children with diabetes in the school and day care setting (position statement). Diabetes Care. 2003;26(suppl 1):S131-S135.

American Diabetes Association. Clinical Practice Recommendations 2003. Diabetes Care. 2003;26(suppl).

American Diabetes Association. Management of diabetes at diabetes camps (position statement). Diabetes Care. 2003;26(suppl 1):S136-S138.

Consensus Guidelines 2000 for the Management of Type 1 Diabetes Mellitus in Children and Adolescents. International Society for Pediatric and Adolescent Diabetes; 2000.

Daneman D. Childhood, adolescence, and diabetes: a delicate developmental balance. Diabetes Spectrum. 1989;2:225-243.

Donaghue KC, Fairchild JM, Craig ME, et al. Do all prepubertal years of diabetes duration contribute equally to diabetes complications? Diabetes Care. 2003;26:1224-1229.

Giordano BP, Petrila AT, Mamien CR, et al. Transferring responsibility for diabetes self-care from parent to child. Pediatr Health Care. 1992;6(Sep-Oct):5.

Holzmeister LA. Medical nutrition therapy for children and adolescents with type 1 diabetes mellitus. Diabetes Spectrum. 1997;10:268-275.

Kleinberg S. Educating the Chronically Ill Child. Rockville, Md: Aspen Publishers; 1982.

Lorenz R, Wysocki T. The family and childhood diabetes. Diabetes Spectrum. 1991;4:261-292.

Petrillo M. Emotional Care of Hospitalized Children. Philadelphia: JB Lippincott Co.; 1980.

Plotnick LP, Clark LM, Brancati FL, Erlinger T. Safety and effectiveness of insulin pump therapy in children and adolescents with type 1 diabetes. Diabetes Care. 2003;26:1142-1146.

Pond JS, Peters ML, Pannell DL, Rogers CS. Psychosocial challenges for children with insulin-dependent diabetes mellitus. Diabetes Educ. 1995;21:297-299.

Sharp AR. Nutrition therapy for children and adolescents with diabetes. In: Franz MJ, Bantle JP, eds. American Diabetes Association Guide to Medical Nutrition Therapy for Diabetes. Alexandria, Va: American Diabetes Association; 1999:211-228.

Vandagriff J, Marrero D, Ingersoll GM, Fineberg NS. Parents of children with diabetes: what are they worried about? Diabetes Educ. 1992;18:299-302.

Learning Assessment: Post-Test Questions

Type 1 Diabetes in Youth

2

1 Type 1 diabetes is caused by:
A Obesity
B Insulin resistance
C Immune-mediated beta cell destruction
D Strong family history

2 Which is a clinical feature which suggests type 2 diabetes?
A Normal body weight
B Acanthosis nigricans
C Necrobiosis lipoidica diabeticorum
D Ketonuria

3 Which is not a goal of therapy for children and adolescents with diabetes?
A Normal growth
B Higher glycemic targets than non-diabetic levels
C Minimal acute or chronic complications
D Positive adjustment to diabetes

4 Most children require approximately the following units of insulin per kilogram of body weight:
A 0.5
B 1.0
C 1.5
D 2.0

5 Which of the following is an appropriate choice when treating hypoglycemia in an infant?
A 4 oz undiluted baby fruit juice
B 1 large tube of glucose gel
C 5 tsp Karo syrup
D 2 Tb honey

6 Which of the following metabolic changes occurs during puberty which leads to deterioration of glycemic control?
A Increased insulin resistance
B Decreased insulin resistance
C Decreased epinephrine responses
D Elevated ketone production

7 A child should be expected to inject his or her insulin by what age?
A Age 8
B Age 10
C Age 12
D No set age: individually determined

8 Infants with diabetes are best fed:
A Soy milk only
B On demand
C On a flexible 3- to 4-hour schedule
D Cereal mixed with milk in the bottle

9 Young children can be helped to express their feelings through:
A Reading
B Play therapy
C Active play
D Singing

10 Poor glycemic control can do all of the following except:
A Delay the onset of puberty
B Cause poor growth
C Cause irregular menstrual cycles
D Cause acne

11 Young children with diabetes do well when given:
A No sugar at all
B Extra insulin before a party
C Choices
D Plenty of water

12 Ketoacidosis in adolescents can be caused by the following except:
A Excessive intake of sweets
B Emotional disturbances
C Insulin omission
D Illness

See next page for answer key.

Post-Test Answer Key

Type 1 Diabetes in Youth   2

1	C	7	D
2	B	8	C
3	B	9	B
4	B	10	D
5	A	11	C
6	A	12	A

A Core Curriculum for Diabetes Education
Diabetes in the Life Cycle and Research

Type 2 Diabetes in Youth

Susan L. Sullivan, RN, BSN, CDE
Driscoll Children's Hospital
Corpus Christi, Texas

Stephanie H. Gerken, RD, LD, CDE
International Diabetes Center
Minneapolis, Minnesota

Introduction

1 Type 2 diabetes is increasingly prevalent in children and adolescents. Despite the wealth of knowledge and experience treating type 2 diabetes in adults, we are just beginning to understand this disease in children.

2 The epidemic of childhood obesity in the United States has been associated with the increased prevalence of type 2 diabetes in children. However, as with adults, both heredity and environmental factors are associated with the diagnosis of type 2 diabetes in children.

3 Insulin resistance is a key factor in type 2 diabetes in youth. In addition to type 2 diabetes, other clinical findings associated with insulin resistance include obesity, acanthosis nigricans, obstructive sleep apnea, hypertension, dyslipidemia, and polycystic ovary syndrome.

4 Treatment of type 2 diabetes in youth is similar to that used in adults, which includes lifestyle modifications and medications. However, the research behind these treatments in youth is still underway. Diagnostic, treatment, and management guidelines are continuing to evolve as evidence-based data become available. Intervention strategies that incorporate food/meal planning and physical activity are emphasized. Research in pharmacologic therapy available for this population is lacking.

5 Children and adolescents who have type 2 diabetes should be monitored for the development of long-term complications. As with adults, it is important to look at other comorbidities such as hyperlipidemia and hypertension when developing a treatment plan. The full effects of this serious health problem are not likely to become evident until these children reach adulthood.

6 Self-management diabetes training is a critical component that involves both the child with diabetes and the entire family or caregivers of the child.

7 Thorough, careful assessment of psychosocial issues is a key component of diabetes self-management training for children or adolescents with type 2 diabetes. Consistent support and reinforcement from healthcare providers as well as the child's family and/or caregivers is key to making long-lasting behavior changes in these youth.

8 Continued efforts at prevention are crucial to preventing or delaying type 2 diabetes in youth. A public health approach to preventing type 2 diabetes in youth will continue to be a priority in the future.

Objectives

Upon completion of this chapter, the learner will be able to
1 State the diagnostic criteria for type 2 diabetes in children and adolescents.
2 List screening criteria for type 2 diabetes in children and adolescents.
3 Identify the unique characteristics of type 2 diabetes in children and adolescents.
4 Describe insulin resistance, including associated clinical findings.

5 State the specific goals of diabetes self-management training for youth with type 2 diabetes.

6 Describe the intervention strategies involving nutrition therapy and physical activity in youth with type 2 diabetes and their families.

7 Describe pharmacologic and monitoring recommendations specific to children and adolescents with type 2 diabetes.

8 Describe the psychosocial issues associated with type 2 diabetes in children and adolescents.

9 Explain the role of the family and/or caregivers in the treatment of type 2 diabetes in children and adolescents.

Diagnosis and Screening of Type 2 Diabetes in Children and Adolescents

1 There has been a significant increase in the number of children and adolescents who are being diagnosed with type 2 diabetes. This increase has paralleled the higher incidence of obesity that is occurring in this age group.

2 Because the exact prevalence of type 2 diabetes in youth is unknown, the Centers for Disease Control and the National Institutes of Health began a 5-year study in 2002 designed to examine the prevalence and status of diabetes mellitus among children and adolescents in the United States.

3 Diagnostic criteria for type 2 diabetes in youth are the same as for adults.[1] The following 3 methods are used to diagnosis diabetes and each must be confirmed on a subsequent day:

   A Symptoms plus casual plasma glucose concentration ≥200 mg/dL (11.1 mmol/L)

   B Fasting plasma glucose concentration ≥126 mg/dL (7.0 mmol/L)

   C Two-hour plasma glucose concentration ≥200 mg/dL (11.1 mmol/L) during an oral glucose tolerance test

4 Ketonuria or ketoacidosis is sometimes present at the time of diagnosis in youth with type 2 diabetes. Up to 33% of children who are diagnosed with type 2 diabetes have ketonuria at the time of diagnosis, and 5% to 25% of children have ketoacidosis at the time of diagnosis.[2]

5 Screening recommendations are based on the American Diabetes Association's consensus statement, Type 2 Diabetes in Children and Adolescents.[2]

   A Screening is recommended for individuals who have a body mass index (BMI) >85th percentile for age and sex, weight for height >85th percentile, or weight >120% of ideal body weight. In addition, 2 or more of the following factors must be present:
   - A family history of first- or second-degree relatives with type 2 diabetes
   - Belong to ethnic groups at higher risk for type 2 diabetes (Native Americans, African Americans, Hispanic Americans, Asians, and South Pacific Islanders)
   - Show signs of insulin resistance (acanthosis nigricans, hypertension, dyslipidemia, or polycystic ovary syndrome)

   B Screening should be done starting at age 10 years or at the onset of puberty, whichever occurs earlier

   C Screening may be considered in other high-risk youths who

- Have a family history of first- or second-degree relatives with type 2 diabetes
- Belong to ethnic groups at higher risk for type 2 diabetes (Native Americans, African Americans, Hispanic Americans, Asians, and South Pacific Islanders)
- Show signs of insulin resistance (acanthosis nigricans, hypertension, dyslipidemia, or polycystic ovary syndrome)

Characteristics of Type 2 Diabetes in Children and Adolescents

1 Youth are usually preteen or older at the time of diagnosis. However, there are reports of diagnosis as early as age 4 years in Pima Indian children.[3]

2 Type 2 diabetes is associated with an increased familial tendency compared with type 1 diabetes. Children and adolescents who are diagnosed with type 2 diabetes are more likely to have adult family members and relatives who have type 2 diabetes.

3 There are a disproportionate number of Native American, African American, Hispanic American, Asian, and South Pacific Islander children and adolescents who are diagnosed with type 2 diabetes.

4 Obesity is a very common finding in children and adolescents who are diagnosed with type 2 diabetes, especially when compared with children and adolescents who are diagnosed with type 1 diabetes.

A Many factors can contribute to the increase in obesity and type 2 diabetes in children, but the most significant factors are increased energy intake and decreased energy output.[3,4]

B More food availability, increased advertising, larger portions of all foods, and increased frequency of eating out are just some of the factors that have increased the intake of energy per person.

C Societal changes account for the decreased amount of physical activity needed for daily living and increased amount of time spent in sedentary activities such as watching television, playing video games, and participating in computer activities.

5 The underlying feature of type 2 diabetes in children and adolescents is insulin resistance, which is defined as a subnormal biological response to a given concentration of insulin.[5] With insulin resistance, muscle, liver, and adipose tissue become less sensitive to insulin.

A Insulin resistance occurs when insulin action is blocked or reduced, causing the ineffective use of insulin. In response to this compromised insulin action, the pancreas produces additional insulin to keep blood glucose levels normal. This results in higher-than-normal endogenous insulin levels in the blood and a condition called hyperinsulinemia.

B The insulin resistance syndrome is characterized by fasting and/or postprandial hyperglycemia plus 1 or more of the following conditions:

- Hypertension based upon age-specific criteria; systolic readings initially greater than diastolic readings
- Dyslipidemia (hypertriglyceridemia and decreased HDL cholesterol)

- Obesity (age-adjusted abnormal weight for height, or body mass index [BMI] >25)
- Menstrual disturbances and hirsutism secondary to ovarian hyperandrogenism[3]

C Insulin resistance is likely an inherited condition for many persons, but there are other possible causes such as fetal exposure to maternal diabetes or obesity and certain medications. Insulin resistance is also associated with puberty.

Clinical Findings in Children and Adolescents Associated With Insulin Resistance

1 Obesity is defined in pediatrics as age-adjusted abnormal weight for height or BMI. Accurate measurements of height and weight should be plotted on gender-specific growth charts to determine the age-appropriate percentile for height, weight, and BMI (see Figures 3.1 to 3.4[6]).

   A In persons with insulin resistance, the ability to produce and store fat may even be greater than normal. Insulin facilitates lipogenesis, the process by which fat cells store unused energy as fat. When insulin levels are high, the extra fuel from food is stored as body fat rather than being used as a source of energy. In this way, hyperinsulinemia contributes to additional weight gain.

   B High insulin levels can also cause rapid growth of muscle, bone, and other tissues. It is common for children with insulin resistance to be heavier, taller, and appear more mature for their years compared with other children the same age.

   C High insulin levels may increase the appetite and cause people to consume larger portions of food before feeling full. As a result, there is speculation that people with insulin resistance have higher energy intakes than those without insulin resistance.

2 Acanthosis nigricans (AN) is a skin condition that signals high insulin levels in the body. The characteristic of hyperpigmented velvety patches of darkened skin over parts of the body that bend or that rub against each other are thought to be caused by the higher than normal insulin levels in the bloodstream.

   A AN is typically found around the neck, under the armpits, along the waistline, in the groin area, and on the knuckles, elbows, and toes. Some children with more severe cases may have thick polyps, called skin tags, around the neck, and/or darkened areas around the nose, eyes, and cheeks (see Figures 3.5[7]).

   B AN is often misidentified as "dirt" or poor hygiene; AN is not a skin infection or other skin disease, but rather a marker of insulin resistance. However, the amount and severity of AN does not reflect the severity of insulin resistance.

   C Darker skinned persons with insulin resistance are more likely to show AN than lighter skinned persons with the same problem. In lighter skinned persons with AN, the skin area may actually appear tan and velvety instead of dark and rough, making AN more difficult to diagnose.

   D There is no skin treatment that will cure AN. Lesions may regress by treating the underlying cause of insulin resistance, but it can take months or years to do so.

3 Hypertension in youth with type 2 diabetes is associated with hyperinsulinemia and obesity. The precise mechanisms have not yet been defined in children and adolescents.

   A To determine the diagnosis of hypertension, the American Heart Association recommends that blood pressure should be interpreted based upon age, gender, and height[8] (see Figures 3.6 to 3.9[9]).

Figure 3.1. Growth Chart for Boys Ages 2 Years to 20 Years

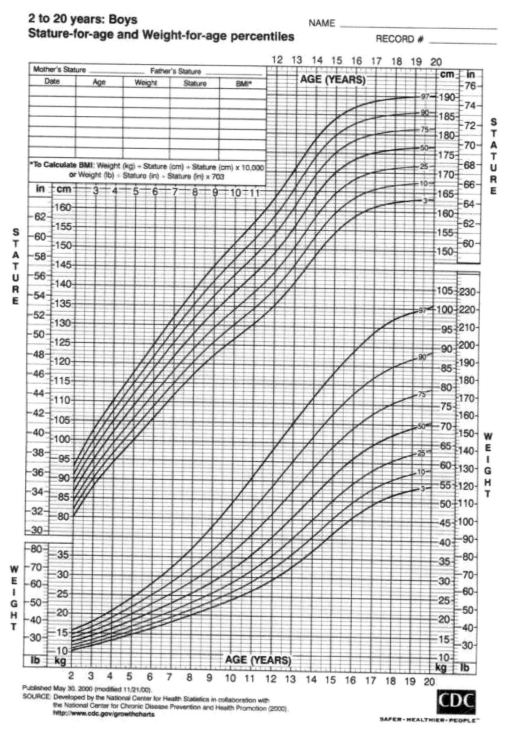

Source: National Center for Health Statistics and National Center for Chronic Disease Prevention and Health Promotion.[6]
Web site: cdc.gov.growthcharts

Figure 3.2. Body Mass Index Chart for Boys Ages 2 Years to 20 Years

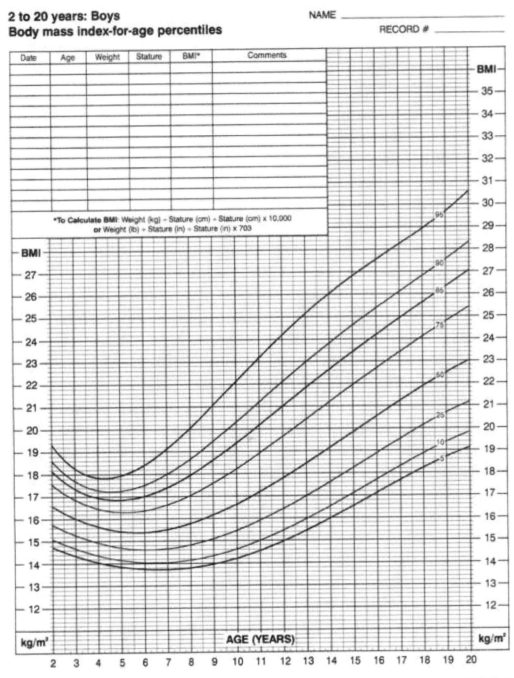

2 to 20 years: Boys
Body mass index-for-age percentiles

NAME _____
RECORD # _____

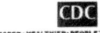

Published May 30, 2000 (modified 10/16/00).
SOURCE: Developed by the National Center for Health Statistics in collaboration with
the National Center for Chronic Disease Prevention and Health Promotion (2000).
http://www.cdc.gov/growthcharts

Source: National Center for Health Statistics and National Center for Chronic Disease Prevention and Health Promotion.[6]

Figure 3.3. Growth Chart for Girls Ages 2 Years to 20 Years

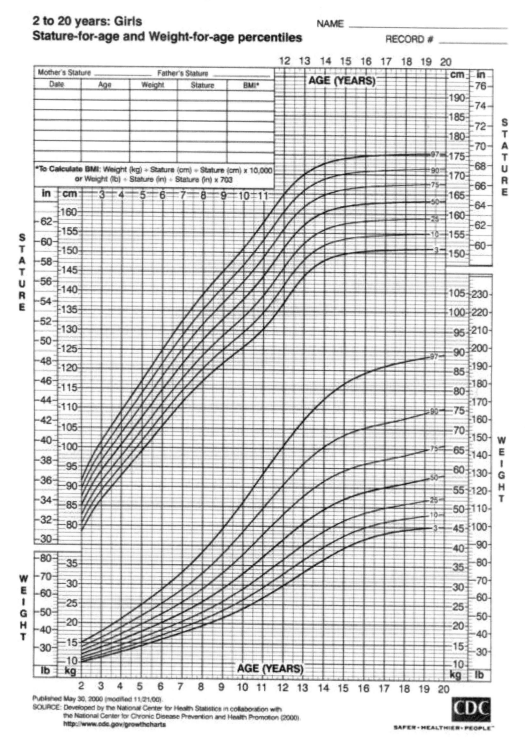

2 to 20 years: Girls
Stature-for-age and Weight-for-age percentiles

NAME _____

RECORD # _____

Published May 30, 2000 (modified 11/21/00).
SOURCE: Developed by the National Center for Health Statistics in collaboration with
the National Center for Chronic Disease Prevention and Health Promotion (2000).
http://www.cdc.gov/growthcharts

CDC
SAFER · HEALTHIER · PEOPLE™

Source: National Center for Health Statistics and National Center for Chronic Disease Prevention and Health Promotion.[6]

Figure 3.4. Body Mass Index Chart for Girls Ages 2 Years to 20 Years

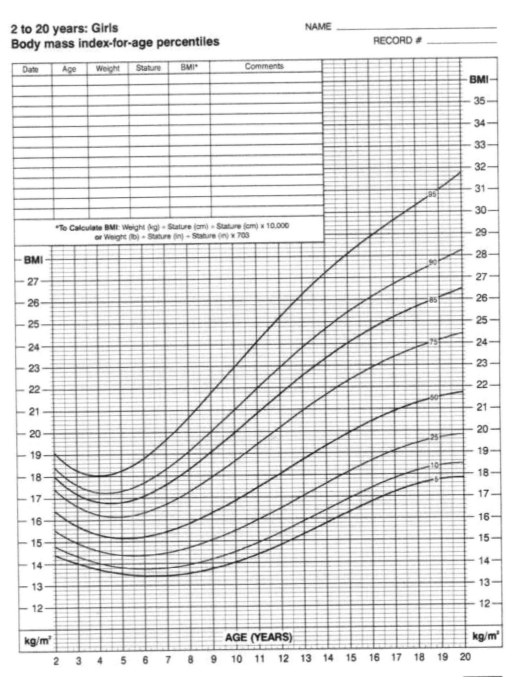

Published May 30, 2000 (modified 10/16/00).
SOURCE: Developed by the National Center for Health Statistics in collaboration with the National Center for Chronic Disease Prevention and Health Promotion (2000).
http://www.cdc.gov/growthcharts

Source: National Center for Health Statistics and National Center for Chronic Disease Prevention and Health Promotion.[6]

Figure 3.5. Examples of Acanthosis Nigricans

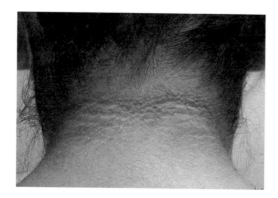

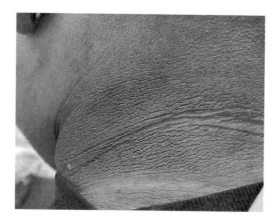

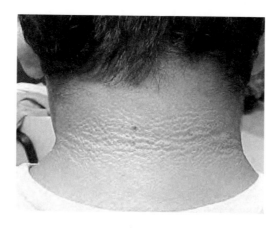

Source: Driscoll Children's Hospital Diabetes Center.[7]

Figure 3.6. Blood Pressure Levels for Boys Ages 1 to 17 Years by Percentiles of Height

BLOOD PRESSURE LEVELS FOR THE 90TH AND 95TH PERCENTILES OF BLOOD PRESSURE FOR BOYS AGE 1 TO 17 YEARS BY PERCENTILES OF HEIGHT

Age	Height Percentiles* → BP†	Systolic BP (mm Hg)							Diastolic BP (mm Hg)						
		5%	10%	25%	50%	75%	90%	95%	5%	10%	25%	50%	75%	90%	95%
1	90th	94	95	97	98	100	102	102	50	51	52	53	54	54	55
	95th	98	99	101	102	104	106	106	55	55	56	57	58	59	59
2	90th	98	99	100	102	104	105	106	55	55	56	57	58	59	59
	95th	101	102	104	106	108	109	110	59	59	60	61	62	63	63
3	90th	100	101	103	105	107	108	109	59	59	60	61	62	63	63
	95th	104	105	107	109	111	112	113	63	63	64	65	66	67	67
4	90th	102	103	105	107	109	110	111	62	62	63	64	65	66	66
	95th	106	107	109	111	113	114	115	66	67	67	68	69	70	71
5	90th	104	105	106	108	110	112	112	65	65	66	67	68	69	69
	95th	108	109	110	112	114	115	116	69	70	70	71	72	73	74
6	90th	105	106	108	110	111	113	114	67	68	69	70	70	71	72
	95th	109	110	112	114	115	117	117	72	72	73	74	75	76	76
7	90th	106	107	109	111	113	114	115	69	70	71	72	72	73	74
	95th	110	111	113	115	116	118	119	74	74	75	76	77	78	78
8	90th	107	108	110	112	114	115	116	71	71	72	73	74	75	75
	95th	111	112	114	116	118	119	120	75	76	76	77	78	79	80
9	90th	109	110	112	113	115	117	117	72	73	73	74	75	76	77
	95th	113	114	116	117	119	121	121	76	77	78	79	80	80	81
10	90th	110	112	113	115	117	118	119	73	74	74	75	76	77	78
	95th	114	115	117	119	121	122	123	77	78	79	80	80	81	82
11	90th	112	113	115	117	119	120	121	74	74	75	76	77	78	78
	95th	116	117	119	121	123	124	125	78	79	79	80	81	82	83
12	90th	115	116	117	119	121	123	123	75	75	76	77	78	78	79
	95th	119	120	121	123	125	126	127	79	79	80	81	82	83	83
13	90th	117	118	120	122	124	125	126	75	76	76	77	78	79	80
	95th	121	122	124	126	128	129	130	79	80	81	82	83	83	84
14	90th	120	121	123	125	126	128	128	76	76	77	78	79	80	80
	95th	124	125	127	128	130	132	132	80	81	81	82	83	84	85
15	90th	123	124	125	127	129	131	131	77	77	78	79	80	81	81
	95th	127	128	129	131	133	134	135	81	82	83	83	84	85	86
16	90th	125	126	128	130	132	133	134	79	79	80	81	82	82	83
	95th	129	130	132	134	136	137	138	83	83	84	85	86	87	87
17	90th	128	129	131	133	134	136	136	81	81	82	83	84	85	85
	95th	132	133	135	136	138	140	140	85	85	86	87	88	89	89

*Height percentile determined by standard growth curves.
†Blood pressure percentile determined by a single measurement.

Source: National Institutes of Health.[9]

Figure 3.7. Blood Pressure Graph of 95th Percentile by Height and Age for Boys

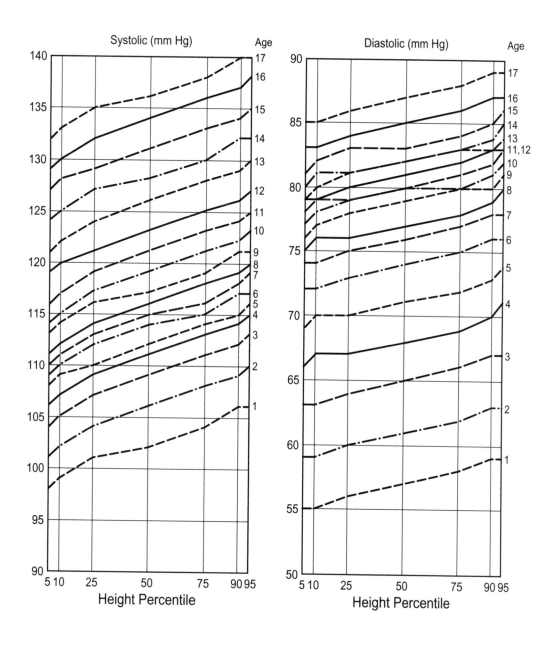

Source: National Institutes of Health.[9]

Figure 3.8. Blood Pressure Levels for Girls Ages 1 to 17 Years by Percentiles of Height

BLOOD PRESSURE LEVELS FOR THE 90TH AND 95TH PERCENTILES OF BLOOD PRESSURE FOR GIRLS AGE 1 TO 17 YEARS BY PERCENTILES OF HEIGHT

Age	Height Percentiles* → BP† ↓	Systolic BP (mm Hg)							Diastolic BP (mm Hg)						
		5%	10%	25%	50%	75%	90%	95%	5%	10%	25%	50%	75%	90%	95%
1	90th	97	98	99	100	102	103	104	53	53	53	54	55	56	56
	95th	101	102	103	104	105	107	107	57	57	57	58	59	60	60
2	90th	99	99	100	102	103	104	105	57	57	58	58	59	60	61
	95th	102	103	104	105	107	108	109	61	61	62	62	63	64	65
3	90th	100	100	102	103	104	105	106	61	61	61	62	63	63	64
	95th	104	104	105	107	108	109	110	65	65	65	66	67	67	68
4	90th	101	102	103	104	106	107	108	63	63	64	65	65	66	67
	95th	105	106	107	108	109	111	111	67	67	68	69	69	70	71
5	90th	103	103	104	106	107	108	109	65	66	66	67	68	68	69
	95th	107	107	108	110	111	112	113	69	70	70	71	72	72	73
6	90th	104	105	106	107	109	110	111	67	67	68	69	69	70	71
	95th	108	109	110	111	112	114	114	71	71	72	73	73	74	75
7	90th	106	107	108	109	110	112	112	69	69	69	70	71	72	72
	95th	110	110	112	113	114	115	116	73	73	73	74	75	76	76
8	90th	108	109	110	111	112	113	114	70	70	71	71	72	73	74
	95th	112	112	113	115	116	117	118	74	74	75	75	76	77	78
9	90th	110	110	112	113	114	115	116	71	72	72	73	74	74	75
	95th	114	114	115	117	118	119	120	75	76	76	77	78	78	79
10	90th	112	112	114	115	116	117	118	73	73	73	74	75	76	76
	95th	116	116	117	119	120	121	122	77	77	77	78	79	80	80
11	90th	114	114	116	117	118	119	120	74	74	75	75	76	77	77
	95th	118	118	119	121	122	123	124	78	78	79	79	80	81	81
12	90th	116	116	118	119	120	121	122	75	75	76	76	77	78	78
	95th	120	120	121	123	124	125	126	79	79	80	80	81	82	82
13	90th	118	118	119	121	122	123	124	76	76	77	78	78	79	80
	95th	121	122	123	125	126	127	128	80	80	81	82	82	83	84
14	90th	119	120	121	122	124	125	126	77	77	78	79	79	80	81
	95th	123	124	125	126	128	129	130	81	81	82	83	83	84	85
15	90th	121	121	122	124	125	126	127	78	78	79	79	80	81	82
	95th	124	125	126	128	129	130	131	82	82	83	83	84	85	86
16	90th	122	122	123	125	126	127	128	79	79	79	80	81	82	82
	95th	125	126	127	128	130	131	132	83	83	83	84	85	86	86
17	90th	122	123	124	125	126	128	128	79	79	79	80	81	82	82
	95th	126	126	127	129	130	131	132	83	83	83	84	85	86	86

*Height percentile determined by standard growth curves.
†Blood pressure percentile determined by a single measurement.

Source: National Institutes of Health.[9]

Figure 3.9. Blood Pressure Graph of 95th Percentile by Height and Age for Girls

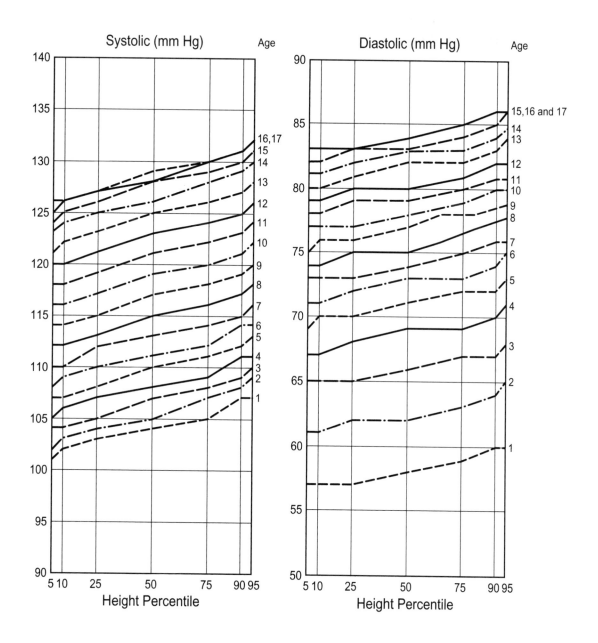

Source: National Institutes of Health.[9]

- Three separate blood pressure readings should be taken on 3 separate days.
- Resting blood pressure measurements are used.
- Values that are above the 95th percentile for children of similar sex, age, and weight indicate hypertension.

B Increased physical activity and weight management are key initial approaches to managing hypertension in youth with type 2 diabetes.

C The following pharmacologic treatment recommendations are from the American Diabetes Association's consensus statement on type 2 diabetes in children.[2]

- Angiotensin-converting enzyme (ACE) inhibitors comprise the first-line therapy for managing hypertension in youth. ACE inhibitors also are the first-line therapy for microalbuminuria.
- Second-choice medications for treating hypertension in youth include ß-blockers, calcium antagonists (long-acting), and low-dose diuretics.
- Although ß-blockers may be used in this age group, there is concern that these medications may mask hypoglycemic symptoms.
- Combination therapy is indicated if normotension is not achieved using these medications as monotherapy.

4 Dyslipidemia is often identified in children and adolescents with type 2 diabetes. For adults with type 2 diabetes, dyslipidemia far outweighs all other risk factors for cardiovascular disease, and this may be true as well for children with type 2 diabetes.[2]

A Lipid screening (total cholesterol, LDL cholesterol, and triglyceride profile) is recommended for all children who have diabetes.[10]

B Nonpharmacologic treatment strategies for dyslipidemia include increased physical activity and reduced dietary fat intake with an emphasis on weight management.

C Cholestyramine and colestipol are currently the only medications approved by the Food and Drug Administration (FDA) for treating hypercholesterolemia in children.

5 Because obstructive sleep apnea (OSA) is often unrecognized and can impact treatment outcomes, the presence or absence of symptoms of OSA should be assessed in obese children and adolescents who have been diagnosed with type 2 diabetes.[3]

A OSA is characterized by pauses or stoppages in the breathing pattern (apneas) during sleep. These pauses in respiration can occur as often as 30 or more times per hour. When breathing is interrupted during sleep, the oxygen level in the brain can fall to dangerously low levels. The low level of oxygen causes the child or adult to partially awaken to begin breathing normally. The person generally will not remember this. These frequent interruptions interfere with getting an adequate night's sleep.

B OSA also can cause an increase in the carbon dioxide level in the blood, which can lead to such serious problems as failure to grow in small children, heart failure in older children and adults, delayed mental development, and even death in some cases. The length of the sleep interruption does not need to be very long; young children have had serious problems caused by frequent stoppages lasting only 3 to 4 seconds each.

C Overweight persons may have difficulty breathing normally during sleep. They may breathe loudly (snore) and may temporarily stop breathing for short periods of time during sleep because of the weight of body tissues in the neck. The episodes of apnea occur during the early stages of deep sleep. When such an episode occurs, the person awakens and then starts breathing normally again. However, the person has been prevented from getting the proper level of deep sleep. These apneas may occur repeatedly throughout the night.

D Children and adolescents who have OSA may experience any or all of the signs and symptoms listed in Table 3.1.

Table 3.1. Signs and Symptoms of Obstructive Sleep Apnea

- Loud breathing and snoring at night
- Daytime sleepiness (falls asleep in the car during short trips)
- Headaches upon awakening
- Restless sleep (moves excessively during sleep)
- Needs multiple pillows to keep the head raised during sleep
- Increased bedwetting
- Hyperactivity and aggressive behaviors at school
- Poor school performance

- OSA is commonly a factor in poor school performance. Children with OSA are always tired and often do not like to exercise and play as much as other children, which can make weight management even more challenging.
- OSA is often confused with attention deficit hyperactivity disorder (ADHD) and, as a result, it is common for OSA to be misdiagnosed as ADHD.
- Children with suspected OSA should be referred to a pediatric sleep specialist. The sleep specialist will perform a sleep study to confirm or deny the diagnosis and determine the severity of the problem. Sleep studies are painless, noninvasive evaluations that only require the person to fall asleep for several hours while breathing patterns, heart rate and rhythm, and brain wave patterns are monitored through EEG and EKG sensors that are placed on the body. This study can be done in a hospital or a special sleep study center.

E The best treatment for OSA is weight loss, but this may take several years to accomplish if it is the only treatment. During that time, the child's health and school performance can be severely damaged. One treatment often used is the removal of the tonsils and adenoids, which allows better breathing at night. Some children may need to wear a special mask over their nose that is connected to a small tube through which air is pumped to help them breath more effectively at night. The choice of treatment is determined based on the severity of the problem.

6 Polycystic ovary syndrome (PCOS) is a reproductive disorder characterized by hyperandrogenism and ovulatory dysfunction without delay in puberty. Oligomenorrhea or amenorrhea is a common complaint. Clinical findings may include hirsutism, alopecia, and acne. Often there is a family history of infertility and oligomenorrhea.[3]

A Treatment options include weight loss and oral contraceptives with low androgen activity and antiandrogens. The use of metformin may normalize ovulatory function in PCOS, but can increase the risk of unplanned pregnancy.

B Psychological counseling and screening for depression should be considered as part of the treatment plan.

Treatment Goals and Diabetes Self-Management Training for Youth With Type 2 Diabetes

1 Treatment goals for type 2 diabetes in youth include

  A Normal growth and development

  B Euglycemia

  C Weight reduction, if indicated

  D Decreased risk of comorbidities associated with insulin resistance

  E Prevention of long-term complications

2 Diabetes self-management training (DSMT) must be viewed as a lifetime process rather than an intensive learning session.

  A Self-monitoring of blood glucose (SMBG) is an essential component of DSMT that involves the person with diabetes performing regular preprandial and postprandial blood glucose testing.[3] The timing and frequency of SMBG should be tailored to the individual.

  B A written record of the blood glucose results should be kept to discuss with the healthcare team and used to evaluate therapy. (See Chapter 5, Monitoring, in Diabetes Management Therapies for discussion of keeping paper records versus using memory/data managers.)

Medical Nutrition Therapy for Youth With Type 2 Diabetes

1 Assessment and intervention strategies involving lifestyle modifications with food and physical activity choices are crucial in the treatment plan for youth with type 2 diabetes. The intervention strategies need to involve the entire family or child's caregivers for continued lifelong success.

2 The Centers for Disease Control published growth charts in 2000 and new body mass index-for-age charts (Figures 3.1 to 3.4) that can be used to can help define a child's percentile of body mass index (BMI) at diagnosis and at continued follow-up appointments.[6]

  A BMI can also be determined by the following formulas:

    • Weight in kilograms/(height in meters)^2 (kg/m^2)

    • (Weight in pounds/height in inches) x 70^3

  B The BMI-for-age for the 85th percentile to 95th percentile for children and adolescents is defined as at risk for overweight.[6]

  C The BMI-for-age for >95th percentile for children and adolescents is defined as overweight.[6]

  D It is important to be sensitive when weighing patients. To maintain privacy, place the scales in the clinic rooms or give the option of doing a blind-weight (stepping backwards on the scale) if the child or adolescent is very nervous or sensitive about the subject.

3 Preparing a comprehensive history of food/nutrition intake and physical activity and/or assessing food records can help identify current energy intake and output. This information is important for determining the behavior change goals that will be tailored to the individual.

A Knowing the specific amounts of food eaten, the duration and type of physical activity performed, and the amount of time spent in sedentary activities can contribute to a better understanding of the issues of concern.

B Points of concern that can usually be identified include, but are not limited to, the following categories:
- High-calorie, high-fat snacks
- High-calorie, high-fat drinks
- Increased amount of sedentary activity
- High percentage of meals and snacks eaten outside of the home
- Low intake of fruits and vegetables
- Irregular meal and snack times
- Disordered type of eating

C Assessing cultural, environmental, and personal circumstances of the child and family can help determine the proper treatment goals related to food and activity.[3,11]

D The child's and family's readiness to change and the level of independence of the child should be assessed.

4 Specific weight goals should be individualized. When weight loss is necessary, the most appropriate method remains modest calorie restriction, incorporating a balanced intake of macronutrients and micronutrients, with increased physical activity.[3]

A The primary weight goal is to prevent further weight gain.

B Dietary restriction may be appropriate for adults but is not appropriate for a growing child. Restricting calories should not interfere with obtaining the crucial nutrients required for optimal growth and development.

C In multidisciplinary weight-reduction programs (modest calorie restriction with increased physical activity) for obese adolescents, the majority of the participants were able to sustain normal growth velocity while effectively decreasing body weight.[12]

D The term diet should be avoided when discussing changes to food choices because this term implies a temporary solution and not a lifelong change.

5 Successful treatment with nutrition therapy and changes in physical activity/exercise is characterized by

A Cessation of excessive weight gain with normal linear growth

B Near-normal fasting blood glucose levels (<126 mg/dL [7.0 mmol/L]) and near-normal A1C values (less than 7% in most laboratories)[2]

C Proper control of and treatment for other associated diagnoses, such as hypertension and dyslipidemia

6 Nutrition education is a crucial part of therapy for children and adolescents with type 2 diabetes. Meal plan goals should be based on consuming foods from all food groups, with special attention to portion sizes and food preferences, emphasizing a whole-diet approach.

A At the time of diagnosis, it is important to decrease or eliminate from the diet excessive amounts of high-carbohydrate foods (eg, extra-large desserts) and drinks (eg, regular soda and juice).

B Meal plan recommendations should be culturally appropriate, sensitive to family resources, and available to all caregivers.

C Measurable, achievable food and nutrition goals should be established with the child and family or caregivers to help normalize blood glucose levels. These goals should also reflect changes that can affect other comorbidities such as dyslipidemia and hypertension.

D The importance of consuming certain nutrients needed for optimal growth, such as calcium and vitamins, should be addressed.

E Ongoing nutrition instruction should be established to focus on specific topics, such as cooking techniques, eating out, and low-fat eating (see Table 3.2 in Key Educational Considerations).

F Food records or journals can be used to help individuals and their families establish behavior changes and evaluate goals.

7 Special attention to the emotional connection between food and/or weight status should be evaluated and monitored. A child's self-esteem can be affected by weight alterations and the diagnosis of a chronic disease.

A Ongoing medical nutrition therapy can help a child overcome habits such as eating out of boredom, fear, isolation, and/or other stressors.

B Dieting can have a significant impact on psychological health, especially for adolescents, during this time of rapid physical, psychological, and social development. Several studies have correlated adolescent problem behavior with dieting status.[12]

C Developing an awareness of hunger and fullness cues can help children with their behavior change goals.

D It is important to emphasize to children and adolescents that their self-worth has nothing to do with their weight status or diagnosis of diabetes.

Physical Activity

1 Emphasis should be placed on decreasing the amount of sedentary activity and setting specific physical activity goals.

A The first priority is to decrease the amount of sedentary activity. Assistance should be given in identifying options for replacing the sedentary activities.

B Increased exercise/physical activity, which increases lean muscle mass, has been shown to help decrease insulin resistance and encourage weight control and weight loss in adults.[13]

2 Identifying activities in which children and adolescents are interested can increase their participation in exercise and physical activity (see Table 3.3 in Key Educational Considerations).

3 Specific achievable physical activity goals should be set initially and revised as the goals are met.

4 Children and adolescents treated with insulin or an insulin secretagogue should be taught to recognize and treat hypoglycemia and adjust medications if necessary for increased participation in physical activities.

5 To match the physiologic function of the child, non weight-bearing activities should be encouraged for children who are 150% to 200% of their ideal body weight (IBW) or >97th percentile for BMI and strongly recommended for those who are >200% of IBW and >95th percentile for BMI, when starting an exercise program.[14]

Pharmacologic Treatment

1 The goal of pharmacologic treatment is to normalize levels of blood glucose and A1C. The choice of an oral glucose-lowering agent, insulin regimen, or combination is based on the clinical situation and individualized to the specific child.

2 Safety and effectiveness of metformin has been established for children ages 10 years and older. Dosage and safety in children under age 10 years has not been established.

A The manufacturer recommends a starting dose of metformin of 500 mg twice daily given with meals. Dosage adjustments are made in increments of 500 mg to a total of 2000 mg per day. The maximum dose for children ages 10 to 16 years is 2000 mg per day. The maximum dose of metformin for adolescents ages 17 years and older is 2500 mg per day.

B An alternate dosing method is to start with a single 250-mg dose of metformin with the largest meal.[15] The dosage is increased weekly by 250 mg, and metformin is then taken with the morning and evening meals.

3 Although there are currently a significant number of pediatric pharmacologic studies in progress, no oral agent besides metformin is currently approved by the FDA for pediatric use. In the near future, other agents are likely to be added to the list of pharmacologic agents approved for pediatric use.

4 Because the pathophysiology of type 2 diabetes in children and adolescents appears to be similar to that of type 2 diabetes in adults, it is reasonable to assume that the currently available glucose-lowering agents will be effective in children.[2]

5 When an oral agent is being considered, the child should be assessed for ability to swallow pills. It may be necessary to choose a pharmacologic agent that can be crushed, such as glimepiride (Amaryl), rosiglitazone maleate (Avandia), or glyburide (Diabeta).

6 Insulin provides the most effective way to quickly normalize blood glucose levels. A wide variety of insulin regimens are available.

A When clinically indicated, insulin therapy should be initiated. Oral agents can be added and the insulin dose decreased when blood glucose levels are under control.

B If it is necessary to initiate insulin therapy at the time of diagnosis, ketones should be monitored due to the possibility that the actual diagnosis may be type 1 diabetes and the patient may be in the honeymoon phase of the disease.

Monitoring

1 Self-monitoring of blood glucose (SMBG) should be part of the initial training at the time of diagnosis. Currently, there are no evidence-based studies on the specific frequency of testing in children and adolescents with type 2 diabetes. The following guidelines are based upon the American Diabetes Association's consensus statement, Type 2 Diabetes in Children and Adolescents.[2] SMBG should be performed as follows:

A During periods of acute illness

B When symptoms of hyperglycemia or hypoglycemia are present

C Periodically if on insulin or sulfonylureas to detect asymptomatic hypoglycemia

D At least 3 times per day if on insulin

E Tailored to individual needs (usually fasting and postprandial)

2 Although not specific to the child or adolescent who has type 2 diabetes, the American Association of Clinical Endocrinologists (ACE) developed the following recommendations for glucose goals: [16]

A Preprandial plasma glucose of 110 mg/dL (6.1 mmol/L) or less

B Postprandial plasma glucose of 140 mg/dL (7.8 mmol/L) or less

3 The American Diabetes Association consensus statement, Type 2 Diabetes in Children and Adolescents, recommends normalization of blood glucose and A1C levels as the ideal goal of treatment.[2]

A The normal fasting plasma glucose level is <126 mg/dL (7.0 mmol/L)

B The normal A1C value is less than 7% (in most laboratories)

4 Individuals with diabetes should be monitored for complications, regardless of their age.

A A dilated eye exam and microalbuminuria screening should be performed annually.[2]

B Although there is a general agreement that other screenings should be performed, including blood pressure screening, lipid screening, foot examinations, and macrovascular disease screening, the frequency of these screenings has not been clearly defined.

Psychosocial Issues

1 Because the family environment influences the lifestyle behaviors of the child with type 2 diabetes, it is often necessary to work with the entire family on lifestyle changes.

A Many children with type 2 diabetes have first-degree family members who also have type 2 diabetes, diagnosed or undiagnosed.[2,11] However, these other family members may not be actively pursuing healthy lifestyle management. In such cases, the child who is being told to "Do as I say, not as I do" may become frustrated or alienated.

B The family of a child with type 2 diabetes will often show lifestyle characteristics such as a high-fat diet, minimal physical activity, and incidences of binge eating.[11]

C The prevalence of obesity is lowest among children who watch 1 hour or less of television per day and a highest among those who watch 4 hours or more of television per day.[17]

D Television viewing can affect an individual's energy balance by providing a greater opportunity to consume more calories, a lower metabolic rate that is associated with sedentary activity, a decreased opportunity for movement, and the influence of advertisements for high-fat foods.

2 Children and adolescents with type 2 diabetes should be assessed for the presence of clinical depression and/or low self-esteem, both of which can have an impact on diabetes self-management and metabolic control.

3 Although youth with type 2 diabetes may not verbally express concerns about long-term complications of diabetes, they may have been exposed to family members who have developed long-term complications and may fear that those complications will happen to them.

4 Classmates of children who are obese can be extremely cruel in teasing and name-calling, which may hinder the child's social interactions, school performance, and self-esteem.

5 Certain developmental issues may need to be evaluated, such as dealing with feelings about being different due to having diabetes (eg, testing blood glucose in the school setting).

6 Adolescence is a time of increased risk taking and decreased parental control.

7 The treatment plan must allow for cultural adaptation if it is to be successful.

Prevention of Type 2 Diabetes in Youth

1 Prevention efforts target the general population and involve a public health approach to developing and implementing school and community-based programs that are directed at improving overall nutrition and physical activity for all children and their families.[2-4,18]

2 Recent data indicate that there may be a significant number of obese children with undiagnosed impaired glucose tolerance or frank type 2 diabetes.[19]

Key Educational Considerations

1 The diagnosis of type 2 diabetes in children and adolescents has increased significantly since the late 1980s.

2 Because the occurrence of type 2 diabetes in this population is relatively new, there are limited data specific to type 2 in children and adolescents on which to base practice recommendations. In the absence of clinical data, experience with adults is being used as a guide for many of the recommendations.

3 The key treatment modality for type 2 diabetes in youth is lifestyle change, which involves increasing physical activity, choosing healthy foods, and improving eating habits. Family involvement plays a vital role in implementing successful lifestyle changes. See Tables 3.2 and 3.3 for a summary of educational strategies for children and adolescents with type 2 diabetes.

4 Pharmacologic therapy may be necessary in the management of type 2 diabetes in children or adolescents who have type 2 diabetes, but should be used with caution due to the potential of unknown long-term effects.

5 Family dynamics, developmental issues, cultural aspects, and treatment goals must all be considered when providing DSMT to the child or adolescent who has type 2 diabetes.

Table 3.2. Nutrition Education Strategies for Youth With Type 2 Diabetes

- Establish set times for meals and snacks; encourage the family to eat together.
- Encourage children and adolescents to eat breakfast.
- Reinforce the idea that all foods are okay; there are no good foods or bad foods.
- Encourage consumption of low-calorie beverages most of the time and drinking only water between meals, particularly for those who tend to get a lot of their daily calories from beverages.
- Teach how to recognize proper portion sizes for various types of foods, especially for snack foods.
- Introduce 1 new fruit or vegetable each week so children will have more choices from which to accomplish the goal of consuming 5 servings of fruits and vegetables per day. New foods may have to be introduced several times before children become familiar with them and ask for them.
- Emphasize eating low-fat dairy products with a goal of consuming 3 servings per day.
- Provide guidance for choosing healthy foods for school lunches.
- Limit eating out to less than 3 times per week.
- Identify the family's attitudes toward food, eating, and physical activity and encourage a more positive relationship between their attitudes and these lifestyle behaviors.

Table 3.3. Physical Activity Education Strategies for Youth With Type 2 Diabetes

- Encourage youths to just keep moving because any type of activity is better than none.
- Focus on more unstructured play for younger children and a physical activity goal of 40 to 60 minutes of physical activity per day for adolescents.
- Teach the youth how to make specific exercise goals, such as walking for the duration of a favorite music CD or walking around the house while talking on the phone.
- Use pedometers or other gadgets to peak interest in exercise.
- Focus on involving the family in physical activities.
- Encourage the youth to work towards a goal of less than 2 hours' sedentary activity daily.
- Emphasize choosing activities that can be done with others rather than exercising in isolation; encourage any extracurricular activities.
- Suggest taking 5-minute activity breaks every 30 minutes while watching TV, playing video games, or sitting at the computer.
- Establish reward systems that are not food related for achieving physical activity goals.
- Identify the family's attitudes towards physical activity, food, and eating, and encourage a more positive relationship between these attitudes and lifestyle behaviors.
- Prepare a selection of practical and enjoyable family activities, and help the family to establish a realistic time commitment, including a schedule of when the entire family can be active together.

Self-Review Questions

1 What are the diagnostic criteria for type 2 diabetes in children and adolescents?

2 What screening criteria are used for type 2 diabetes in children and adolescents?

3 What are unique characteristics of type 2 diabetes in children and adolescents?

4 What casual factors have been associated with the increase in obesity and type 2 diabetes in children and adolescents?

5 What is the definition of "at risk for overweight" and "overweight" for children and adolescents based on the CDC's body mass index-for-age charts?

6 What is insulin resistance?

7 What are the 6 clinical findings associated with insulin resistance?

8 What are 5 treatment goals?

9 How has the American Diabetes Association defined successful treatment with a child who has type 2 diabetes?

10 What are the recommendations for monitoring long-term complications specific to type 2 diabetes in youth?

11 What areas of concern regarding food and activity can be identified after a comprehensive assessment with children or adolescents with type 2 diabetes and for their family or caregiver?

12 Which oral agents are approved for use in children ages 10 years and older?

13 When should SMBG be performed in the child or adolescent with type 2 diabetes?

14 What psychosocial issues are associated with type 2 diabetes in children and adolescents?

Learning Assessment: Case Study 1

Sarah is a quiet, unsmiling, obese 11-year-old Hispanic preteen who just been diagnosed with type 2 diabetes and referred for DSMT. Her physician has ordered insulin injections twice daily (a rapid-acting/intermediate insulin mix of 75/25 with 50 units to be given before breakfast and 40 units to be given before dinner), and SMBG 5 times per day (before meals, 2 hours after breakfast, and at bedtime). A return appointment is scheduled at the physician's office in 1 month for evaluation of treatment and to possibly start metformin. Her A1C level is 9.7%.

Sarah's mother and a grandmother, who are both overweight, accompany Sarah to her appointment. The family history includes type 2 diabetes in both grandmothers, and numerous aunts and uncles on both sides of the family, and her mother had gestational diabetes with her last pregnancy. Sarah's mother denies having diabetes, but has not been tested since her last pregnancy 8 years ago. Both of Sarah's grandfathers have died of diabetes-related complications. Sarah's mother tells you that the family does not want Sarah to start insulin because insulin "made one of her aunts go blind." The presence of acanthosis nigricans is noted on Sarah's neck, knuckles, and elbows. Sarah's mom apologizes for her daughter's "dirty" skin and says that she tries repeatedly to wash her skin but can not get it clean.

Sarah is doing very poorly in school and has trouble staying awake in class. Her mother reports that the children in school tease Sarah about her weight, and Sarah starts to cry.

Questions for Discussion

1 What are the priorities for this DSMT session?

2 What concerns will you want to address at future sessions?

3 What additional information will you need that may require additional referrals?

Discussion

1 The priority for this session is for Sarah to start insulin administration and SMBG instruction. Issues that will have to be addressed include the following:

A SMBG
- Determine whether Sarah is able and willing to perform SMBG. If so, she will need instruction as well as her mother and grandmother.
- Make arrangements for Sarah to perform SMBG at school.

B Insulin administration
- Determine who will supervise and administer the insulin.
- Initially you may want to recommend that Sarah's mother and grandmother give all injections.

C Psychosocial issues
- Reassure the family that insulin does not cause blindness and provide a brief explanation as to the role of hyperglycemia in long-term complications such as blindness.
- Encourage family participation in the educational sessions and interventions.

2 Other concerns for Sarah and her family that you may want to address at future sessions include the following:

A Nutrition management
- A major goal of nutrition therapy will be weight management.
- Family participation and involvement are necessary to support Sarah.
- Cultural/ethnic food preferences need to be incorporated into the meal plan.
- Meals and snacks at school need to be assessed and included in the meal plan.

B Increased physical activity
- Encourage Sarah to identify activities in which she would like to participate.
- Encourage Sarah's family to participate in physical activities with Sarah.

C Acanthosis nigricans (AN)
- Explain that AN is a skin condition that signals high insulin levels in the body. It is believed that the higher-than-normal insulin levels in the bloodstream cause the growth of darkened skin over parts of the body that bend or that rub against each other. AN is not the result of poor hygiene, and it can not be scrubbed clean.
- Remind Sarah and her mother that AN is not a skin infection or disease. There is no skin treatment that will make AN quickly disappear, but treatment of the underlying cause can lighten the skin and make the condition less noticeable.

D If Sarah is started on metformin, she will need to monitor blood glucose levels carefully for the possible need to decrease the insulin dose and potentially discontinue the insulin.

E Sarah's mother should be tested for type 2 diabetes.

3 Other areas in which additional information is needed that may require interventions include the following:

A Hypertension

- Because Sarah has type 2 diabetes, she should be assessed for hypertension.
- Age, gender, and height are required to accurately determine if Sarah has hypertension.

B Dyslipidemia

- Sarah's screening should include a total cholesterol, LDL cholesterol, and triglyceride profile.
- Initial treatments include increased physical activity and medical nutrition therapy.

C School performance

- Sarah should be screened for possible depression, an undiagnosed learning disability, and/or OSA.
- If Sarah is diagnosed with depression, pharmacologic treatment as well as counseling may be indicated.
- If screening indicates that Sarah may have OSA, a referral to a pediatric sleep specialist should be considered.

Learning Assessment: Case Study 2

Richard is a very pleasant 15-year-old adolescent referred for DSMT. His physician is treating him with metformin and referred him for diabetes education. His current screening measurements are as follows: A1C 8.1%, cholesterol 215 mg/dL, triglycerides 239 mg/dL, LDL cholesterol 140 mg/dL, HDL cholesterol 25 mg/dL, height 5 ft 10 in, and weight 310 lb.

Family history reveals that Richard's father has type 2 diabetes and a recent heart attack but has never attended any formal education for either condition. Both parents continue to smoke in the home but are trying to quit. His mother is most involved in Richard's care. Lately, Richard has been very concerned about his father's health and also confused because there is a girl at his school who has diabetes but takes "shots."

A typical day for Richard begins by either eating breakfast at school or grabbing a regular soda if he is running late, or often, not eating at all. Lunch at school consists of items from the ala carte line, such as a burger and fries or pizza. Richard is part of the football team and tries to lift weights during the off-season. However, he has no other structured activity on a regular basis. After school he comes home and either does his homework, plays on the computer, or watches television. Both parents are usually not home until after 5:30 PM. His mother does most of the cooking and is asking for specific menus that she could follow. She is feeling overwhelmed about what to prepare for Richard yet also cooks meals that her husband will like since he is partial to fried foods. Richard has expressed some interest in cooking.

Questions for Discussion

1 What are your major concerns about Richard's lifestyle?

2 What is Richard's BMI? Where is he on the BMI growth charts?

3 What is the A1C goal for Richard?

4 How would you prioritize and start the education process?

Discussion

1 There are many concerns regarding Richard and his family's lifestyle that will need to be prioritized. Some concerns include not eating breakfast, drinking regular soda, eating high-fat meals at school and home, being sedentary after school on a regular basis, the high-fat cooking at home, being exposed to second-hand smoke, and Richard's emotional stress/concern for his father's health.

2 Richard's BMI is 44.5, which places him at the >95th percentile.

3 Richard's A1C goal should be less than 7%.

4 As an education team, it is important to help Richard understand the difference between type 1 and type 2 diabetes and to explain why he is taking a certain medication and when to take it.

5 The level of nutrition education should be based on how open Richard is to change. A first step to positive change will be to decrease the amount of high-carbohydrate foods and drinks. It will be important to show Richard and his family some healthier food options to replace their current high-calorie, high-fat foods as well as ways to decrease portion sizes. Examples of fruits and vegetables should be introduced along with ways to incorporate them into the meals at home, preferably at breakfast and dinner.

6 Decreasing the amount of time spent in sedentary activity is one of the most important goals. Exploring different activity options based on his interests will help Richard increase his daily physical activity and achieve the goal of less than 2 hours of watching television and playing video games or computer activities. By building on his interest in football, future goals should be established and reinforced to establish a regular physical activity routine for Richard. Activities for the entire family should also be encouraged.

7 Blood glucose testing should be introduced with specific recommendations, such as testing in the fasting state, before the main meal, and 2 hours after the main meal. For Richard, this testing schedule would probably be before dinner and 2 hours after dinner.

8 Educating the entire family can help establish long-lasting behavior changes and facilitate support for Richard. Psychology or counseling interventions may help Richard deal with his concerns for his dad as well as help the family dynamics in terms of changing lifestyle.

References

1 The Expert Committee on the Diagnosis and Classification of Diabetes Mellitus. Report of the Expert Committee on the Diagnosis and Classification of Diabetes Mellitus. Diabetes Care. 2003;26(suppl 1):S5-S20.

2 American Diabetes Association. Type 2 diabetes in children and adolescents (consensus statement). Diabetes Care. 2000; 23:381-389.

3 Ponder SW, Sullivan S, McBath G. Type 2 diabetes mellitus in teens. Diabetes Spectrum. 2000;13:95-105.

4 Rosenbloom AL, Joe JR, Young RS, Winter WE. Emerging epidemic of type 2 diabetes in youth. Diabetes Care. 1999;22: 345-354.

5 Shirn ML, Geffner ME. Insulin resistance in children. Endocrinologist. 1999;9:270-276.

6 Growth charts (2000). Developed by the National Center for Health Statistics in collaboration with the National Center for Chronic Disease Prevention and Health Promotion. Available at: http://www.cdc. gov/growthcharts. Accessed March 19, 2003.

7 Stuart C. Photographs of acanthosis nigricans. Available at: http://www.driscoll-childrens.org/Greystone/diabetes/pated.html. Corpus Christi, Tex: Driscoll Children's Hospital. Accessed March 19, 2003.

8 American Heart Association. Scientific statement. Cardiovascular health in children: a statement for health professionals from the Committee on Atherosclerosis, Hypertension, and Obesity in the Young (AHOY) of the Council on Cardiovascular Disease in the Young, American Heart Association. Circulation. 2002;106:143-160.

9 National Institutes of Health. Update on the Task Force Report (1987) on High Blood Pressure in Children and Adolescents: A Working Group Report from the National High Blood Pressure Education Program. Bethesda, Md: National Institutes of Health; 1996. NIH publication 96-3790. Available at: http://www.nhlbi.nih.gov/health/prof/heart/hbp/hbp_ped.pdf. Accessed March 21, 2003.

10 American Association of Clinical Endocrinologists. Medical guidelines for clinical practice for the diagnosis and treatment of dyslipidemia and prevention of atherogenesis (2002 amended version). Endocr Pract. 2000;6:1-52.

11 Hamiel OP, Standiford D, Hamiel D, et al. The type 2 family: a setting for development and treatment of adolescent type 2 diabetes mellitus. Arch Pediatr Adolesc Med. 1999;153:1063-1067.

12 Daee A, Robinson P, Lawson M, et al. Psychologic and physiologic effects of dieting in adolescents. South Med J. 2002;95:1032-1041.

13 Després J-P, Couillard C, Bergeron J, LaMarche B. Regional body fat distribution, the insulin resistance-dyslipidemic syndrome, and the risk of type 2 diabetes and coronary heart disease. In Ruderman N, Devlin JT, Schneider SH, Kriska A, eds. Handbook of Exercise in Diabetes. Alexandria, Va: American Diabetes Association; 2002;197-234.

14 Sothern M, Schumacher H, Von Almen T, Carlisle L, Udall J. Committed to kids: an integrated, 4-level approach to weight management in adolescents. J Am Diet Assoc. 2002;102 (3 suppl):S81-S85.

15 Mazze RA, Robinson R, Simonson G, et al. Detection and Treatment of Metabolic Syndrome and Type 2 Diabetes in Children and Adolescents: Quick Guide. 1st ed. Minneapolis, Minn: International Diabetes Center; 2002.

16 American Association of Clinical Endocrinologists. The American Association of Clinical Endocrinologists medical guidelines for the management of diabetes mellitus: The AACE system of intensive diabetes self-management—2002 Update. Endocr Pract. 2002;8(suppl 1):40-82.

17 Crespo CJ, Smit E, Trojano RP, et al. Television watching, energy intake, and obesity in US children. Arch Pediatr Adolesc Med. 2001;155:360-365.

18 American Diabetes Association. The prevention or delay of type 2 diabetes (position statement). Diabetes Care. 2003;26 (suppl 1):S62-S69.

19 Sinha R, Fisch G, Teague B, et al. Prevalence of impaired glucose tolerance among children and adolescents with marked obesity. N Engl J Med. 2002; 346:802-810.

Suggested Readings

Berg Frances M. Children and Teens Afraid to Eat: Helping Youth in Today's Weight-Obsessed World. Healthy Weight Publishing Network. 2001.

Betschart-Roemer J. Type 2 Diabetes in Teens: Secrets for Success. New York: John Wiley & Sons; 2002.

International Diabetes Center. Being Healthy Rocks! Minneapolis, Minn: International Diabetes Center; 2002.

Mazze RA, Robinson R, Simonson G, et al. Detection and Treatment of Metabolic Syndrome and Type 2 Diabetes in Children and Adolescents: Quick Guide. 1st ed. Minneapolis, Minn: International Diabetes Center; 2002.

Sothern M. Trim Kids: The Proven 12-Week Plan That Has Helped Thousands of Children Achieve a Healthier Weight. New York: Harper Resource; 2001.

Child-Friendly Internet Resources

www.bam.gov. Bam! Body and Mind. Atlanta, Ga: US Dept of Health and Human Services, Centers for Disease Control and Prevention. Accessed June 11, 2003.

www.childrenwithdiabetes.com. Hamilton, Ohio: Diabetes123/Children with Diabetes/ Diabetes Monitor. Accessed June 11, 2003.

www.diabetes.org/wizdom. Alexandria, Va: American Diabetes Association. Accessed June 11, 2003.

www.VERBnow.com. Atlanta, Ga: US Dept of Health and Human Services, Centers for Disease Control and Prevention. Accessed June 11, 2003.

Learning Assessment: Post-Test Questions

Type 2 Diabetes in Youth

3

1 The skin condition known as acanthosis nigricans:
  A Is a diagnostic criteria for the youth with type 2 diabetes
  B Signals high insulin levels in the body
  C Can be treated with 2% hydrocortisone topical cream
  D Reflects the level of insulin resistance

2 The only medication that currently has FDA approval for use in children with type 2 diabetes who are ages 10 years and older is:
  A Glimepiride
  B Glyburide
  C Metformin
  D None of the above

3 All of the following conditions are commonly associated with type 2 diabetes in youth except:
  A Cystic fibrosis
  B Hypertension
  C Dyslipidemia
  D Obesity

4 When comparing type 1 and type 2 diabetes in children, the youth who has type 2 diabetes is more likely to:
  A Have first- or second-degree relatives who also have diabetes
  B Be overweight
  C Show signs of insulin resistance (acanthosis nigricans, hypertension, and dyslipidemia)
  D All of the above

5 What is the definition of successful nutrition therapy of type 2 diabetes in youth?
  A Decrease of symptoms and blood glucose levels <200 mg/dL
  B Cessation of excessive weight gain with normal linear growth
  C Near-normal fasting blood glucose levels (<126 mg/dL) and near-normal A1C values (less than 7%)
  D B and C

6 The primary weight management goal for youth with type 2 diabetes is to:
  A Restrict daily energy intake by 500 calories
  B Follow a weight-loss diet until the weight goal is achieved
  C Stop weight gain through modest energy restriction and increased physical activity
  D Increase the amount of physical activity per day to avoid energy restriction

7 When setting behavior change goals with the youth and the youth's family or caregivers, it is important to:
  A Assess cultural, environmental, and personal circumstances of the family
  B Explore the youth's and family's readiness to change and/or level of independence of the youth
  C Determine if there are other psychosocial issues that will interfere with the youth's success
  D All of the above

8 What are some of the casual factors that have contributed to the increase in childhood obesity as well as type 2 diabetes?
  A Increased portion sizes and greater availability of food
  B Autoimmune viruses
  C Increased sedentary lifestyle
  D A and C

9 The definition of overweight for children and adolescents is
  A >85th percentile of body mass index
  B >50th percentile of body mass index
  C >95th percentile of body mass index
  D >100th percentile of body mass index

10 Based on a food/nutrition history of a youth with type 2 diabetes, which areas of increased concern should be considered in developing an individualized care plan?
  A The youth does not know carbohydrate counting
  B The youth drinks large amounts of juice each day
  C The youth watches television or plays games on the computer after school each day
  D B and C

See next page for answer key.

Post-Test Answer Key

Type 2 Diabetes in Youth

3

1	B		6	C
2	C		7	D
3	A		8	D
4	D		9	C
5	D		10	D

A Core Curriculum for Diabetes Education
Diabetes in the Life Cycle and Research

Pregnancy With Preexisting Diabetes

Carol J. Homko, RN, PhD, CDE
Temple University Hospital
Philadelphia, Pennsylvania

Karin R. Sargrad, MS, RD, CDE
Temple University Hospital
Philadelphia, Pennsylvania

Introduction

1 Diabetes mellitus is one of the most commonly encountered complications of pregnancy, affecting more than 150 000 pregnancies in the United States annually.[1]

2 The outlook for pregnant women with diabetes and their children has improved dramatically over the last 25 years due to improvements in diabetes care such as the use of self-monitoring of blood glucose and intensive insulin therapy to normalize maternal metabolism throughout the gestation period, better fetal monitoring, and advances in neonatal intensive care.

3 The perinatal mortality rate of infants of women with diabetes has decreased dramatically from 25% of live births in the 1960s to a near-normal 2% of live births since the 1980s.[2,3]

4 Despite these recent advances in care, women with diabetes and their infants remain at greater risk for a number of complications, most notably congenital malformations, which account for 40% to 50% of the perinatal deaths in these infants. To prevent these anomalies, euglycemia must begin in the preconception period and continue throughout the period of organogenesis.

5 The fetal risks and infant morbidity observed in the infant of the diabetic mother are related to the severity of the maternal hyperglycemia and consequent fetal hyperinsulinism. To prevent these short-term and long-term metabolic and growth complications, glycemic control must be maintained throughout pregnancy. This is best accomplished through the provision of multidisciplinary team care and targeted self-management education.

6 Topics that are addressed in this chapter include the metabolism of normal pregnancy and the alterations that occur in maternal diabetes, potential maternal and neonatal complications, the essentials of preconception counseling and care, and diabetes management and education.

Objectives

Upon completion of this chapter, the learner will be able to

1 Identify how gestational diabetes differs from type 1 or type 2 diabetes that existed prior to pregnancy.

2 Identify risk factors associated with a poor outcome in a pregnancy complicated by diabetes.

3 Describe normal maternal metabolism during pregnancy.

4 List neonatal complications.

5 List potential maternal complications.

6 Explain the relationship between preconception glucose control and the incidence of congenital anomalies and spontaneous abortions.

7 State potential maternal complications for the patient with pregestational diabetes.

8 State blood glucose guidelines for pregnancy.

9 State 4 nutrients whose requirements increase substantially during pregnancy.

10 Describe 2 important topics to discuss with patients during preconception counseling.

11 Identify strategies to achieve blood glucose levels.

12 Identify specific patient education needed for self-management during pregnancy.

13 List 2 components of postpartum care and education for women with diabetes.

Definition of Diabetes in Pregnancy

1 The types of diabetes that occur during pregnancy can be divided into 2 groups.

   A The first group consists of women with preexisting diabetes, either type 1 diabetes or type 2 prior to pregnancy (pregestational).

   B The second group consists of women who develop gestational diabetes, which is defined as carbohydrate intolerance of variable severity with the onset or first recognition during pregnancy.[4] (See Chapter 5, Gestational Diabetes, for more information.)

2 Approximately 0.2% to 0.3% of all pregnancies occur in women with insulin-treated diabetes diagnosed prior to pregnancy.[1] Another 2% of all women in the United States of childbearing age have undiagnosed type 2 diabetes. Type 2 diabetes is increased among individuals of African, Latino, and American Indian ancestry. Type 2 diabetes comprises 65% of all pregnancies complicated by established diabetes.[5-8]

Classification Systems for Pregnancy Complicated by Diabetes

1 Various classification systems have been developed to identify risk factors in women who are pregnant and have diabetes.

2 The White classification system was for many years the most widely applied system for assessing the risk factors of pregnancy complicated by diabetes.[9]

   A White observed that the age of onset of maternal diabetes, duration, and the presence of vascular complications all had an important impact on the outcome of pregnancy.

   B In terms of outcome measures, problems with the White classification include omission of any mention of glycemic control and guidelines regarding insulin treatment for gestational diabetes. For these reasons, many diabetes and pregnancy programs rely on narrative descriptions of women with both preexisting and gestational diabetes to more closely predict maternal and neonatal outcomes.

3 Pederson et al[10] offered another classification system for poor pregnancy outcomes. They noted 5 prognostically "bad" signs of pregnancy associated with unfavorable outcomes: ketoacidosis, pyelonephritis, pregnancy-induced hypertension, poor clinic attendance, and self-neglect.

4 Both White's classifications and Pederson's prognostically "bad" signs have been used to identify patients at risk for poor pregnancy outcomes.

5 Buchanan and Coustan[11] offer another classification system which takes into account glycemia, the presence of diabetic vascular complications, and the type of diabetes (Table 4.1). These factors appear to be more important predictors of perinatal outcome than either the age at onset or the duration of maternal diabetes.

6 From a management standpoint, pregnancies complicated by diabetes are generally separated into 2 groups: those with and those without vascular complications.

Table 4.1. Classification of Diabetes During Pregnancy

Pregestational Diabetes	Risks
Type of maternal diabetes	
Type 1	• Ketoacidosis
Type 2	• Obesity, hypertension
Metabolic control and timing	
Early pregnancy	• Birth defects, spontaneous abortions
Later pregnancy	• Hyperinsulinemia, overgrowth, stillbirth, polycythemia, respiratory distress syndrome
Maternal vascular complications	
Retinopathy	• Worsening during pregnancy
Nephropathy	• Edema, hypertension, intrauterine growth retardation
Atherosclerosis	• Maternal death
Gestational diabetes	
Fetal risks	• Hyperinsulinemia and macrosomia, possibility of stillbirth
Maternal risks	• Hypertensive disorders in pregnancy, diabetes following pregnancy
Metabolic control	
Fasting plasma glucose <105 mg/dL (Class A^1; diet-controlled)	
Fasting plasma glucose >105 mg/dL (Class A^2; insulin treated)	

Source: Adapted from Buchanan and Coustan.[11]

Normal Metabolism

1 An understanding of the metabolic changes that occur in a nondiabetic pregnancy is necessary to be able to normalize metabolism for the best possible outcome in a diabetic pregnancy.

2 Fuel metabolism during early gestation:

A The fetus depends upon the mother for an uninterrupted supply of fuel. To meet fetal needs, the following maternal adaptations occur:[12]

- Increased tissue glycogen storage and peripheral glucose utilization, enhanced hepatic glucose production
- A shift toward production of free fatty acids and ketones
- Pancreatic cell hypertrophy with resultant increased insulin response to glucose
- Decreased maternal alanine (gluconeogenic amino acid) leading to hypoglycemia and lower fasting blood glucose levels than in the nongravid state

B There is a passive diffusion of glucose across the placenta.

C Hyperemesis and food intolerance may occur.

D The early months of a nondiabetic pregnancy can be described as a period of maternal anabolism during which maternal fat storage takes place.

3 Fuel metabolism during late gestation:

A The metabolic changes related to pregnancy increase progressively during the second and third trimesters. Late pregnancy is characterized by accelerated growth of the fetus, sharply rising blood levels of several diabetogenic hormones, including human placental lactogen and estrogens, and increasing resistance to the multiple action of insulin.[13-15]

B Changes occur in both the fasting and fed states.

- The fasting state of pregnancy is characterized by a more rapid diversion to fat metabolism (accelerated starvation).[16] It consists of an earlier than normal switch from predominately carbohydrate to predominately fat utilization. This results in an increased risk for diabetic ketoacidosis (DKA) and fasting ketosis.
- Whenever food is withheld, concentrations of free fatty acids and ketones reach higher levels in pregnant women than in nongravid women, again increasing the risk for DKA.
- Although fasting and 24-hour mean glucose levels are reduced, food ingestion results in higher and more prolonged plasma glucose concentrations in pregnant women compared with nongravid women.[17] This more sustained, postprandial hyperglycemia enhances transplacental delivery of glucose to the fetus and promotes growth of the fetus. (Maternal insulin and glucagon do not cross the placenta.)
- During late pregnancy, a woman's basal insulin levels are higher than nongravid levels, and food ingestion results in a twofold to threefold increase in insulin secretion.[17]

Perinatal Complications

1 There are increased rates of perinatal complications in pregnancies complicated by diabetes. These complication rates can be correlated to the level of maternal glycemia.

A Complications can result from high glucose levels during the first trimester (ie, congenital malformations and spontaneous abortions).

B Metabolic complications can be seen secondary to maternal hyperglycemia in the second and third trimester after the fetal pancreas has begun to function. These include neonatal hypoglycemia, macrosomia, increased childhood rates of obesity and impaired glucose tolerance, stillbirth, respiratory distress syndrome (RDS), hyperbilirubinemia, hypocalcemia, and polycythemia.

2 First-trimester hyperglycemia can result in a number of complications including congenital malformations and spontaneous abortions in pregnant women with diabetes.

A Congenital malformations often develop before the woman knows she is pregnant; fetal organogenesis occurs during the first 8 weeks of gestation.[18]

- The incidence of congenital malformations is 6% to 13% in pregnancies complicated by preexisting diabetes where glycemic control is not established prior to conception. This rate of congenital malformations is 2 to 3 times greater than the 2% to 3% rate for the general population.[18-23]

- Studies of maternal glycosylated hemoglobin levels at the end of the first trimester as an index of glycemia during organogenesis generally reveal an anomaly risk of 2% to 5% in women with diabetes who have normal to moderately elevated levels.[20-22] When levels are markedly elevated, the malformation rate rises substantially, reaching as high as 20% to 40% in some studies.[21-23]

- The types of birth defects that occur in infants of women with poorly controlled diabetes during organogenesis are varied but most often involve the cardiovascular, central nervous, and skeletal systems (see Table 4.2). The defects are commonly multiple, more severe, and more often fatal than those in the general population.

- Congenital heart defects are the most common birth defect seen in infants of mothers with type 1 diabetes, occurring in 4% of all diabetic pregnancies.[18] Transposition of the great vessels, ventricular septal defects, and coarctation of the aorta are other common cardiac defects.

B Spontaneous abortion rates have also been found to correlate with first-trimester glycosylated hemoglobin values. These rates have been reported to be as high as 30% to 60%, depending on the degree of hyperglycemia at the time of conception (Figure 4.1).[24] In the Diabetes in Early Pregnancy Project (DIEP)[25] and a study by Greene et al,[22] the frequency of spontaneous abortions was similar to the frequency expected in nondiabetic pregnancies when first-trimester glycosylated hemoglobin levels were in the normal to moderately elevated ranges. Once the glycosylated hemoglobin value was 3 standard deviations above the norm, the risk for spontaneous abortion increased more and more steeply as the levels increased further from normal.

3 The association between glycemic control and birth defects prompted several studies of preconception management in women with diabetes. Fuhrmann et al,[26,27] Steel et al,[28] and Kitzmiller et al[29] have reported a virtual elimination of excess anomalies in studies designed to achieve very good glycemic control prior to conception. The results of these studies suggest that it may be possible to eliminate the high rate of congenital malformations by achieving a normalized A1C value prior to conception. Therefore, planned pregnancies are extremely important for women with diabetes.

4 Second- and third-trimester hyperglycemia results in increased neonatal metabolic complications.

A Hypoglycemia in the neonate, the most common metabolic complication, is defined as plasma glucose values less than 35 mg/dL (1.92 mmol/L) in term infants and less than 25 mg/dL (1.37 mmol/L) in preterm infants.[30]

Table 4.2. Congenital Malformations in Infants of Diabetic Mothers (Type 1 Diabetes)

Anomaly	Gestational Age After Last Menstrual Period
Sacral agenesis (Caudal regression)	5 weeks
Spina bifida, hydrocephalus, or other CNS defect	6 weeks
Anencephalus	6 weeks
Heart anomalies	
Transposition of great vessels	7 weeks
Ventricular septal defect	8 weeks
Atrial septal defect	8 weeks
Anal/rectal atresia	8 weeks
Renal anomalies	
Agenesis	7 weeks
Cystic kidney	7 weeks
Ureter duplex	7 weeks
Situs inversus	6 weeks

Source: Reprinted with permission from Mills et al.[18]

Figure 4.1. Major Malformations and Spontaneous Abortions According to First-Trimester A1C

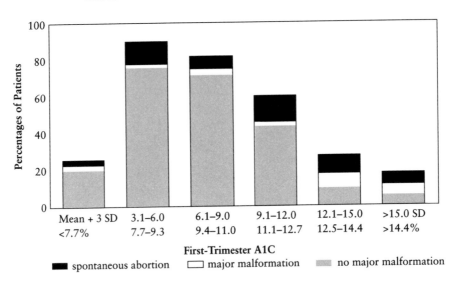

Source: Adapted from Jovanovic.[24]

- When blood glucose levels are elevated during pregnancy, the fetus receives larger amounts of glucose, amino acids, and fatty acid fuels than are required for normal growth and development. The increased delivery of these nutrients stimulates fetal growth and maturation of normally immature pancreatic beta cells in the fetus.
- At delivery, when the maternal blood supply is eliminated, the fetus continues to produce excess amounts of insulin that may result in neonatal hypoglycemia.
- The peak incidence of neonatal hypoglycemia is 6 to 12 hours after birth, but if severe it can persist for several days or more.
- The clinical signs of hypoglycemia in the newborn include tremor, tachypnea, episodes of cyanosis, convulsion, weak or high-pitched cry, and episodes of sweating.
- Because prolonged and severe hypoglycemia may be associated with neurological sequelae, treatment is advised for plasma glucose levels of less than 40 mg/dL (2.2 mmol/L). However, the most efficient and safest treatment is prevention by the early initiation of oral feedings.

B Macrosomia (abnormally large body size) in the neonate is generally defined as a weight of 4000 g or greater.[31] It should be noted that there is no widely agreed-upon weight definition. Any evaluation of fetal weight must be considered in the context of gestational age.

- A fetus with a gestational age of 32 weeks and an estimated fetal weight of 3800 g or > 90% for gestational age is nonetheless considered large for gestational age (LGA) and also has an increased perinatal morbidity similar to a fetus with macrosomia. LGA is the most common clinical definition of macrosomia.
- In the general population, macrosomia occurs in 10% of all pregnancies, and a fetus with a weight of 4500 g occurs in only 1% of all pregnancies. In pregnancies complicated by diabetes, the incidence of macrosomia is between 20% and 32%, making macrosomia the most common complication of diabetes during pregnancy.
- Macrosomic and LGA fetuses have increased demands for oxygen. When the demands for oxygen exceed the supply, asphyxia results. This reaction may account for the increased death rate in macrosomic fetuses in the late third trimester. Thus, close follow-up and fetal surveillance are needed.
- The development of macrosomia in late pregnancy is highly correlated with maternal glycemia as explained by the Pederson hypothesis.[19] The hypothesis states that maternal hyperglycemia leads to fetal hyperglycemia, which in turn stimulates the fetal pancreas to produce excessive amounts of insulin (a growth factor for fetal tissue).
- Fetal macrosomia is evidenced by the enlargement of the abdominal and chest circumference compared with the head circumference. These infants tend to have almost twice as much body fat as infants of a nondiabetic mother, with their fat cells being increased both in size and number. Organomegaly is also present and there is considerable disproportionality between head and shoulder size. Increased skin fold thickness and a fetal fat line are specific to infants of mothers with poor glucose control and can be seen on ultrasound. In 2 separate studies,[32,33] ultrasonographic evidence of these fetal morbidities confirmed poor glucose control and was associated with an A1C level of 6.3% or greater (normal equals 4.4% to 6.4%).
- Most of the perinatal morbidity associated with pregnancies complicated by diabetes result from the traumatic delivery of a macrosomic infant. Macrosomia is a risk factor for shoulder dystocia, which can lead to birth trauma such as Erb

palsy. A cesarean section is judicious when the estimated fetal weight is in excess of 4500 g.[34]

C Stillbirth is a complication of a diabetic pregnancy that can be dramatically reduced when glycemic control is maintained throughout pregnancy and delivery and sophisticated fetal monitoring tests are employed. The precise cause of stillbirths in pregnancies complicated by diabetes is still not known. However, chronic intrauterine hypoxia is a likely explanation.

D Respiratory distress syndrome (RDS) now is an infrequent complication of a diabetic pregnancy.

- In the past, obstetricians commonly induced preterm delivery, which often resulted in RDS because the infant's lungs were not fully mature.
- Because of blood glucose monitoring and new approaches to care resulting in improved glycemic control, sophisticated fetal monitoring, and the ability to document fetal lung maturity, most babies can now be delivered close to term (38 to 40 weeks), thereby eliminating the problems of preterm delivery.

E Hypocalcemia, hyperbilirubinemia, and polycythemia occur more frequently in infants of mothers with less-than-optimal glucose control during the third trimester of pregnancy. These problems are infrequent in babies whose mothers maintained glycemic control and who were delivered at term (37 to 40 weeks' gestation). The pathogenesis of hypocalcemia is not well understood. Polycythemia is related to increased levels of erythropoietin (which correlate directly with maternal insulin levels), and hyperbilirubinemia results from the breakdown of the excess red blood cells that are needed during pregnancy.

F Poor maternal glucose control and ketonemia have been associated with neuropsychological defects in the offspring of women with diabetes. [35-38]

Maternal Complications

1 The incidence of total hypertensive complications, including pregnancy-induced hypertension, preeclampsia, and chronic hypertension is increased among women with diabetes.[39] A large Scandinavian report found the combined incidence of preeclampsia and pregnancy-induced hypertension to be 4 times higher among women with overt diabetes as compared to controls.[40] In addition, the incidence of these complications is greater in women with vascular disease than among those without vasculopathy. An association between poor glycemic control and preeclampsia and pregnancy-induced hypertension has been reported by several investigators.[41,42]

2 Hydramnios are significantly more common among women with pregestational diabetes. The etiology of hydramnios among diabetic pregnancies has not been established, but is believed to be related to increased fetal urine production. Increasing amniotic fluid volume has been associated with increased output of fetal urine measured sonographically.

3 More recent studies have not found an increased incidence of pyelonephritis but do report a significantly higher incidence of infectious postoperative complications among women with pregestational diabetes.

4 Studies indicate that preterm delivery occurs at an increased rate among women with overt diabetes. The risk of preterm delivery has been found to be significantly affected by the mother's blood pressure state. Green and associates[43] found that the relative risk (RR) of preterm delivery for normotensive diabetic women was 2.08 RR and rose to 5.19 RR among hypertensive women.

5 The rate of delivery by cesarean section has been shown to be increased among women with diabetes. Given the increased likelihood of both obstetrical and medical complications, this difference is understandable. However, some of this increase is believed to be related to differences in patterns of physician decision-making.

Preconception Counseling and Care

1 Preconception care in the US remains the exception rather than the rule, despite the fact that clinical trials over the last decade have demonstrated its effectiveness in reducing the incidence of malformations.

A In Copenhagen between 1982 and 1986, 76% of women with diabetes sought care prior to conception.[44]

B In contrast, in the California Diabetes and Pregnancy Program (CDAPP), only 7% of women sought preconception care between 1982 and 1986.[45]

C In Maine between 1987 and 1990, 34% of eligible women sought care prior to conception.[46]

D A multi-center study involving 5 institutions in Michigan found that 37% of women sought preconception care with the proportion of women seeking this care varying from 15% to 50%.[47]

2 The economics of preconception care were examined in 2 separate studies.[48,49] In the first study by Elixhauser et al,[47] the costs of preconception care for women with established diabetes were $1721 per enrolled patient, and the benefit-cost ratio was 1.87. In other words, for every dollar spent on preconception care, $1.87 was gained. A second study by Scheffler and colleagues[48] examined actual hospital charges and lengths of stay, comparing women from the CDAPP who enrolled prior to 8 weeks' gestation versus after 8 weeks' gestation. A savings of $7 253 for each enrolled patient was realized, and the benefit-cost ratio for the program was between $5 and $6. This suggests that for every dollar spent on preconception care, $5 to $6 was recovered in direct medical costs.

3 Preconception care for women with preexisting diabetes ideally begins 3 to 6 months prior to conception to allow sufficient time to evaluate the mother's health status and to normalize or maximize glycemic control, thereby offering the best chance for the unborn child.

4 Two percent of women of childbearing age have unrecognized type 2 diabetes.

A Women of childbearing age who have risk factors for diabetes need to be tested before they attempt conception.

B Provide counseling for women with diabetes of childbearing age about the potential risks of an unplanned pregnancy. Appropriate contraception also needs to be emphasized and offered.

C Women with type 2 diabetes need to make the transition from oral glucose-lowering agents to insulin before conception. The safety of all currently available oral agents has not been established in pregnancy and may lead to prolonged neonatal hypoglycemia and are therefore not recommended. However, a study in women with gestational diabetes mellitus has found glyburide to be a safe and clinically effective alternative to insulin.[50] (For more information on oral glucose-lowering agents during pregnancy, see Chapter 5, Gestational Diabetes, in Diabetes in the Life Cycle and Research.)

5 Neonatal and maternal problems may develop if blood glucose control is not maintained prior to and throughout gestation and if skilled obstetrical care is not available. For this reason, team management by an endocrinologist, obstetrician/perinatologist, nurse educator, dietitian, and social worker is highly desirable. In addition, women with diabetes who have complications require special attention by the appropriate medical subspecialist.

6 Topics that are important to discuss with each patient and her significant other include fertility, spontaneous abortion rates, incidence of congenital anomalies, incidence of diabetes in offspring, and the effects of pregnancy on existing complications.
 A The discussion of risks needs to be done with sensitivity to the distress that it may cause. Offer realistic but positive messages. Discuss psychosocial concerns and offer support as an integral part of care and education.
 B The increased financial burden of a pregnancy with diabetes also needs to be discussed (eg, testing and fetal surveillance, diabetes supplies, and the potential for lost time from work).
 C The following information is helpful for discussing these issues with patients:
 • There is no evidence to suggest that women with diabetes are less fertile than nondiabetic women.
 • The risk of spontaneous abortion in women with diabetes appears to be no greater than the risk for nondiabetic women when glycemic control is good to fair.[13,23] Spontaneous abortion rates increased dramatically in these studies when glycosylated hemoglobin levels were markedly elevated.
 • Results from one long-term follow-up study[51] indicated a net cumulative risk of 2% for type 1 diabetes in children born to mothers with type 1 diabetes. In contrast, the prevalence of type 1 diabetes in the offspring of type 1 fathers is reported to be 6%.[52] The risk for offspring of mothers with type 2 diabetes is not precisely known but is related to ethnic origin and the presence or absence of obesity. The empiric risk for offspring to develop diabetes or some form of glucose intolerance is 33%.[46] Frequently, diabetes or impaired glucose tolerance of the offspring is not manifested until adulthood.
 • An essential preconception consideration is achieving optimal diabetes control prior to and throughout early pregnancy.
 • With normal or near-normal glycosylated hemoglobin levels in early pregnancy the risk of birth defects is reduced to a level similar to that in the general population. However, a perfectly healthy baby cannot be guaranteed because the risk in the general population is still 2% to 3%.[19-21,25]
 • Women with markedly elevated glycosylated hemoglobin levels need to be informed that they may be at higher risk for an infant with a congenital mal-

formation and that the risk may be as high as 20% to 40%. While this is difficult for patients to hear, it is important for them to know.

- When counseling about birth defects, offer maternal serum alpha-fetoprotein screening for neural tube defects and ultrasonographic evaluation for central nervous system, heart, renal, and skeletal anomalies. It must be emphasized that none of these tests is 100% sensitive for detecting fetal malformations.

7 The following preconception protocol is recommended prior to discontinuing contraception.

A A thorough assessment is needed to detect any vascular complications, including a dilated retinal examination; a 24-hour urine collection for creatinine, creatinine clearance, and microalbumin; thyroid function tests; and an EKG. Any detected complications need evaluation by the appropriate subspecialist as indicated on an individual basis.

B Discontinue oral agent if applicable.

C Provide food/nutrition assessment and counseling to modify the meal plan to meet the current needs in anticipation of pregnancy.

- The dietary intake of calcium, iron, and folic acid are particularly important, as is the assessment of supplement use.
- Start folic acid supplement. Assess folic acid intake to ensure adequate (600 µg) but not excessive amounts are being consumed (>1000 µg). Since 1998, folic acid has been added to most enriched flour and grain products, making excessive folic acid intake a concern due to the potential masking of vitamin B12 deficiencies. Currently folic acid fortification safety data for the general population (including pregnant women and fetuses) does not exist.[53]

D Assess diabetes self-management skills.

- Observe self-monitoring of blood glucose to assess technique and accuracy and to make sure that the meter is accurate.
- Observe insulin dose and administration technique. Assess injection sites for lipohypertrophy.
- Provide education about hypoglycemia to the patient and her significant other including prevention of hypoglycemia, oral carbohydrate intake, and the administration of glucagon.

E Achieve A1C levels within or close to the normal range and acceptable mean blood glucose levels. Recommended glucose targets include fasting plasma glucose levels of less than 110 mg/dL and 2-hour postprandial plasma glucose levels less than 155 mg/dL. The A1C value should be within 2 standard deviations of the mean for the nondiabetic range prior to conception.

F Continue contraception until glucose goals are attained.

- Patients may have already discontinued contraception by the time they present for preconception care. Reinforce the importance of maintaining contraception until normal or near-normal glucose values have been achieved.
- Basal body temperatures at this time are helpful to maximize the opportunity for conception and to accurately date conception.

G Obtain a serum pregnancy test if menses does not occur within 15 to 18 days following ovulation.

8 Women with diabetic retinopathy as well as the other vascular complications of diabetes present additional concerns.

  A Counsel women who have diabetic retinopathy about the effect of pregnancy on their eyes. All women with type 1 diabetes for 5 years or more, or type 2 diabetes at diagnosis, require a thorough dilated ophthalmologic evaluation.[54] This may necessitate preconception fluorescein angiography as dye studies are generally contraindicated during pregnancy. These evaluations need to be completed prior to counseling if possible and certainly prior to attempting conception. Laser therapy, if indicated, also needs to be completed prior to conception.

  B The severity of retinopathy is related to the duration of diabetes,[55] the level of glycemia,[56] the patient's age at diagnosis,[55] the presence of proteinuria, and higher diastolic blood pressures.

   • The Kroc study[57] demonstrated that retinopathy progresses when diabetes control is rapidly achieved. It is therefore advisable to normalize blood glucose levels in the presence of retinopathy over a period of 6 to 9 months.[58] Women with retinopathy need close ophthalmologic follow-up prior to conception.

   • Rosenn et al[59] found that pregnancy-induced or preexisting chronic hypertension was the most important risk factor associated with progression of retinopathy in pregnancy.

  C Pregnancy per se is an independent risk factor that accelerates retinopathy. Pregnancy is associated with a marked elevation in placental lactogen and other hormones that cause vascular changes and may in fact accelerate retinopathy.

  D Nonproliferative (background) retinopathy does not generally threaten vision and is not considered a contraindication to pregnancy (see Chapter 7, Eye Disease and Adaptive Diabetes Education for Visually Impaired Persons, in Diabetes and Complications). When a woman has background retinopathy at the start of her pregnancy, there is a 16% to 50% risk of progression during the pregnancy (Table 4.3).[59-67] In most situations, background retinopathy that occurs during pregnancy regresses after delivery.[61]

  E Earlier data showed that women with proliferative eye disease who had photocoagulation prior to pregnancy encountered a low risk (approximately 5%) of significant disease progression during gestation.[61] Rosenn et al,[59] however, reported risk of progression as high as 63% for women with proliferative retinopathy.

   • Women with untreated proliferative retinopathy have the greatest risk of progression,[61] and pregnancy is contraindicated until they receive laser photocoagulation to stabilize their eye disease.

   • Because retinopathy is known to regress postpartum, the need for photocoagulation during pregnancy continues to be controversial. Most centers treat patients with significant neovascularization rather than risk retinal hemorrhage.

   • The mode of delivery is an important consideration as ophthalmologists warn women with proliferative retinopathy to avoid the Valsalva maneuver. Many obstetricians recommend a cesarean delivery or a vacuum-extracted vaginal delivery to avoid pushing during a vaginal delivery.

Table 4.3. Progression of Diabetic Retinopathy in Pregnancy Stratified by Initial Retinal Findings

Author, Year	No. of Pregnancies	No. (%) With Progression Given the Initial Findings		
		None	Background	Proliferative
Horvat et al, 1980[60]	160	13/118 (11)	11/35 (31)	1/7 (14)
Moloney and Drury, 1982[61]	53	8/20 (40)	15/30 (50)	1/3 (33)
Dibble et al, 1982[62]	55	0/23 (0)	3/19 (16)	7/13 (54)
Ohrt, 1984[63]	100	4/50 (8)	15/48 (31)	1/2 (50)
Rosenn et al, 1992[59]	154	18/78 (23)	28/68 (41)	5/8 (63)
Chew, 1995[64]	155	4/39 (10)	31/101 (31)	*
Axer-Siegel, 1996[65]	65	10/38 (25)	17/22 (77)	2/5 (40)
Lovestam-Adrian, 1997[66]	55	10/39 (26)	3/14 (21)	5/12 (42)
Lapolla, 1998[67]	16	0/9 (0)	1/7 (14)	0/0 (0)

*Women with proliferative retinopathy were excluded from analysis.
Source: Adapted from Jovanovic-Peterson et al.[54]

9 Diabetic nephropathy is the complication of diabetes most likely to affect pregnancy outcomes.[68-72] In 2 studies,[68,69] 61% and 27%, respectively, of women with nephropathy were undiagnosed until they were examined during pregnancy (see Chapter 8, Nephropathy, in Diabetes and Complications, for more information).

A It is recommended that a thorough evaluation of renal function be part of routine preconception care for all women with type 1 diabetes of greater than 5 years' duration or at diagnosis with type 2 diabetes. This evaluation includes a 24-hour urine collection for creatinine, creatinine clearance, and microalbumin performed in a reference laboratory because of technical problems encountered with the albumin assay. Established nephropathy is staged and counseling should be provided concerning the potential risks to both maternal and fetal well-being.

B Because the use of ACE inhibitors is contraindicated during pregnancy, Kitzmiller et al[71] and others have recommended methyldopa as a first-line agent for hypertension control. Prazosin or clonidine can be added if additional therapy is necessary in early pregnancy; diltiazem can be added at the end of the first trimester. Blood pressure control often worsens as pregnancy progresses.

C Preeclampsia is the most frequent, serious complication of maternal nephropathy. Combs et al[72] found that the rate of preeclampsia in women with diabetes depended on the initial level of proteinuria. Preeclampsia occurred in 7% of women with proteinuria of <190 mg per day, 31% with proteinuria of 190 to 499 mg per day, and 38% with proteinuria of >500 mg per day. This increased risk of preeclampsia with proteinuria >190 mg per day persisted after controlling glycemia, parity, and diabetes complications.

D In general, the chances for a successful outcome are good for women with diabetic nephropathy. Studies have shown that the perinatal survival rate in this group has been between 89% and 100% (Table 4.4).[73-76] However, the course of pregnancy is not necessarily easy.

- There are increased risks for pregnancy-induced hypertension and/or a progression of already existing hypertension, intrauterine growth retardation resulting in small-for-gestational-age infants, preterm deliveries secondary to fetal distress, and a tenfold increase in the incidence of stillbirth over women with diabetes but without nephropathy.[68-72]
- Preterm delivery and stillbirth are most likely related to the fact that women with diabetes, hypertension, and chronic proteinuria have a high frequency of atherotic lesions in the uterine arteries that compromise the oxygenation of the fetus.

Table 4.4. Diabetic Nephropathy, Perinatal Survival, and Congenital Malformations in 4 Series Over 15 Years

	Kitzmiller (1981)[73] Boston	Grenfell (1986)[74] London	Reece (1998)[75] New Haven	Pierce (1992)[76] California
Years of study	1975–1978	1974–1984	1975–1984	1986–1990
Infants	27	23	31	39
Fetal deaths*	2	0	2	1
Neonatal deaths	1	0	0	0
Perinatal survival	88.9%	100%	93.5%	97.4%
Major anomalies	3 (11.1%)	1 (4.3%)	3 (9.7%)	3 (7.7%)

*Elective and spontaneous abortions excluded.
Source: Adapted from Kitzmiller.[77]

E Studies over the last decade have addressed the long-debated question of what effect pregnancy has on the natural history of renal disease.[68,76-79] Conclusions from these studies indicate that renal function deteriorates after pregnancy in women with overt nephropathy, but the rate of deterioration is not different (10 mL/min/year decrease in creatinine clearance) than would be expected without pregnancy.

- A later study by Miodovnik and colleagues[79] demonstrated that pregnancy in women with diabetes does not increase the risk for the subsequent development of diabetic nephropathy. Results from this study also supported the findings from the earlier studies that pregnancy does not accelerate the progression of renal disease in women who already have nephropathy.
- It is important to counsel women with nephropathy and their partners that diabetic nephropathy worsens over time and women with this condition must consider the possibility of a future complicated by dialysis or renal transplantation.

10 Significant coronary artery disease is 2 to 4 times more common in patients with overt diabetic nephropathy than in those without nephropathy. Prior to conception, it is recommended that women with overt nephropathy be given a comprehensive physical examination with a thorough history and an electrocardiogram.

A Manske et al[80] found virtually no significant coronary disease among people with diabetes and end-stage renal disease as long as their age was less than 45 years, their duration of diabetes was less than 25 years, and there were no ST-T wave changes in the electrocardiogram. In the presence of any of these risk factors, exercise tolerance testing is needed.

B Pregnant women with diabetes and coronary artery disease have a maternal mortality rate of 25% to 50% based on limited data.[81] These women along with their partners must be advised of the considerable risk of pregnancy.

11 Diabetic neuropathy with severe gastroparesis may lead to significant nausea, vomiting, hypoglycemia or hyperglycemia, and problems with maternal and, indirectly, fetal nutrition. Metoclopramide can be used for women with symptoms of gastroparesis to improve comfort, nutritional status, and glucose control; symptoms of diarrhea are safely treated with loperamide during pregnancy.[81]

Care and Education During Pregnancy

1 Care and education are focused on achieving and maintaining excellent blood glucose levels to maximize chances for a positive outcome. Glucose metabolism in a normal pregnancy provides the reference point for glycemic control. Lower fasting and preprandial blood glucose levels are normal during the second and third trimesters of pregnancy.

2 Because of the greater tendency for maternal ketosis during fasting and the possible adverse effects of ketones on the fetus, periods of fasting during pregnancy need to be avoided to help prevent ketonemia.[82,83] Food is best consumed in small, frequent meals and snacks, including 3 meals and 2 to 4 snacks daily.

3 Because of the increased resistance to insulin during the latter half of pregnancy, increasing doses of rapid-acting or short-acting insulin with meals often are necessary. In addition, larger amounts of intermediate- or long-acting insulin or increased basal rates are needed to maintain insulin levels overnight. It is not unusual for a woman's insulin requirement to increase twofold to threefold during the course of pregnancy.

Medical Nutrition Therapy in Pregnancy

1 No general consensus exists regarding optimal nutrition guidelines in pregnancy for women with diabetes. Because no evidence exists to indicate otherwise, it is generally assumed that nutritional guidelines for pregnant women with type 1 and type 2 diabetes are similar to recommendations for pregnant women who do not have diabetes.

A An individualized prenatal food/meal plan is important prepregnancy to optimize blood glucose control.

B Goals of nutrition therapy during pregnancy are to provide adequate maternal and fetal nutrition throughout pregnancy, to assist in appropriate gestational weight gain that is neither subnormal nor excessive, and to minimize blood glucose excursions.

C Energy requirements increase in the latter half of pregnancy. Of particular concern during pregnancy are requirements for protein, carbohydrate, calcium, iron, and folate. The Institute of Medicine of the National Academies' Dietary Reference Intakes 2002 updated previous recommendations for energy intake and nutrients for women during pregnancy. [84]

2 The National Academy of Science in 1990 established recommended ranges for total weight gain for pregnant women based on prepregnancy body mass index (BMI) (Table 4.5).[85]

A Weight gain by women who give birth to healthy infants is highly variable. Obese women have significantly heavier babies independent of weight gain. It is generally recommended that obese women gain a minimum equivalent to the products of conception, 15 lb (6.8 kg), although lower weight gains are often compatible with optimal birth weight.[86]

B Recommended weight gain is approximately 1 lb per week (0.3 to 0.7 kg) during the second and third trimester; overweight women can gain at half that rate. Gains of less than 2 lb per month (0.9 kg/month) or more than 6.5 lb per month (3 kg per month) for normal-weight women warrant further evaluation.[85]

Table 4.5. Recommended Ranges of Total Weight Gain for Pregnant Women[85]

Weight-for-Height Category	Recommended Total Weight Gain
Underweight (BMI <19.8)	28–40 lb (12.7–18.2 kg)
Normal weight (BMI 19.8–26.0)	25–35 lb (11.2–15.9 kg)
Overweight (BMI 26.0–29.0)	15–25 lb (6.8–11.3 kg)
Obese (BMI >29)	~15 lb (6.8 kg)
Twin Gestation	35-45 lb
Triplet Gestation	45-55 lb

*BMI = weight/height^2

3 Adequate calories are needed to provide for weight gain in underweight and normal-weight women and for weight maintenance or minimum weight gain in obese women. Weight loss is contraindicated.

A The 2002 Dietary Reference Intakes have updated estimated energy requirements (EER) during pregnancy.[84] The EER for pregnancy is derived from the sum of the total energy expenditure of the woman in the nonpregnant state plus the median change in total energy expenditure of 8 kcal per week due to pregnancy plus the mean energy deposition during pregnancy of 180 kcal per day (energy costs from the amount of protein and fat deposited during pregnancy).

- The EERs for pregnancy are the following:
  - 1st trimester = Adult EER + 0
  - 2nd trimester = Adult EER + 160 kcal (8 kcal/wk x 20 wk) + 180 kcal
  - 3rd trimester = Adult EER + 272 kcal (8 kcal/wk x 34 wk) + 180 kcal
- The 2002 Dietary Reference Intakes also calculate EER for the nonpregnant state.[84] The predictive equations for EER were developed for adult women from age, height, weight, and physical activity level (PAL) and were determined by using the individual's observed basal energy expenditure. A table of EER for women (and men) is included in the text of the DRI publication. For example, a 30 year old woman with a height of 65 inches, depending on weight (BMI) and PAL will have an EER of 1800 kcal (sedentary) to 2800 kcal (very active). The EER shows the range of possible energy needs and shows the effect of activity level.
- The updated EER for pregnancy is slightly higher than the previous recommendation, which was to determine caloric requirements based on prepregnancy weight and add an additional 300 calories per day for the last 2 trimesters.
- Successful pregnancy outcomes, however, have been reported with lower energy intakes.[87] Therefore, a preferred method is to take a detailed food/nutrition history, prepare an individualized food/meal plan, follow up with food records, and monitor weight gain.

B During the first trimester, energy requirements do not differ from prepregnancy. However, hormonal changes during this time can cause blood glucose levels to be erratic and the food/meal plan may need to be adjusted. At the beginning of the second trimester, the food/meal plan is adjusted to provide for the additional energy needs.

C Every attempt should be made to avoid ketonemia either from ketoacidosis or accelerated starvation ketosis in all pregnant women.[88]

4 The Recommended Dietary Allowance (RDA) for protein for pregnancy is in addition to the RDA for the nonpregnant woman.[84]

A The RDA for women 19 to 50 years is 0.80 g/kg/day or 46 g per day of protein.

B The RDA for pregnancy in all age groups is 1.1 g/kg/day of protein or an additional 25 g per day of additional protein.

C The additional protein need during pregnancy is due to protein deposition during pregnancy. The RDA for pregnancy is only for the second half of pregnancy. For the first half of pregnancy protein requirements are the same as before pregnancy. For twin pregnancies a protein intake of an additional 50 g per day during the second trimester of pregnancy is suggested, along with sufficient energy to utilize the protein as efficiently as possible.[84]

5 The Dietary Reference Intakes 2002 for the first time determined an RDA for carbohydrate.[84] It is the amount that should be sufficient to fuel central nervous system cells without having to rely on a partial replacement of glucose by ketoacids.

A For women ages 19 to 50 years this was determined to be 130 g per day of carbohydrate.

B In order to assure provision of the fetal brain with glucose (approximately 33 g/day) as a fuel as well as to supply the glucose fuel requirement for the mother's brain, independent of utilization of ketoacids (or other substrates), the RDA for pregnancy is 175 g per day of carbohydrate.

C Although the recommendation for carbohydrate intake in gestational diabetes may be slightly lower than in a nonpregnant state, there is no need to lower carbohydrate intake during pregnancy with preexisting diabetes. The amount should be individualized based on the woman's preference and covered with an appropriate amount of mealtime rapid-acting or short-acting insulin.

- Teach women insulin-to-carbohydrate ratios so appropriate insulin doses can be given for meal and snack carbohydrate amounts.
- Carbohydrate is generally less well tolerated at breakfast; increased levels of cortisol and growth hormone appear to contribute to morning glucose intolerance. Therefore, the insulin-to-carbohydrate ratio at breakfast may be larger than for other meals.

6 During pregnancy, the distribution of the energy intake and carbohydrate in the food/meal plan is based on the woman's food and eating habits, blood glucose records, and the expected physiological effects of pregnancy on her body.[89]

A Insulin can be matched to food intake, but maintaining consistency of times and amounts of food eaten are essential to avoid hypoglycemia due to the continuous fetal draw of glucose from the mother. Frequent smaller meals and snacks are often helpful.

B A snack at bedtime is important to prevent overnight starvation ketonuria and/or ketonemia and to decrease the potential for overnight hypoglycemia.

C Monitoring blood glucose levels, blood or urine ketones, appetite, and weight gain can guide the registered dietitian in developing an appropriate individualized meal plan and in making adjustments to the meal plan throughout the pregnancy.[89]

7 The Dietary Reference Intakes use the following definitions for nutrient intake and intake recommendations for micronutrients during pregnancy.[90]

A Recommended Dietary Allowance (RDA): the average daily dietary nutrient level sufficient to meet the nutrient requirement of nearly all (97% to 98%) healthy individuals in a particular life stage and gender group.

B Adequate Intake (AI): the recommended average daily intake level based on approximations of estimates of nutrient intake by a group of apparently healthy people that are assumed to be adequate—used when an RDA cannot be determined.

C Tolerable Upper Intake Level (UL): the highest average daily nutrient intake level that is likely to pose no risk of adverse health effects to almost all individuals in the general population. As intake increases above the UL, the potential for risk of adverse effects may increase.

D Pregnant women require 1000 to 1300 mg per day of calcium (AI) to calcify fetal bones and teeth. This need is most dramatic in the third trimester (Table 4.6).

E The iron requirement increases substantially in pregnancy. There is no increased need in the first trimester, but the need doubles in the second and third trimester for a total of 27 to 45 mg/day (RDA) (Table 4.6).

F Folate requirements increase dramatically during pregnancy from 400 to 600 µg per day (RDA) (Table 4.6). Because folate supplementation has been associated with a decrease in neural tube defects, folate supplementation is recommended before contraception is stopped.

Table 4.6. Dietary Reference Intakes (DRIs) for Pregnant and Lactating Women[90]

	Calcium (mg/d)		Iron (mg/d)		Folate (µg/d)	
	AI	UL	RDA	UL	RDA	UL
Pregnancy						
<18 years	1300	2500	27	45	600*	800
19–30 years	1000	2500	27	45	600*	1000
31–50 years	1000	2500	27	45	600*	1000
Lactation						
<18 years	1300	2500	10	45	500	800
19–30 years	1000	2500	9	45	500	1000
31–50 years	1000	2500	9	45	500	1000

AI = Adequate Intakes   UL = Tolerable Upper Intake Level   RDA = Recommended Dietary Allowances
*As dietary folate equivalents (DFE)

8 Other nutrition related issues during pregnancy are nonnutritive sweeteners, alcoholic beverages, morning sickness, and fish intake.

   A The Food and Drug Administration (FDA) has approved 5 nonnutritive sweeteners: saccharin, aspartame, acesulfame K, sucralose, and neotame. All were shown to be safe when consumed by the public including people with diabetes and during pregnancy.[89] (For additional information on nonnutritive sweeteners, see Chapter 1, Medical Nutrition Therapy, in Diabetes Management Therapies.)

   B As with nondiabetic women, women with diabetes should avoid alcoholic beverages during pregnancy.

   C Morning sickness can present a challenge. The following recommendations may be helpful:
   • Eating dry crackers or toast before rising.
   • Consuming small frequent meals.
   • Avoiding caffeine and foods that are spicy or fatty.
   • Drinking fluids between meals rather than with meals.
   • Taking prenatal vitamins anytime other than morning.
   • Avoiding hypoglycemia because it aggravates morning sickness. Checking blood glucose levels when nausea appears at unpredictable times and always carrying treatment for potential reactions.
   • If vomiting occurs after taking the premeal rapid-acting or short-acting insulin dose, administration of 0.15 mg of glucagon subcutaneously increases blood glucose 30 to 40 mg/dL and can help prevent hypoglycemia until the vomiting wanes. This increase in glucose level generally lasts 1 to 2 hours so the glucagon dose may need to be repeated until the peak mealtime insulin action has subsided. Advise any woman with continued vomiting to contact her healthcare team.[24,91]

   D The Food and Drug Administration has recommended that pregnant women and women of child-bearing age avoid eating shark, swordfish, mackerel, and tilefish. These fish often contain high levels of methylmercury, a potent human neurotoxin, which readily crosses the placenta and has the potential to damage the fetal nervous system.[92]

9 Physical activity can have a beneficial effect on blood glucose levels as well as overall well-being during pregnancy.

A Pregnancy generally is not a time for a woman who was previously sedentary to initiate strenuous activity. However, walking is possible for most women; a 15- to 20-minute walk can lower blood glucose by 20 to 40 mg/dL.

B Active women can continue to do similar activity during pregnancy but need to limit exercise periods to less than 30 minutes to help prevent hypoglycemia. In addition, women should be taught to palpate their uterus during physical activity and stop if they detect contractions. They should also be cautioned against becoming dehydrated, overheated, tachycardia (heart rate >140 bpm), or dyspneic.

C As with physical activity for any person with diabetes, planning, adjustments, and education for safety (eg, always carrying additional carbohydrate in case of hypoglycemia) are needed.

Glucose Goals During Pregnancy

1 At the present time, there is lack of agreement regarding precise glucose thresholds and the best timing of those determinations. Table 4.7 summarizes the range of plasma glucose targets recommended by various experts, including the American Diabetes Association.[24, 93-95] Until consensus is reached, glycemic profiles should be individualized in women with preexisting diabetes.

A When defining glycemic goals during pregnancy, it is important to recognize that these targets are not always attainable. In Kitzmiller's successful preconception study,[29] 90% of the patient population achieved mean blood glucose levels of 104 to 160 mg/dL (5.8 to 8.9 mmol/L) during organogenesis, which was substantially higher than the recommended goals. Even with these blood glucose ranges there was no excess of congenital anomalies.

B Discussing and establishing glucose goals with the woman and her partner is one of the most important aspects of both preconception and prenatal care. They need to understand the costs, benefits, barriers, and strategies of glycemic control in order to determine safe and realistic goals. If a woman has impaired glucose counterregulation or hypoglycemia unawareness, preprandial blood glucose levels less than 100 mg/dL (5.6 mmol/L) may not be safe. Hypoglycemia has not been found to be teratogenic in human studies,[21,27,28,96] although animal studies suggest otherwise.[97]

2 Neonatal complications other than congenital malformations are associated with the level of glycemia throughout pregnancy. The fetal pancreas begins to function at approximately 13 weeks' gestation. Elevations of glucose beyond this point stimulate fetal hyperinsulinism,[98] which accelerates fetal growth beyond normal (macrosomia). Neonatal hypoglycemia, hyperbilirubinemia, and hypocalcemia have all been associated with maternal hyperglycemia.

3 Several authors[98,99] have reported lowered rates of macrosomia, neonatal hypoglycemia, and cesarean deliveries when glucose values were monitored postprandially rather than preprandially.

Table 4.7. Blood Glucose Goals in Diabetic Pregnancy

	During Pregnancy	Preconception
Fasting	65 to 100 mg/dL (3.6 to 5.6 mmol/L)	
Premeal	65 to 115 mg/dL (3.6 to 6.4 mmol/L)	80 to 110 mg/dL (4.4 to 6.1 mmol/L)
1-h postprandial	<145 mg/dL (<8.1 mmol/L)	
2-h postprandial	<135 mg/dL (<7.5 mmol/L)	<155 mg/dL (<8.8 mmol/L)
2 h to 6 h	65 to 135 mg/dL (3.6 to 7.5 mmol/L)	

Source: Adapted from Jovanovic,[24] Kitzmiller,[94] and American Diabetes Association.[95]

Insulin Requirements During Pregnancy

1 Many patterns of insulin administration can be used to achieve the desired ranges of glycemia.

A Because only human insulin with its faster absorption is used during pregnancy, the vast majority of women with diabetes will require 3 injections to achieve glucose goals: intermediate- and rapid-acting or short-acting insulin in the morning, rapid-acting insulin at lunch, rapid-acting or short-acting insulin at dinner, and intermediate-acting insulin at bedtime. Intermediate-acting insulin before dinner is not advised because of the increased risk of overnight hypoglycemia during pregnancy.

B Other women may achieve their goals with short-acting insulin prior to meals and intermediate-acting insulin at bedtime.

C New rapid-acting insulin analogs with peak hypoglycemic action 1 to 2 hours after injection offer the potential for improved postprandial glucose control. The long-acting insulin analog, glargine, which is peakless and provides insulin in a basal pattern for 24 hours, may also prove to be beneficial during pregnancy. However, limited studies on insulin analog safety during pregnancy are available and their ability to improve perinatal outcomes has yet to be established.

2 Still others will benefit from insulin pump therapy, which can be particularly helpful during pregnancy.[100] Insulin pump therapy lowers the amount of circulating basal insulin, thereby decreasing the incidence of premeal hypoglycemia while efficiently controlling the more dramatic rise in postprandial glucose common during pregnancy.[101] Frequent and severe hypoglycemia is an indication for pump therapy.

A Other advantages of insulin pump therapy during pregnancy include more rapid and predictable insulin absorption, enhanced lifestyle flexibility, and simplified morning sickness management.[102] In addition, women continuing on insulin pump therapy postpartum have been shown to have significantly lower A1C levels 1 year following delivery as compared to women receiving multiple daily injections of insulin.[103]

B Pregnant women using insulin pumps require extensive education to avoid complications that could arise from any interruption in insulin delivery. In the third trimester there is an increased risk of DKA. Marcus and colleagues[104] recommended using 0.2 units/kg of NPH or lente insulin at bedtime in addition to the usual basal rate in order to reduce the incidence of DKA to <0.5% during pregnancy.

C Insulin pump therapy is best initiated before conception, but successful therapy can and should be started at any point if glycemic control is suboptimal.

3 Keeping activity and timing and content of meals as constant as possible will help as women learn their own glucose patterns. As they become more knowledgeable and the glucose patterns normalize, greater flexibility is possible and the insulin dosage can be varied to keep up with changing insulin requirements.

4 Insulin requirements are estimated based on current weight, gestational age, blood glucose monitoring results, and caloric intake. Generally, 0.6 units/kg/day total daily dose during preconception, increasing to 0.7 units at 6 weeks' gestation, 0.8 units at 16 weeks' gestation, 0.9 units at 26 weeks' gestation, and 1.0 units at 36 weeks' gestation are recommended (Table 4.8).[105] Women who are >150% of desirable body weight may need 1.5 to 2.0 units/kg secondary to insulin resistance due to obesity.

A Adjustments need to be made cautiously in the first trimester because of the significant incidence of hypoglycemia.

B Kimmerle and colleagues[106] reported a hypoglycemic rate as high as 41%; 84% of these episodes occurred before 20 weeks' gestation and 77% occurred during sleep. Women with a previous history of severe hypoglycemia were at particular risk. Diamond et al[107] suggested that impaired counterregulatory responses in women with type 1 diabetes may be responsible for this increased rate.

C Provide education to all patients regarding hypoglycemia prevention and treatment, including instructing family members in the use of glucagon.

Table 4.8. Insulin Requirements Throughout Gestation

	Units/kg
Preconception	0.6
First trimester	0.7
Second trimester	0.8
Third trimester	0.9 to 1.0
Postpartum	<0.6

Source: Adapted from Jovanovic and Peterson.[105]

Monitoring During Pregnancy

1 Diabetes control is monitored through blood glucose levels, ketone measurements, and glycosylated hemoglobin concentrations. In addition, some centers have successfully measured glycosylated serum protein levels to evaluate short-term glycemic control.[108]

2 Self-monitoring of blood glucose is needed before each meal and before the bedtime snack. Additionally, postprandial measurements (1 or 2 hours after the start of a meal or snack) are used to evaluate the effectiveness of rapid-acting or short-acting insulin, and 3 AM levels are helpful to detect asymptomatic hypoglycemia or evaluate unexplained fasting hyperglycemia.

   A Verifiable data are preferred to document blood glucose results. Pregnant women are no different than nonpregnant women in their abilities to fabricate data.

   B Along with the use of memory meters, detailed record keeping is useful to help women with diabetes identify their glucose patterns.

3 Urine monitoring for ketones in the first morning urine specimen, or blood testing for ketones, is needed daily, any time the blood glucose level exceeds 200 mg/dL (10.0 mmol/L), during illness, or when the person is unable to eat as a result of nausea and/or vomiting. The glucose value at which a woman will spill ketones is lower during pregnancy, and therefore the risk of DKA is greater. Testing for ketones is needed because of the increased tendency toward fat catabolism during pregnancy. Ketones cross the placenta if the patient has ketonemia and may be potentially harmful to the fetus. A fetal loss rate of approximately 30% has been reported with maternal acidosis and coma. In addition, studies have demonstrated an association between elevated plasma ketone levels and lower IQ scores in offspring.[82,83]

   A The presence of ketones with normal or low blood glucose levels is suggestive of starvation ketones and usually indicates inadequate food intake.

   B The presence of ketones in the face of mildly elevated blood glucose levels may indicate incipient ketoacidosis.

   - The main cause of ketoacidosis is infection.
   - Ketoacidosis in pregnancy is associated with a high perinatal mortality rate.
   - ß-sympathomimetic therapy such as ritodrine or terbutaline used to treat premature labor has been reported to cause deterioration of blood glucose control and ketosis in pregnant women with diabetes.[109] These agents should not be the first line of therapy for women with diabetes; if they are used, blood glucose levels must be carefully monitored.
   - Ketoacidosis has been reported in pregnancy with normal glucose values.

4 A1C measurements may be obtained monthly. Ideally, A1C levels will be in the mid-normal range throughout pregnancy (~5%). Relatively mild elevations of A1C have been associated with increased fetal morbidity.[32]

5 Hospitalization may be indicated whenever a woman with diabetes who has not been using intensive management prior to pregnancy becomes pregnant. Other indications for hospitalization include a lack of self-management skills, nausea and vomiting that prevent adequate energy intake, deterioration of blood glucose control that is unresolved with close telephone contact, hyperglycemia with ketones, nonadherence, and any obstetric complications such as preeclampsia or premature labor.[110]

Monitoring of the Fetus During Pregnancy

1 Fetal ultrasonography in the first or early second trimester allows confirmation of gestational age and helps to verify the absence of any malformations. A fetal echocardiogram in midpregnancy is used to screen for congenital heart defects. Serial ultrasounds thereafter are used to assess fetal growth, measure the amniotic fluid volume, and evaluate the state of the placenta (Table 4.9).[111]

Table 4.9. Fetal Testing Timeline for Women With Preexisting Diabetes

	Tests	Number of Weeks Into the Pregnancy
First trimester	Early ultrasound to date the pregnancy	8 weeks
Second trimester	Alpha-fetoprotein test	15 to 18 weeks
	Comprehensive ultrasound	18 to 22 weeks
	Fetal echocardiogram	20 to 22 weeks
Third trimester	Kick counting	26 weeks
	Nonstress test	If there are complications, twice a week starting at 28 weeks. If there are no complications, twice a week starting at 32 to 34 weeks.
	Biophysical profile	28 to 32 weeks to begin
	Fetal echocardiogram	32 to 33 weeks if needed
	Amniocentesis to test lung maturity	If birth will be induced before 39 weeks

Source: Adapted with permission from Jornsay.[111]

2 A blood test to screen maternal serum alpha-fetoprotein (MSAFP) levels provides additional information when trying to identify the fetus at risk for a neural tube defect. In women with diabetes, the incidence of neural tube defects is 20 per 1000, which is 10 to 20 times greater than in the general population.[112] Thus, all women with diabetes need referral for targeted ultrasound regardless of their MSAFP test result.

A Neural tube defects develop from defective closure of the neural tube during embryogenesis, which results in anencephaly, encephalocele, and all variants of spina bifida.

B The MSAFP test should be offered between 15 and 18 weeks of gestation (Table 4.9). An elevated result identifies a fetus that may have a neural tube defect or other abnormality.

• There are many conditions that can falsely raise this test result including diabetes, inaccurate conception dates, or multiple gestations.

- Advise patients that the MSAFP is a screening test to identify fetuses that require a closer look and is not diagnostic in and of itself.
- Patients with positive results may be advised to have a further evaluation with ultrasound and/or amniocentesis.

3 Fetal movement recording is an accurate, reliable, and inexpensive way for the pregnant women to assess her baby's overall health. Fetal kick counting, as it is popularly called, is advisable for all pregnant women with diabetes beginning in the early third trimester.

A One method is to keep track of fetal movements over a 12-hour period. If fewer than 10 movements are observed during the 12-hour period, or if it takes progressively longer before the 10 movements are identified, the woman should notify her obstetrician immediately. In many cases, further evaluation of fetal status is indicated.[111]

B Another method is to count fetal movement for several 30-minute or 1-hour periods each day. The patient may be asked to keep written records of fetal movement.

4 The nonstress test (NST) is a safe, noninvasive assessment of the overall health of the fetus. Two transducers are placed on the mother's abdomen; one records the fetal heart rate while the other detects uterine contractions. The fetal heart rate should increase with activity and/or stimulation. This is called a reactive test.

A In some centers, nonstress tests are performed weekly from the gestational age of 32 to 34 weeks, then twice weekly from 36 weeks until delivery (Table 4.9). If a nonstress test is abnormal or nonreactive, a contraction stress test or a biophysical profile may be ordered.

B Earlier and more frequent testing may be necessary for patients who have vascular disease.

5 Weekly contraction stress tests are used by some centers to assess fetal well-being beginning at 32 to 34 weeks. The contraction stress test (CST) is a record of the fetal heart-rate response to mild uterine contractions, which are induced by intravenous pitocin or by nipple stimulation.

A If late decelerations of the fetal heart rate occur following more than 50% of the uterine contractions, the test is considered positive.

B A positive CST may indicate fetal distress and the need for delivery.

6 A biophysical profile is another test to discriminate between fetuses that are well adapted to their intrauterine environment and those in danger of fetal demise (Table 4.9).

A A biophysical profile involves the evaluation of 5 parameters. Ultrasound is used to assess 4 components: fetal breathing, fetal body movement, fetal muscle tone, and amniotic fluid volume. Fetal heart-rate activity is evaluated by means of a non-stress test. Two points are given for the normal observation of each of these 5 parameters. The lowest score is 0 and the highest score is 10. A score of 8 to 10 is desirable; scores lower than 6 generally warrant further evaluation.

B A biophysical profile sometimes is performed when an NST is nonreactive or a CST is positive.

7 If an amniocentesis is performed, it is used to assess fetal lung maturity (Table 4.9). Amniocentesis may be part of the protocol when induction of labor or elective cesarean section is planned prior to 39 weeks.

8 Many pregnancies can safely progress to term as long as fetal health does not appear to be compromised and no maternal complications (such as preeclampsia) are present.

Diabetes Care During Labor and Delivery

1 The goals of managing diabetes during labor are to provide adequate carbohydrate intake to meet maternal energy requirements and to maintain maternal euglycemia.
  A Glucose is administered 2.0 to 2.5 mg/kg/minute by continuous intravenous infusion to meet maternal energy requirements and thus to prevent ketosis.[113] This dosage corresponds to approximately 5 to 10 g per hour in lean individuals.

2 Maternal blood glucose values are measured every 1 to 2 hours, and short-acting insulin is administered by multiple subcutaneous doses or by continuous intravenous infusion as necessary to maintain euglycemia. Maternal euglycemia may help prevent undue stimulation of fetal insulin secretion prior to delivery to prevent neonatal hypoglycemia.[114]
  A Insulin pump therapy has been used successfully during labor and delivery.
  B Regardless of the method, the key to successful intrapartum management is to monitor blood glucose levels frequently and administer insulin and glucose as necessary.

Postpartum Period

1 The postpartum period is characterized by an immediate decrease in insulin requirements.
  A In general, insulin requirements are recalculated at 0.6 unit/kg current weight for nonlactating women and 0.4 unit/kg current weight for lactating women.
  B Occasionally little or no insulin is required during the first 24 to 48 hours following delivery.
  C No reduction in insulin requirements may indicate an underlying infection such as endometritis or a urinary tract infection.

2 Many issues surround the patient in the postpartum period. The role of the educator is to continue to offer support and information during this period of adjustment.
  A The mother needs to learn to balance her own self-care needs with the needs of her infant. Assess for postpartum depression or other psychosocial needs related to diabetes or the demands of motherhood.
  B The risk of hypoglycemia is very significant in the first few weeks postpartum. Review hypoglycemia knowledge and skills with the new mother and her partner, including the need to first care for herself then her baby when hypoglycemic.
  C Provide close follow-up of diabetes control to reestablish her baseline insulin requirement.
  D Offer referral to a registered dietitian concerning weight reduction and/or prevention of hypoglycemia while breastfeeding.

E Offer referral for counseling or other support if the outcome was not positive.

Lactation

1 Provide support and education for women who desire to breastfeed.

 A In most situations, breastfeeding mothers require less insulin because of the calories expended with nursing. Lactating women have reported drops in glucose of 50 to 100 mg/dL over a 30-minute nursing session.

 B All lactating women with diabetes need information about the prevention and prompt recognition and treatment of hypoglycemia.

 C Although achieving desired metabolic control during the establishment of lactation is reported to be a challenge,[115] breastfeeding is recommended for women with pre-existing diabetes. Because breastfeeding may lower blood glucose levels, women may need to eat a snack containing carbohydrate either before or during breastfeeding. Evening or late night snacks may also be required.[115] Approximately the same food/meal plan as that of the third trimester of pregnancy may be appropriate during lactation.

2 The Institute of Medicine Dietary Reference Intakes updated energy and nutrient requirements for lactation.[84]

 A The estimated energy requirement (EER) for lactation is estimated from total energy expenditure, milk energy output, and energy mobilization from tissue stores.[84]

  • Energy requirements for lactating women are met partially by mobilizing of tissue stores, but primarily from the diet. In the first 6 months postpartum, well-nourished lactating women experience an average weight loss of 0.8 kg per month, which is equivalent to 170 kcal per day. Weight stability is assumed after 6 months postpartum.

  • Milk production rates average 0.78 L per day from birth through 6 months of age and 0.6 L per day from 7 through 12 months of age. At 0.67 kcal per g of milk, the milk energy output would be 523 kcal per day, which is rounded to 500 kcal per day, in the first 6 months and 402 kcal per day, which is rounded to 400 kcal per day, in the second 6 months of lactation.

  • EER for lactation is the following:
    1st 6 months = Estimated energy requirement + 500 – 170
       (milk energy output – weight loss)
    2nd 6 months = Estimated energy requirement + 400 – 0
       (milk energy output – weight loss)

 B The RDA protein requirement for lactation is 1.1 g/kg/day or + an additional 25 g/day.[84]

 C The RDA carbohydrate requirement for lactation is 210 g/day.[84]

 D Table 4.6 lists the DRIs for calcium, iron, and folate for lactating women.

3 Oral glucose-lowering agents cannot be used while lactating. Other medications may also affect breast milk.

4 Women with type 2 diabetes whose glucose values are not maintained with medical nutrition therapy alone will need to continue to take insulin throughout lactation.

Contraception and Family Planning

1 The use of contraception in all women with diabetes or a prior history of gestational diabetes cannot be emphasized strongly enough. This is the only way to ensure that preconception care can be provided.

2 Barrier methods of contraception create mechanical and/or chemical barriers to fertilization.

A Barrier methods include diaphragms, male condoms, spermicides, jelly or foam, cervical caps, and female condoms.

B Although these methods pose no health risks to women with diabetes, they are user-dependent, require correct application or insertion before intercourse, and have a high failure rate of 18% to 28%[116-118] in the first year because of improper use. With experience and motivation, these failure rates may be reduced to levels of 2% to 6%.[116]

3 Oral contraceptives remain the most popular form of birth control despite controversy over potential side effects.

A The main reasons for their popularity are their failure rate of generally less than 1% and ease of use.

B Low-dose formulations are preferred and are recommended only for patients without vascular complications or additional risk factors such as smoking or a strong family history of myocardial disease.[117,118]

C Progestin only ("mini-pill") oral contraceptives are an option for women with contraindications to the estrogen component, such as hypertension or thrombosis.

4 An intrauterine device (IUD) is the most effective nonhormonal device.[116]

A It should only be offered to women who have a low risk of sexually transmitted diseases because any infection might place the patient with diabetes at risk for sepsis and ketoacidosis.

B Patient education includes the early signs of sexually transmitted diseases, such as increased and abnormal vaginal discharge; dyspareunia; heavy, painful menses; lower abdominal pain; and fever.[116] Teach patients to seek prompt health care attention if any of these occur.

5 Long-acting progestin-only methods have not been studied in women with diabetes and therefore, cannot be recommended as first-line methods of contraception.

A Hormone injections, such as medroxyprogesterone acetate (eg, Depoprovera®) contain a long-acting progestin; they are administered intramuscularly every 3 months and work by inhibiting ovulation. Deterioration of carbohydrate tolerance has been demonstrated in healthy women.[118]

B A hormone implant (ie, the Norplant® implant), which is a subcutaneously implanted levonorgestrel, is metabolically neutral and therefore, may be indicated for women with a history of poor medication-taking.[116]

6 Permanent sterilization, including tubal ligation and vasectomy, may be considered by the woman or her partner when they desire no more children.

7 Other methods of contraception are periodic abstinence of sexual intercourse (the rhythm method) and other "natural family planning methods" (ie, basal body temperature changes, alternations in cervical mucus). However, it should be noted that these methods are less effective and require a high level of motivation.

8 Emergency contraceptive therapy is also available for women who have had unprotected sexual intercourse, including sexual assault. Methods include use of combination or progestin-only oral contraceptives, danazol, synthetic estrogens and conjugated estrogens, antiprogestins, and the insertion of an intrauterine device.

Key Educational Considerations for Women With Preexisting Diabetes

1 Information needed by women with diabetes in the preconception and/or early postconception period includes the effects of maternal diabetes on her baby. Explain that glucose and ketones cross the placenta, while insulin and glucagon do not. This concept is also quite helpful in helping women to understand the importance of waiting until glycemia is normalized before conceiving.

2 Explain that it is usual for the insulin dose to increase during pregnancy and that she may need a twofold to threefold increase toward the end of pregnancy. Discuss with her that her insulin requirements will increase because the placenta produces hormones that act against insulin, not because her diabetes is more severe. Tell her explicitly that her diabetes is not getting worse.

3 Explain how it may be difficult to accomplish glycemic goals and that her numbers do not need to be perfect to have a normal A1C value and a healthy baby. Be sure to make adjustments for the woman who has problems with hypoglycemia awareness.

4 Table 4.10 is a patient education outline for pregnant women with preexisting diabetes.

5 Offer referral to a registered dietitian for nutritional counseling. It is important that the woman with diabetes understand sick-day rules because hyperemesis can be a problem in early pregnancy. It is also important that she understand the role of snacks in preventing ketonuria.

6 Assess her blood glucose monitoring technique periodically. Verify her meter's accuracy with a laboratory plasma glucose test done simultaneously with a capillary blood glucose reading. Ideally, the capillary value should be within 10% to 15% of the laboratory value.

7 Review the signs, symptoms, causes, treatment, and prevention of hypoglycemia with the women and her partner or other family member. Instruct family members on glucagon administration. Recommended treatment may change from concentrated sources of carbohydrates (eg, orange juice) to milk. Advise her to carry food at all times and provide information on how to obtain diabetes identification.

Table 4.10. Patient Education Outline for Pregnant Women With Preexisting Diabetes

I Prepregnancy counseling
  A Congenital malformations and spontaneous abortion
    1 Risks
    2 Relationship of diabetes control and vasculopathy
  B Impact of pregnancy on chronic complications
  C Appropriate use of contraception and timing of pregnancy
  D Optimization of glucose control
    1 Nutrition counseling
    2 Patient education review
      a Insulin administration
      b Glucose monitoring and pattern management
      c Symptoms and treatment of hypoglycemia

II Patient education for pregnancy
  A General overview
    1 Effects of diabetes on pregnancy
    2 Effects of pregnancy on diabetes
    3 Relationship of diabetes control to improved perinatal outcome
  B Review of self-management skills
    1 Nutrition counseling
    2 Physical activity
    3 Blood glucose monitoring
    4 Insulin: dose adjustments and changing insulin requirements
  C Fetal monitoring
    1 Perinatal testing
    2 Fetal movements counting
  D Preparation for labor and delivery

III Postpartum teaching
  A Postpartum glycemic control
  B Breastfeeding
  C Birth control
  D Appropriate nutrition for mother and infant

8 Review injection sites and the differences in absorption times for different sites. Reassure her that it is fine to use her abdomen.

9 Ask the women about her daily routine and create a schedule together with times for meals, snacks, testing, and insulin injections. If she does not follow a schedule, it is virtually impossible to successfully titrate her insulin dosage to keep up with the changing requirements of pregnancy.

10 Provide written parameters for when to contact healthcare providers. Suggest that she or a family member notify her healthcare provider if any of the following occurs: a marked change in blood glucose levels, presence of ketones, vomiting, hypoglycemia requiring a glucagon injection or any severe episode, fever, vaginal bleeding, severe headache, blurred vision, a decrease in fetal movement (in the second half of pregnancy), uterine contractions, or other pregnancy complications.

11 It is common for the mother to lose interest in her own self-management following the birth of her baby and months of intensive monitoring. Remind her that she worked hard to have a healthy infant and healthy babies need healthy mothers. Careful diabetes management will help ensure future successful pregnancies and reduce the risk for long-term diabetes complications such as retinopathy and/or nephropathy.

12 Work with the mother closely in the postpartum period to avoid maternal hypoglycemia, which can be a safety issue for her infant and/or herself.

Self-Review Questions

1 What are the normal metabolic changes related to pregnancy during the latter half of gestation?
2 Why is it important to achieve optimal diabetes control prior to conception?
3 What are 4 potential neonatal complications that may occur in pregnancies complicated by diabetes mellitus?
4 Why are nonstress tests routinely ordered in pregnant women with diabetes?
5 What are 3 maternal complications associated with diabetes and pregnancy?
6 When and why should pregnant women with diabetes test their urine for ketones?
7 What should preconception counseling emphasize?
8 What are changes in nutritional requirements during gestation?
9 What are 2 methods that might be used to assess fetal status?
10 What are contraceptive options for women with diabetes?

Learning Assessment: Case Study 1

NC is a 29-year-old, newly married woman with type 1 diabetes who presents to the Diabetes in Pregnancy Center for preconception counseling and care. NC was diagnosed with type 1 diabetes at age 10 years and has been in good health with the exception of one episode of DKA at age 12 years when she had the flu. She has never been pregnant and is using a diaphragm with spermicidal cream as her method of contraception. NC denies a history of diabetic nephropathy and claims that she is normotensive. Her history is significant for background retinopathy that was diagnosed 1 year ago.

At this initial visit, a physical examination was also performed. NC's blood pressure was 110/70 and her urine sample tested 1+ for protein on dipstick. Her blood glucose records during the previous 2 weeks were reviewed. She appeared to be in reasonably good diabetes control with fasting blood glucose values ranging from 80 to 130 mg/dL (4.4 to 7.2 mmol/L) and predinner values from 95 to 140 mg/dL (5.3 to 7.8 mmol/L). NC tests her blood glucose levels twice daily. She takes 3 injections per day with short- and intermediate-acting insulin prior to breakfast, short-acting insulin prior to dinner, and intermediate-acting insulin prior to bedtime. NC did not bring her blood glucose meter with her during this initial visit.

Questions for Discussion

1 What are appropriate laboratory tests for this patient?

2 What are potential topics that need to be addressed with her?

3 How would you involve her husband in the education?

Discussion

1 Baseline renal function studies including a 24-hour urine for creatinine clearance, quantitative protein, and microalbumin are needed. A urinalysis to rule out a urinary tract infection, which might have caused the 1+ proteinuria, is also needed.

2 A glycosylated hemoglobin is needed to assess overall glycemic control as well as a rubella titer to assess her immune status. If NC is nonimmune, an inoculation could be administered during this preconception period. If thyroid function tests have not been performed in the last year, these should be done now.

3 In addition to these laboratory tests, referrals to a retinal specialist for a reassessment of her background retinopathy and to the team dietitian to evaluate her nutritional intake, supplement use, weight gain/loss history, and meal plan are needed. If she is interested, the dietitian can work with NC to initiate a physical activity program.

4 Discuss blood glucose goals during preconception and pregnancy with NC and the purpose of blood glucose checks prior to each meal, 1-hour postmeal, and at bedtime. Weekly calls to the diabetes educator are needed so that any necessary insulin and/or meal plan adjustments can be made. Assess NC's understanding and willingness to work towards these targets.

5 Counsel NC to continue her barrier method of contraception. The incidence of congenital malformations is 6% to 13% in diabetic pregnancies when glycemic control is not established prior to conception. Therefore, NC should continue on contraception until blood glucose levels are optimal and the glycosylated hemoglobin level is in the normal or near-normal range.

6 Discuss the topics of fertility, spontaneous abortion rate, incidence of diabetes mellitus in offspring, effects of pregnancy on existing vascular complications, and the incidence of congenital malformations and answer any questions. Assess NC's emotional response throughout the discussion.

7 Ask NC how her husband has coped with her diabetes during their marriage and what he knows about pregnancy and diabetes. Invite NC to bring her husband to her next appointment and all future appointments so that he can learn about diabetes in pregnancy and how to administer glucagon.

8 Additionally, ask NC to bring her glucose meter so her technique and meter accuracy can be assessed. Ask her to bring food intake records for 3 days.

Learning Assessment: Case Study 2

RG is a 26-year-old G2P1000 (ie, second pregnancy, one previous full-term delivery and no living children), obese Hispanic woman with type 2 diabetes who presents to the outpatient Diabetes in Pregnancy Center at 7-3/7 weeks of gestation. RG stated that she was referred to the center by her family practitioner for prenatal care and management of her diabetes.

RG's past obstetric history was significant for gestational diabetes mellitus in her first pregnancy, 2 years earlier. That pregnancy resulted in the delivery of a 9 lb 12 oz (4.4 kg) stillborn son at 38+ weeks of gestation. One year following that delivery, RG was diagnosed with type 2 and started on glyburide 10 mg once a day.

Her medical profile revealed a glycosylated hemoglobin of 10.9% (normal range 4.0% to 6.5%). A urinalysis revealed 4+ glucose, negative protein, and small ketones. Her fasting blood glucose was 150 mg/dL. RG's oral agent was discontinued and she was started on 3 injections per day of insulin because of her fasting glucose levels. She met with the dietitian and they developed a meal plan that included the ethnic foods RG prepares at her husband's request. In addition, RG learned how to monitor capillary blood glucose levels and urine ketone levels.

Questions for Discussion

1 What other information would you like to have received about this patient?

2 What changes in insulin requirements would you anticipate throughout gestation and advancing pregnancy?

3 What types of fetal surveillance do you expect would be utilized in the management of this patient's pregnancy?

4 How can the educator show sensitivity to RG's cultural background?

Discussion

1 It would be important to find out if RG had received an oral glucose tolerance test following the delivery of her stillborn son to determine whether or not she had reverted to normal glucose tolerance or whether the diabetes had remained following that pregnancy. More information surrounding the stillbirth would have been helpful. The absence of obstetric complications suggests, but do not prove, that the stillbirth was related to maternal diabetes. Therefore, RG should be asked the following questions: Was she preeclamptic? Was there a cord accident? Did she have a placental abruption?

    A It is also important to assess her beliefs about why the stillbirth occurred as it will influence how she cares for herself and her current emotional status. In addition, knowing more about her past experiences with gestational diabetes and her self-care practices may provide important insights of value in her education and care.

2 Insulin requirements change dramatically during pregnancy. In the first trimester, insulin sensitivity is enhanced and maternal insulin requirements are approximately 0.7 U/kg of body weight per day. Late gestation is characterized by rising concentrations of several diabetogenic hormones and increased insulin resistance. Therefore, insulin requirements increase to approximately 1.0 U/kg by late gestation. Insulin requirements drop precipitously at delivery as the placenta is no longer secreting insulin antagonists.

3 All women with pregestational diabetes should be evaluated for possible fetal anomalies. A glycosylated hemoglobin should be performed at the first prenatal visit since a significant relationship has been reported between elevated glycosylated hemoglobin levels in early pregnancy and an increased rate of fetal anomalies. Although the risk for delivering an anomalous infant cannot be fully determined by a glycosylated hemoglobin level, an elevated level at least alerts the practitioner to an increased risk for structural defects. Routine screening by maternal serum alpha-fetoprotein is also important since the fetuses of women with diabetes have as high as a 20-fold increased rate of neural tube defects. In addition, routine screening of all diabetic pregnancies by ultrasonic evaluation should begin at approximately 20 weeks of gestation. The evaluation should include a general anatomical survey and a fetal echocardiogram.

4 Women with diabetes are at risk for fetal growth aberrations and frequent scans are performed to identify states of altered growth. In addition, since stillbirth occurs with increased frequency during the third trimester, a program of fetal monitoring will be instituted at about 32 to 34 weeks' gestation. This commonly involves either once or twice weekly nonstress tests or biophysical profiles. Maternal evaluation of fetal movement counts will also be integrated in the surveillance program.

5 Review of weight gain during the first pregnancy should be made. RG should be counseled about appropriate weight gain during this pregnancy.

6 It is important to assess the influence of her culture on the care of her pregnancy and her diabetes.
   A Ask, "Are there cultural or religious practices that affect how you care for yourself or your pregnancy?"
   B It is also important to assess the use of alternative therapies (eg, herbs, vitamins) for pregnancy.

References

1 Engelgau MM, Herman WH, Smith PJ, German RR, Aubert RE. The epidemiology of diabetes and pregnancy in the US, 1988. Diabetes Care. 1995;18:1029-1033.

2 Weintrob N, Karp M, Hod M. Short- and long-range complications in offspring of diabetic mothers. J Diabetes Complications. 1996;10:294-301.

3 Schwarz R, Teramo KA. Effects of diabetic pregnancy on the fetus and newborn. Semin in Perinatal. 2000;24:120-135.

4 Metzger BE, Coustan DR, Organizing Committee. Summary and recommendations of the Fourth International Workshop-Conference on Gestational Diabetes Mellitus. Diabetes Care. 1998;21(suppl 2):B161-B167.

5 Marshall JA, Hamman RF, Baxter J. et al. Ethnic differences in risk factors associated with prevalence of non-insulin dependent diabetes mellitus. The San Luis Valley diabetes study. Am J Epidemiol. 1993; 137:706-718.

6 Feig DS, Palda VA. Type 2 diabetes in pregnancy: A growing concern. Lancet. 2002;359:1690-92.

7 Omori Y, Minei S, Testo T, et al. Current status of pregnancy in diabetic women: A comparison of pregnancy in IDDM and NIDDM mothers. Diabetes Res Clin Pract. 1994;24(suppl):S273-S78.

8 Harris SB, Caulfield L, Sugamori ME, et al. The epidemiology of diabetes in pregnant Native Canadians. Diabetes Care. 1997;20: 1455-1525.

9 White P. Pregnancy complicating diabetes. Am J Med. 1949;7:609-616.

10 Pedersen J, Pedersen LM, Andersen B. Assessors of fetal perinatal mortality in diabetic pregnancy: analysis of 1,332 pregnancies in the Copenhagen series, 1946-1972. Diabetes. 1974;23:302-305.

11 Buchanan TA, Coustan DR. Diabetes mellitus. In: Burrows GN, Ferris TF, eds. Medical Complications During Pregnancy. 4th ed. Philadelphia: WB Saunders; 1994:29-61.

12 Homko CJ, Sivan E, Reece EA, Boden G. Fuel metabolism during pregnancy. Semin Reprod Endocrinol. 1999;17:119-125.

13 Sivan E, Homko CJ, Whittaker PG, Reece EA, Boden G. Free fatty acids and insulin resistance during pregnancy. J Clin Endocrinol and Metabolism. 1998;83:2338-2342.

14 Sivan E, Homko CJ, Chen X, Reece EA, Boden G. Effect of insulin on fat metabolism during and after normal pregnancy. Diabetes. 1999; 48:834-838.

15 Sivan E, Chen X, Homko CJ, Reece EA, Boden G. A longitudinal study of carbohydrate metabolism in healthy, obese pregnant women. Diabetes Care. 1997; 20:1470-1475.

16 Metzger BE, Ravnikar V, Vilelsis RA, Freinkel N. "Accelerated starvation" and the skipped breakfast in late normal pregnancy. Lancet. 1982;1:588-592.

17 Phelps RL, Metzger BE, Freinkel N. Carbohydrate metabolism in pregnancy. XVII. Diurnal profiles of plasma glucose, insulin, free fatty acids, triglycerides, cholesterol, and individual amino acids in late normal pregnancy. Am J Obstet Gynecol. 1981;140:730-736.

18 Mills JL, Baker L, Goldman AS. Malformations in infants of diabetic mothers occur before the seventh gestational week: implications for treatment. Diabetes. 1979;28:292-293.

19 Simpson JL, Elias S, Martin AO, et al. Diabetes in pregnancy. Northwestern University series (1977-1981): Prospective study of anomalies in offspring of mothers with diabetes mellitus. Am J Obstet Gynecol. 1983;146:263-270.

20 Mills JL, Knopp RH, Simpson JL, et al. Lack of relation of increased malformation rates in infants of diabetic mothers to glycemic control during organogenesis. N Engl J Med. 1988;318:671-676.

21 Miller E, Hare JW, Cloherty JP, et al. Elevated maternal hemoglobin A1c in early pregnancy and major congenital anomalies in infants of diabetic mothers. N Engl J Med. 1981;304:1331-1334.

22 Greene MF, Hare JW, Cloherty JP, et al. First-trimester hemoglobin A1 and risk for major malformation and spontaneous abortion in diabetic pregnancy. Teratology. 1989;39:225-231.

23 Ylinen K, Aula P, Stenman UH, et al. Risk of minor and major fetal malformations in diabetics with high hemoglobin A1c values in early pregnancy. Br Med J. 1984;289:345-346.

24 Jovanovic-Peterson L, ed. Medical Management of Pregnancy Complicated by Diabetes. 3rd ed. Alexandria, Va: American Diabetes Association; 2000:7.

25 Mills JL, Simpson JL, Driscoll SG, et al. Incidence of spontaneous abortion among normal women and insulin-dependent diabetic women whose pregnancies were identified within 21 days of conception. N Eng J Med. 1988;319:1617-1623.

26 Fuhrmann K, Reiher H, Semmler K, et al. Prevention of congenital malformations in infants of insulin-dependent diabetic mothers. Diabetes Care. 1983;6:219-223.

27 Fuhrmann K, Reiher H, Semmler K, Glockner E. The effect of intensified conventional insulin therapy before and during pregnancy on the malformation rate in offspring of diabetic mothers. Exp Clin Endocrinol. 1984;83:173-177.

28 Steel JM, Johnstone FD, Hepburn DA, Smith AF. Can prepregnancy care of diabetic women reduce the risk of abnormal babies? Br Med J. 1990;301:1070-1074.

29 Kitzmiller JL, Gavin LA, Gin GD, et al. Preconception care of diabetes: Glycemic control prevents congenital anomalies. JAMA. 1991;265:731-736.

30 Cornblath M, Schwartz R. Disorders of Carbohydrate Metabolism in Infancy. Philadelphia: WB Saunders; 1976.

31 Reece EA, Friedman AM, Copel J, Kleinman CS. Prenatal diagnosis and management of deviant fetal growth and congenital malformations. In Reece EA, Coustan DR, eds. Diabetes Mellitus in Pregnancy. 2nd ed. New York; Churchill-Livingston; 1995.

32 Wyse LJ, Jones M, Mandel F. Relationship of glycosylated hemoglobin, fetal macrosomia, and birthweight macrosomia. Am J Perinatol. 1994;11:260-262.

33 Morris MA, Grandis AS, Litton JC. Glycosylated hemoglobin concentration in early gestation associated with neonatal outcome. Am J Obstet Gynecol. 1985; 153:651-654.

34 Coustan DR. Delivery: timing, mode and management. In: Reece EA, Coustan DR, eds. Diabetes Mellitus in Pregnancy. 2nd ed. New York: Churchill-Livingston; 1995:353-360.

35 Jovanovic-Peterson L, Peterson CM, Reed GF, et al. Maternal postprandial glucose levels and infant birth weight: The Diabetes in Early Pregnancy Study. Am J Obstet Gynecol. 1991;164:103-111.

36 Silverman BL, Rizzo TA, Cho NH, Metzger BE. Long-term effects of the intrauterine environment. Diabetes Care. 1998;21 (suppl. 2):B124-149.

37 Rizzo TA, Dooley SL, Metzger BE, Cho NH, Ogata ES, Silverman BL. Prenatal and perinatal influences on long-term psychomotor development in offspring of diabetic mothers. Am J Obstet Gynecol. 1995;173:1753-1758.

38 Rizzo TA, Metzger BE, Dooley SL, Cho NH. Early malnutrition and child neurobehavioral development: insights from the Study of Children of Diabetic Mothers. Child Dev. 1997;68:26-38.

39 Cousins L. Obstetric complications. In: Reece EA, Coustan DR, eds. Diabetes Mellitus in Pregnancy. 2nd ed. New York: Churchill-Livingston; 1995:287-302.

40 Hanson U, Persson B. Outcome of pregnancies complicated by type 1 insulin-dependent diabetes in Sweden: acute pregnancy complications, neonatal mortality and morbidity. Am J Perinatol. 1993;10:330-337.

41 Combs CA, Rosenn B, Kitzmiller JL, et al. Early pregnancy proteinuria in diabetes related to preeclampsia. Obstet Gynecol. 1993;82:801-805.

42 Rosenn B, Miodovnik M, Combs CA, et al. Poor glycemic control and antepartum obstetric complications in women with insulin-dependent diabetes. Int J Gynaecol Obstet. 1993;43:21-25.

43 Greene MF, Hare JW, Krache M, et al. Prematurity among insulin-requiring diabetic gravid women. Am J Obstet Gynecol. 1989;161:106-110.

44 Damm P, Molsted-Pedersen L. Significant decrease in congenital malformations in the newborn infants of an unselected population of diabetic women. Am J Obstet Gynecol. 1989;161:1163-1167.

45 Cousins L. The California Diabetes and Pregnancy Program: a statewide collaborative program for the preconception and prenatal care of diabetic women. Clin Obstet Gynecol. 1991;5:443-459.

46 Willhoite MB, Bennert HW Jr, Palomaki GE, et al. The impact of preconception counseling on pregnancy outcomes. The experience of the Maine Diabetes and Pregnancy Program. Diabetes Care. 1993;16:450-455.

47 Janz HK, Herman WH, Becker MP, et al. Diabetes and pregnancy: factors associated with seeking pre-conception care. Diabetes Care. 1995;18:157-165.

48 Elixhauser A, Weschler JM, Kitzmiller JL, et al. Cost-benefit analysis of preconception care for women with established diabetes mellitus. Diabetes Care. 1993;16:1146-1157.

49 Scheffler RM, Feuchtbaum LB, Phibbs CS. Prevention: the cost-effectiveness of the California Diabetes and Pregnancy Program. Am J Public Health. 1992;82:168-175.

50 Langer O, Conway DL, Berkus M, Elly M, Xenakis J, Gonzales O. A comparison of glyburide and insulin in women with GDM. NEJM. 2000;343:1134-1138.

51 Warram JH, Krolewski AS, Kahn CR. Determinants of IDDM and perinatal mortality in children of diabetic mothers. Diabetes. 1988;37:1328-1334.

52 Kobberly J, Tallil H. Empirical risk figures for first degree relatives of non-insulin-dependent diabetics. In: Genetics of Diabetes Mellitus. Proceedings of the Serone Symposia. Vol 47. London: Academic Press; 1982:201.

53 Shane B. Folate fortification: enough already? Am Journal of Clin Nutr. 2003; 77:8-9.

54 Jovanovic-Peterson L, Peterson CM. Diabetic retinopathy. In: Reece EA, Coustan DR, eds. Diabetes Mellitus in Pregnancy. 2nd ed. New York: Churchill-Livingston; 1995:303-314.

55 Klein R, Klein BE, Moss SE, et al. Retinopathy in young-onset diabetic patients. Diabetes Care. 1985;8:311-315.

56 The Diabetes Control and Complications Trial Research Group. The effect of intensive treatment of diabetes on the development and progression of long-term complications in insulin-dependent diabetes mellitus. N Engl J Med. 1993;329:977-986.

57 The Kroc Collaborative Study Group. Diabetic retinopathy after two years of intensified insulin treatment. Follow-up of the Kroc Collaborative Study. JAMA. 1988;260:37-41.

58 Laatikainen I, Teramo K, Hieta-Heikurainen H, Koivisto V, Pelkonen R. A controlled study of the influence of continuous subcutaneous insulin infusion treatment on diabetic retinopathy during pregnancy. J Intern Med. 1987;221:367-376.

59 Rosenn B, Miodovnik M, Kranias G, et al. Progression of diabetic retinopathy in pregnancy: association with hypertension in pregnancy. Am J Obstet Gynecol. 1992;166:1214-1218.

60 Horvat M, Maclean H, Goldberg L, Crock GW. Diabetic retinopathy in pregnancy: a 12-year prospective survey. Br J Opthclmol. 1980;64:398-403.

61 Moloney JB, Drury MI. The effect of pregnancy on the natural course of diabetic retinopathy. Am J Ophthalmol. 1982;93:745-756.

62 Dibble CM, Kochenour NK, Worley RJ, et al. Effect of pregnancy on diabetic retinopathy. Obstet Gynecol. 1982;59:699-704.

63 Ohrt V. The influence of pregnancy on diabetic retinopathy with special regards to the reversible changes shown in 200 pregnancies. Acta Ophthalmol. 1984;62:603-616.

64 Chew EY, Mills JL, Metzger BE, et al. Metabolic control and progression of retinopathy. The Diabetes in Early Pregnancy Study. National Institute of Child Health and Human Development Diabetes in Early Pregnancy Study. Diabetes Care. 1995;18:631-637.

65 Axer-Siegel R, Hod M, Fink-Cohen S, et al. Diabetic retinopathy during pregnancy. Ophthalmology. 1996;103:1815-1819.

66 Lovestam-Adrian M, Agardh CD, Aberg A, Agardh E. Preeclampsia is a potent risk factor for deterioration of retinopathy during pregnancy in Type 1 diabetic patients. Diabetic Med. 1997;14:1059-1065.

67 Lapolla A, Cardone C, Negrin P, et al. Pregnancy does not induce or worsen retinal and peripheral nerve dysfunction in insulin-dependent diabetic women. J Diabetes Complications. 1998;12:74-80.

68 Reece EA, Coustan DR, Hayslett JP, et al. Diabetic nephropathy: pregnancy performance and fetomaternal outcome. Am J Obstet Gynecol. 1988;159:56-66.

69 Jovanovic R, Jovanovic L. Obstetric management when normoglycemia is maintained in diabetic pregnant women with vascular compromise. Am J Obstet Gynecol. 1984;149:617-623.

70 Reece EA, Winn HN, Hayslett JP, Coulehan JJ, Wan M, Hobbins JC. Does pregnancy alter the rate of progression of diabetic nephropathy? Am J Perinatol. 1990;7:193-197.

71 Kitzmiller JL, Combs CA. Maternal and perinatal implications of diabetic nephropathy. Clin Perinatol. 1993;20:561-570.

72 Combs CA, Rosenn B, Kitzmiller JL, et al. Early-pregnancy proteinuria in diabetes related to preeclampsia. Obstet Gynecol. 1993;82:802-807.

73 Kitzmiller JL, Brown ER, Phillippe M, et al. Diabetic nephropathy and perinatal outcome. Am J Obstet Gynecol. 1981;141:741-751.

74 Grenfell A, Brudenell JM, Doddridge MC, Watkins PJ. Pregnancy in diabetic women who have proteinuria. Q J Med. 1986;59:379-386.

75 Reece EA, Leguizamon G, Homko C. Pregnancy performance and outcomes associated with diabetic nephropathy. Am J Perinatol. 1998;15:413-421.

76 Pierce J. California Diabetes and Pregnancy Program Data System Report, 1992. California Department of Health Services, Maternal and Child Health Branch, Contract 97644.

77 Kitzmiller JK. Diabetic nephropathy. In: Reece EA, Coustan DR, eds. Diabetes Mellitus in Pregnancy. 2nd ed. New York: Churchill-Livingston; 1995:315-344.

78 Hou SH, Grossman SD, Madias NE. Pregnancy in women with renal disease and moderate renal insufficiency. Am J Med. 1985;78:185-194.

79 Miodovnik M, Rosenn BM, Khoury JC, Grigsby JL, Siddiqi TA. Does pregnancy increase the risk for development and progression of diabetic nephropathy? Am J Obstet Gynecol. 1996;174:1180-1191.

80 Manske CL, Thomas W, Wang Y, Wilson RF. Screening diabetic transplant candidates for coronary artery disease: identification of a low risk subgroup. Kidney Int. 1993;44:617-621.

81 Brown FM, Hare JW. Diabetic neuropathy and coronary heart disease. In: Reece EA, Coustan DR, eds. Diabetes Mellitus in Pregnancy. 2nd ed. New York: Churchill-Livingston; 1995:345-351.

82 Churchill JA, Berendes HW. Intelligence of children whose mothers had acetonuria during pregnancy. In: Perinatal Factors Affecting Human Development. Pan American Health Organization Scientific Publication. Washington, DC: Pan American Health Organization; 1969;185:300.

83 Rizzo T, Metzger BE, Burns WJ, Burns K. Correlations between antepartum maternal metabolism and child intelligence. N Engl J Med. 1991;325:911-916.

84 Institute of Medicine of the National Academies. Dietary Reference Intakes: Energy, Carbohydrate, Fiber, Fat, Fatty Acids, Cholesterol, Protein, and Amino Acids. Washington, DC: The National Academies Press; 2002.

85 National Academy of Sciences. Nutrition During Pregnancy. Washington, DC: National Academy Press, 1990.

86 Abrahms BF, Laros RK, Jr. Prepregnancy weight, weight gain and birth weight. Am J Obstet Gynecol. 1986;154:503-509.

87 Durnin JVGA. Energy requirements of pregnancy. Diabetes. 1991;40(suppl 2):152-156.

88 Rizzo TA, Dooley SL, Metzger BE, Cho NH, Ogata ES, Silverman BL. Prenatal and perinatal influences on long-term psychomotor development in offspring of diabetic mothers. Am J Obstet Gynecol. 1995;173:1753-1758.

89 American Diabetes Association. Evidence-based nutrition principles and recommendations for the treatment and prevention of diabetes and related complications (position statement). Diabetes Care. 2003;26(suppl 1):S51-S61.

90 Trumbo P, Schlicker S, Yates AA, Poos M. Dietary reference intakes for energy, carbohydrate, fiber, fat, fatty acids, cholesterol, protein and amino acids. J Am Diet Assoc. 2002;102:1621-1630.

91 Jornsay DL. Managing morning sickness. Diabetes Self-Manage. 1990;10(2):10-12.

92 Evans EC. The FDA recommendations on fish intake during pregnancy. J Obstet Gynecol Neonatal Nurs. 2002; 31:715-720.

93 American College of Obstetricians and Gynecologists. Diabetes and Pregnancy, Technical Bulletin 200. Washington, DC:ACOG; 1994.

94 Kitzmiller JL. Antepartum and intrapartum obstetric care. In: Lebovitz HE. Therapy for Diabetes Mellitus and Related Disorders. 3rd ed. Alexandria, VA: American Diabetes Association; 1998: 36-43.

95 American Diabetes Association. Preconception care of women with diabetes. Diabetes Care. 2003; 26(suppl 1):S91-93.

96 Reece EA, Homko CJ, Wiznitzer A. Hypoglycemia in pregnancies complicated by diabetes mellitus: maternal and fetal considerations. Clinical Obstet Gynecol. 1994;37:50-58.

97 Buchanan TA, Schemmer JK, Freinkel N. Embryotoxic effects of brief maternal insulin-hypoglycemia during organogenesis in the rat. J Clin Invest. 1986;78:643-649.

98 Combs CA, Gunderson E, Kitzmiller JL, et al. Relationship of fetal macrosomia to maternal postprandial glucose control during pregnancy. Diabetes Care. 1992;15:1251-1257.

99 DeVeciana M, Major CA, Morgan MA, et al. Postprandial versus preprandial blood glucose monitoring in women with gestational diabetes mellitus requiring insulin therapy. N Engl J Med. 1995;333:1237-1241.

100 Jornsay DL. Pregnancy and continuous insulin infusion therapy. Diabetes Spectrum. 1998;11:26-32.

101 Rudolf MC, Coustan DR, Sherwin RS, et al. Efficacy of the insulin pump in the home treatment of pregnant diabetics. Diabetes. 1981;30:891-895.

102 Kitzmiller J, Younger D, Hare J, Philips M, Vignati L, Fargnoli B, Grause A. Continuous subcutaneous insulin therapy during early pregnancy. Obstetrics and Gynecology. 1985:66:606-611.

103 Gabbe SG. New concepts and applications in the use of insulin pump during pregnancy. J Matern Fetal Med. 2000;9:42-45.

104 Marcus AO, Fernandez MP. Insulin pump therapy: acceptable alternative to injection therapy. Postgrad Med. 1996:3;125-132, 142-144.

105 Jovanovic L, Peterson CM. Optimal insulin delivery for the pregnant diabetic patient. Diabetes Care. 1982;5(suppl 1):24-37.

106 Kimmerle R, Heinemann L, Delecki A, Berger M. Severe hypoglycemia incidence and predisposing factors in 85 pregnancies of type 1 diabetic women. Diabetes Care. 1992;15:1034-1037.

107 Diamond MP, Reece EA, Caprio S, et al. Impairment of counterregulatory hormone responses to hypoglycemia in pregnant women with insulin-dependent diabetes mellitus. Am J Obstet Gynecol. 1992;166:70-77.

108 Nelson DM, Barrows HJ, Clapp DH, Ortman-Nabi J, Whitehurst RM. Glycosylated serum protein levels in diabetic and nondiabetic pregnant patients: an indicator of short-term glycemic control in the diabetic patient. Am J Obstet Gynecol. 1985;151:1042-1047.

109 Mordes D, Kreutner K, Metzger W, Colwell JA. Dangers of intravenous ritodrine in diabetic patients. JAMA. 1982;248:973-975.

110 Buchanan TA, Unterman TG, Metzger BE. The medical management of diabetes in pregnancy. Clin Perinatal. 1985;12:625-650.

111 Jornsay D. Fetal monitoring: how's your baby doing in there? Diabetes Self-Manage. 1996;13:40-44.

112 Main DM, Mennuti MT. Neural tube defects: issues in prenatal diagnosis and counseling. Obstet Gynecol. 1986;67:1-16.

113 Jovanovic L, Peterson CM. Insulin and glucose requirements during the first stage of labor in insulin-dependent diabetic women. Am J Med. 1983;75:607-612.

114 Landon MB. Diabetes mellitus and other endocrine disorders. In: Gabble SG, Niebyl JR, Simpson JL, eds. Obstetrics: Normal and Problem Pregnancies. New York: Churchill-Livingston; 1991:1097-1136.

115 Murtaugh MA, Ferris AM, Capacchione CM, Reece A. Energy intake and glycemia in lactating women with type 1 diabetes. J Am Diet Assoc. 1998;98:642-648.

116 Kjos SL. Contraception in women with diabetes mellitus. Diabetes Spectrum. 1993;6:80-86.

117 Trussell J, Hatcher RA, Cates W Jr, et al. Contraceptive failure in the United States: an update. Stud Fam Plan. 1990;21:51-54.

118 Kjos SL. Postpartum care of women with diabetes. Clin Obstet Gynecol. 2000;43:46-55.

Suggested Readings

Bailey BK, Cardwell MS. A team approach to managing preexisting diabetes complicated by pregnancy. Diabetes Educator. 1996;22:111-115.

California Diabetes and Pregnancy Program. Sweet Success: Guidelines for Care. Campbell, Calif: Education Program Associates; 1998.

Evers IM, DeValk HW, Mol BE, TerBraak EW, Visser GH. Macrosomia despite good glycemic control in type 1 diabetic pregnancy: results of a nationwide study in the Netherlands. Diabetologia. 2002;45:1484-1489.

Homko CJ, Reece EA. Ambulatory management of the pregnant woman with diabetes. Obstetrics and Gynecology Clinics of North America. 1998;41:584-596.

Jovanovic L, ed. Medical Management of Pregnancy Complicated by Diabetes. 3rd ed. Alexandria, Va: American Diabetes Association; 2000.

Ray JG, O'Brien TE, Chan WS. Preconception care and the risk of congenital anomalies in the offspring of women with diabetes mellitus: A meta-analysis. QJM. 2001;94: 435-444.

Reece EA, Coustan DR, eds. Diabetes Mellitus in Pregnancy. 2nd ed. New York: Churchill-Livingston; 1995.

Rosenn BM, Miodovnik M. Medical complications of diabetes mellitus in pregnancy. Clinical Obstetrics and Gynecology. 2000;43:17-31.

Shils ME, Olson JA, Shike M, Ross AC. Modern Nutrition in Health and Disease. Philadelphia: JB Lippincott; 1999.

Worthington-Roberts BS, Rodwell Williams S. Nutrition in Pregnancy and Lactation. New York: McGraw Hill; 1996.

Learning Assessment: Post-Test Questions

Pregnancy With Preexisting Diabetes

4

1 Which of the following is not true regarding diabetes and pregnancy?

A Insulin may be necessary to achieve euglycemia during pregnancy in women with both type 1 and 2 diabetes

B Women with diabetes with vascular complications should be counseled to avoid pregnancy

C Pregnant women with type 1 or type 2 diabetes are at risk for having a baby with congenital anomalies if they are not in good glycemic control prior to pregnancy

D The incidence of hypertensive complications is increased among pregnant women with diabetes

2 Which of the following statements is true about preconception care?

A Spontaneous abortion rates have been found to correlate with glycosylated hemoglobin values during the first trimester

B Good preconception glucose control can eliminate the risks for congenital anomalies and spontaneous abortion

C Most women in the US with type 1 or type 2 diabetes achieve optimal glycemic control prior to pregnancy

D Major malformations occur after the eighth week of gestation

3 The following metabolic changes are seen during the latter part of pregnancy except:

A Accelerated starvation characterized by higher concentration of ketones during the fasting state

B Prolonged postprandial blood glucose levels that promote fetal growth

C Transplacental delivery of insulin to the fetus promotes fetal growth

D Insulin resistance is related to human placental lactogen, prolactin, and cortisol levels

4 Vaginal delivery is contraindicated in the woman with diabetes who has:

A A macrosomic infant

B Gastroparesis

C Neuropathy

D Untreated proliferative retinopathy

5 Which of the following sets of neonatal complications are not associated with a pregnancy complicated by diabetes?

A Macrosomia and hyperbilirubinemia

B Hydrocephalus and thrombocytopenia

C Hypoglycemia and hyperbilirubinemia

D Macrosomia and hypoglycemia

6 Which of the following has been identified as a predictor of poor perinatal outcome?

A Age of onset of maternal diabetes

B Duration of maternal diabetes

C Presence of vascular complications of diabetes

D Mild nonproliferative retinopathy

7 TS has type 2 diabetes and has been taking metformin for 1 year. Her glycosylated hemoglobin is within normal range. She is using her meal plan but is still 25 pounds overweight. During preconception care, which of the following is the most likely recommendation?

A Do not attempt conception until she has lost 25 pounds

B Discontinue metformin and start her on insulin

C Start on prenatal vitamins

D Discontinue metformin and start her on glyburide

8 Women with diabetes should seek pre-conception counseling 3 to 6 months prior to conception. The main goal of preconception counseling is:

A To normalize A1C levels
B To start calcium supplementation
C To add an oral agent to the existing medication regimen
D To achieve desirable body weight

9 Which 4 nutrient requirements increase significantly during pregnancy?

A Protein, folate, fat, calcium
B Protein, folate, carbohydrate, iron
C Protein, folate, vitamin C, iron
D Protein, folate, iron, calcium.

10 Which of the following is not true when working with women who have type 1 diabetes and who are breastfeeding?

A They are at risk for hypoglycemia
B Their infants are at risk for hyper-glycemia
C Their insulin dosage will need to be adjusted
D The meal plan during lactation is similar to that of the third trimester

See next page for answer key.

Post-Test Answer Key

Pregnancy With Preexisting Diabetes   4

1   B   6   C

2   A   7   B

3   C   8   A

4   A   9   D

5   B   10 B

A Core Curriculum for Diabetes Education
Diabetes in the Life Cycle and Research

Susan A. Biastre, RD, LDN, CDE
Women & Infants Hospital
Providence, Rhode Island

Julie Slocum, RN, MS, CDE
Women & Infants Hospital
Providence, Rhode Island

Introduction

1 The diagnosis of gestational diabetes mellitus (GDM) accounts for nearly 90% of all pregnancies complicated by diabetes.[1] Approximately 7% of all pregnancies are complicated by GDM, resulting in more than 200 000 cases annually.[2] The prevalence may range from 1% to 14% of all pregnancies, depending on the population studied and the diagnostic tests employed.

2 There are long-term and short-term implications of GDM for both the mother and the fetus. When glucose is under tight control in GDM, pregnancy outcomes are improved.[3]

3 Treatment of GDM begins with medical nutrition therapy, monitoring of outcomes, and, when necessary, insulin. The goal of nutrition therapy is to keep the postprandial glucose response in the normal range. Because the balance between the carbohydrate content of the meal and available insulin determines the postprandial glucose response, attention is given to limiting excess carbohydrate in meals.

Objectives

Upon completion of this chapter, the learner will be able to
1 Define gestational diabetes.
2 Explain the metabolic changes associated with the development of GDM.
3 Describe the potential risks of GDM to the fetus and neonate.
4 List the diagnostic criteria for GDM.
5 State guidelines for self-management and potential barriers.
6 Describe nutrition practice guidelines for GDM.
7 Describe criteria for initiation of insulin therapy.
8 List 2 fetal monitoring tests used for routine surveillance in GDM.
9 State postpartum recommendations for women with GDM.

Definition of Gestational Diabetes Mellitus

1 Gestational diabetes mellitus (GDM) is defined as carbohydrate intolerance of varying degrees of severity with onset or first recognition during pregnancy.[3,4]
  A This definition applies regardless if insulin is used as treatment or if the condition persists after pregnancy.
  B Included in this classification are women who may have had undiagnosed type 2 diabetes prior to pregnancy but who are first diagnosed during pregnancy. Approximately 2% of women of childbearing age in the United States have undiagnosed type 2 diabetes.[5]
  C Pregnant women requiring use of exogenous steroids, tocolytics, or other medications or who have medical conditions that alter glucose tolerance may develop GDM.

2 Women with previous GDM should undergo a 2-hour 75-g oral glucose tolerance test at 6 to 12 weeks postpartum. They can be reclassified according to their test results into normal glucose tolerance, pre-diabetes (impaired glucose tolerance), or as having type 2 diabetes.[3,6]

Metabolic Influences During Pregnancy

1 Pregnancy is an insulin-resistant or diabetogenic state (see Chapter 4, Pregnancy With Preexisting Diabetes, in Diabetes in the Life Cycle and Research). In the second and third trimesters of pregnancy, the metabolic changes are pronounced. A combination of increased mobilization of glucose and decreased insulin sensitivity places pregnant women at risk for developing GDM.

  A Insulin resistance is progressive and appears to be related to increased circulating levels of hormones, such as human placental lactogen, prolactin, estrogen, and free and bound cortisol. This action is parallel to fetal and placental growth.

  B In pregnant women, this insulin resistance results in higher and more prolonged plasma glucose concentrations postprandially than in nonpregnant women. Conversely in a fasting state (ie, >5 hours after eating), there is an exaggerated decrease in plasma glucose levels.[7,8]

  C Basal insulin levels increase and insulin secretion in response to food increases twofold to threefold above nonpregnant levels. There is evidence that women who develop GDM secrete less insulin in response to a glucose load than women who do not develop GDM.[9]

2 In the second and third trimesters of pregnancy, pregnant women who are fasting or in a period of food deprivation experience a rapid shift to the products of fat metabolism, with greater rises in plasma and urinary ketones. This condition is called accelerated starvation.

Perinatal Implications of Gestational Diabetes

1 Untreated or poorly treated GDM results in a higher risk of morbidity and mortality for both the mother and the fetus.

  A Today, widespread testing and intensive management appear to be associated with a decrease in complications in both mothers and infants.

  B With appropriate treatment of GDM, the rate of intrauterine death is similar to that in the general population.[1]

2 GDM is associated with many of the same fetal and neonatal complications observed during pregnancy in women with preexisting diabetes. The frequency and severity of perinatal morbidities decrease when GDM is managed intensively.[3]

  A The primary perinatal concern in GDM is excessive fetal growth. Macrosomia is significantly more common in infants of women with GDM than in the general population.[10]

  B There is an increased rate of infant shoulder dystocia and traumatic birth due to disproportional enlargement of the trunk and shoulders. Other morbidities observed in infants are hypoglycemia, hypocalcemia, polycythemia, and hyperbilirubinemia.

  C GDM with onset late in pregnancy is not associated with an increased incidence of congenital malformations. There is some evidence that GDM diagnosed for the first time during pregnancy with fasting plasma glucose levels >120 mg/dL (6.7 mmol/L) may indicate that preexisting diabetes was present and may be associated with a rate of anomalies greater than that in the general population.[11]

3 Maternal risks of hypertension, preeclampsia, polyhydramnios, and surgical delivery are increased in a pregnancy complicated by GDM.[3]

Long-Term Implications of Gestational Diabetes Mellitus

1 Women with previous GDM are at increased risk for the development of diabetes, usually type 2 diabetes, after pregnancy.[2] Obesity and other risk factors for insulin resistance enhance the risk of type 2 diabetes, while markers of islet cell–directed autoimmunity are associated with an increased risk of type 1 diabetes.

A The risk of subsequent diabetes is greatest in women with GDM who are diagnosed early in the pregnancy, exhibit the highest rates of hyperglycemia during the pregnancy, and are obese.[4,12]

B Many women will develop GDM in a subsequent pregnancy. This rate has been reported to range from 30% to 50%. Some studies have found that the risk factors for subsequent GDM include insulin use in the index pregnancy, obesity, and weight gain between pregnancies. One study suggested that modification of fat intake before and during pregnancy may reduce this risk.[12]

2 There are also long-term health risks for the offspring of women with GDM.

A The risk of obesity is increased in the offspring of women with GDM. After age 5, the children of women with GDM have a higher body mass index than the children of women who did not have GDM.[13] This trend toward obesity continues into adolescence.

B Infants born to women with GDM also have higher rates of impaired glucose tolerance and type 2 diabetes.[13]

C Altered metabolic substrates during pregnancy may affect the intellectual and neurological development of the offspring of women with GDM who were in poor glycemic control during the pregnancy.[3]

Diagnosis of Gestational Diabetes

1 There is general agreement among experts that the prevalence of GDM is increasing globally.[3] Currently, no worldwide uniform standards exist for the detection and diagnosis of GDM. This lack of standards has interfered with dispelling the controversy regarding the clinical importance of GDM and its impact on women and offspring. These issues have been addressed in the Summary and Recommendations of the Second, Third, and Fourth Workshop-Conferences on Gestational Diabetes.[3,14,15] As a result, an international multicenter study, the Hyperglycemia and Adverse Outcome (HAPO) Study, is being conducted for the purpose of clarifying the associations between various levels of glucose intolerance during pregnancy and macrosomia, cesarean section rate, and hypertension among women of different cultures and ethnic groups.

2 The Second and Third International Workshop-Conferences on Gestational Diabetes Mellitus made the recommendation that all pregnant women be screened for glucose intolerance.[14,15]

3 There are specific factors that place some women at low risk for developing glucose intolerance, and it may not be cost effective to screen this low-risk group.[3] Therefore, the current recommendation by both the Fourth International Conference-Workshop on Gestational Diabetes Mellitus[3] and the Expert Committee on the Diagnosis and Classification of Diabetes Mellitus[4] is for selective rather than universal screening. The following are screening recommendations for GDM:

A Every pregnant women should have a risk assessment at her first prenatal visit for the development of abnormal glucose tolerance.

B Women at low risk for GDM do not need to be routinely screened. Low-risk women must have all of the following criteria:
- Age <25 years
- Weight normal before pregnancy
- No first-degree family history of diabetes
- Member of an ethnic group with a low prevalence of GDM
- No history of abnormal glucose tolerance
- No history of poor obstetric outcome

C Women at average risk for GDM and women who have not been identified as having abnormal glucose tolerance prior to the 24th week of gestation should have a screening test for GDM between the 24th and 28th weeks of gestation.

D Women at high risk for GDM should be screened as early as possible in the pregnancy. The clinical characteristics of being at high risk for GDM are
- Marked obesity
- Personal history of GDM
- A strong family history of diabetes
- Glycosuria
- Member of an ethnic group with a high prevalence of type 2 diabetes. These groups include Hispanic, African American, Mexican, Native American, South or East Asian, Pacific Island, or indigenous Australian ancestry, especially when residing in westernized countries or in an urban setting.

4 A fasting plasma glucose level >126 mg/dL (7.0 mmol/L) or a casual plasma glucose of >200 mg/dL (11.1 mmol/L) outside the context of a formal glucose challenge is suggestive of diabetes and warrants evaluation as quickly as possible.[2]

5 Women at average risk and high risk who have not already been diagnosed with glucose intolerance by the 24th week of gestation should be evaluated for GDM between the 24th and 28th weeks of gestation. Evaluation may be done in 1 or 2 steps.

6 In the United States the diagnostic criteria are fairly well standardized into a 2-step approach.

A A screening test (glucose challenge test) that measures plasma or serum glucose is done 1 hour after a 50-g oral glucose load without regard for time of day or time of last meal. If a plasma or serum glucose level meets or exceeds the threshold (>130 mg/dL [7.2 mmol/L] or >140 mg/dL [7.8 mmol/L], respectively), an oral glucose tolerance test (OGTT) is performed.[2]

B A diagnosis of GDM is made with a 100-g oral glucose load after an overnight fast. Using a 3-hour test, if 2 or more plasma or serum glucose levels meet or exceed the threshold, a diagnosis of GDM is made. Alternatively, the diagnosis can be made using a 75-g oral glucose load. The glucose threshold values for both tests are listed in Table 5.1.[2] The 75-g glucose load test is not as well validated as the 100-g OGTT.

7 Another diagnostic approach used throughout the world and supported by the World Health Organization (WHO) is based on the method and criteria used in non-pregnant adults for diagnosing diabetes outside of pregnancy.[16] The WHO method also uses a 75-g glucose load and interposes an intermediate diagnostic category of impaired glucose tolerance between a diagnosis of normal and GDM. This 1-step approach may be cost effective in high-risk women or populations.

8 With either the 75-g OGTT or the 100-g OGTT, it is recommended that the test be performed after an overnight fast of at least 8 hours but no longer than 14 hours. For 3 days prior to the test the woman should consume an unrestricted diet (>150 g carbohydrate per day) and maintain unrestricted physical activity. Women need to remain seated and not smoke during the test.

Table 5.1. Diagnosis of GDM With a 100-g or 75-g Oral Glucose Load

Time (h)	100-g Oral Glucose Load	75-g Oral Glucose Load
Fasting	95 mg/dL (5.3 mmol/L)	95 mg/dL (5.3 mmol/L)
1	180 mg/dL (10.0 mmol/L)	180 mg/dL (10.0 mmol/L)
2	155 mg/dL (8.6 mmol/L)	155 mg/dL (8.6 mmol/L)
3	140 mg/dL (7.8 mmol/L)	

Two or more of the venous plasma concentrations must be met or exceeded for a positive diagnosis.
Source: American Diabetes Association.[2]

Management of Gestational Diabetes Mellitus

1 The goals of managing GDM are the same as for preexisting diabetes in pregnancy: normalize metabolism and achieve tight metabolic control to reduce perinatal morbidity and improve pregnancy outcomes while meeting the nutritional needs of pregnancy and achieving appropriate weight gain (see Chapter 4, Pregnancy With Preexisting Diabetes, in Diabetes in the Life Cycle and Research). These goals are achieved by using medical nutrition therapy, insulin therapy, if required, and close maternal and fetal surveillance.

2 Using a team approach with the woman as the center of the team can enhance the achievement of outcome goals. Those involved in the care of a woman with GDM, in addition to her primary care provider, might include a registered dietitian, registered nurse, social worker, exercise physiologist, and others required to meet the woman's medical, physical, and mental needs.

Medical Nutrition Therapy for Gestational Diabetes

1 Medical nutrition therapy (MNT) is the primary treatment for the management of GDM. All women should receive nutrition therapy upon diagnosis of GDM, by a registered dietitian when possible.[2]

2 Medical nutrition therapy for GDM primarily involves a carbohydrate-controlled food/meal plan that promotes adequate nutrition with appropriate weight gain, normoglycemia, and the absence of ketones.[17] For some women with GDM, modest energy and carbohydrate restriction may be appropriate.[18]

3 The clinical outcomes of MNT in GDM are to
A Achieve and maintain normoglycemia
B Provide adequate energy to promote appropriate gestational weight gain and avoid maternal ketosis
C Provide food with the nutrients necessary for maternal and fetal health
D Decrease pregnancy-related discomforts such as hypoglycemia, nausea, vomiting, constipation, heartburn, pica, and ptyalism.

4 Timing of the intervention and evaluation is critical in GDM due to the time-limited nature of the problem. Once a referral for MNT has been made, the initial intervention should begin as soon as possible. Timing of follow-up visits is equally important. A summary of the visit schedule recommended in the nutrition practice guidelines for GDM is shown in Table 5.2.[17]

Table 5.2. Summary of Visit Schedule to Provide Medical Nutrition Therapy

Type of Visit	Timing of Visit
Referral contact/make appointment Have client begin food records	Within 48 hours of referral
Initial visit	Within 1 week of receiving referral
Second visit	1 week after the initial visit
Third visit	1 to 3 weeks after second visit
Subsequent follow-up visit(s)	2 to 3 weeks after third visit Follow until delivery
Postpartum visits*	After 6 weeks postdelivery

*At 6 to 12 weeks postdelivery, a review of glucose tolerance and the postpartum nutrition plan is recommended.
Source: American Dietetic Association.[17]

5 A nutrition assessment is completed at the initial visit. Data are gathered to assist in designing a food/meal plan that will achieve the clinical goals and that is appropriate for the individual woman. The assessment includes the following:

A Medical and obstetrical histories

B Anthropometric data: height, current weight, prepregnancy weight and body mass index (weight/height^2), and weight-gain goal for pregnancy

C Lab data: glucose challenge test, oral glucose tolerance test, hemoglobin, hematocrit, blood pressure, blood or urine ketones, and A1C

D Lifestyle factors: type of work and schedule, education level, family, cultural/ethnic/religious issues, financial concerns, use of food assistance, and substance use

E Gastrointestinal issues: appetite, eating disorders, discomforts, allergies, intolerances, cravings, aversions, and pica

F Food recall: meal and snack time, food choices, portions, preparation methods, and preferences

G Exercise patterns and limitations

H Infant feeding plans

6 A summary of nutrient recommendations for gestational diabetes is listed in Table 5.3.[17,19]

7 Keeping food records along with results of fasting and postmeal blood glucose levels is essential for helping the woman and dietitian assess the effectiveness of nutrition therapy.

A Self-monitoring of blood glucose (SMBG) guides nutrition therapy.[17] The blood glucose information from SMBG shows the glycemic effects of foods and can be used to make alterations in the food/meal plan based upon an individual woman's response.

B The balance between the amount and type of carbohydrate in foods and available insulin and the distribution of carbohydrate determine postprandial blood glucose levels.[17]

8 The energy level of the food/meal plan should be individualized, based on assessment, and take into consideration prepregnancy weight, physical activity level, and pregnancy weight gain to date.

A The 2002 Dietary Reference Intakes[19] make the following recommendations for energy requirements during pregnancy:

- First trimester: no extra calories required
- Second and third trimester: total energy expenditure (TEE) of woman in non-pregnancy state + 8 kcal/week for additional TEE during pregnancy + 180 kcal/day for energy deposition during pregnancy
- For example the energy requirements during pregnancy for a woman consuming 2 000 kcal prior to pregnancy and in the 30th week of pregnancy would be: 2 000 + 240 (8 x 30) + 180 = 2 420 kcal/day

B However, energy recommendations should be based on actual intake rather than relying on formulas. Energy recommendations should be monitored by following weight-gain patterns, evaluating results of ketone testing, assessing appetite, and reviewing food records.

Table 5.3. Nutrient Recommendations for Gestational Diabetes

Calories	Sufficient to promote adequate weight gain and avoid ketones.
Carbohydrate	Based on effect of intake on blood glucose levels; distributed throughout the day in frequent feedings and distribution in smaller portions, but in sufficient amounts to avoid ketonemia and ketonuria. The Recommended Dietary Allowance (RDA) for carbohydrate requirements during pregnancy is 175 g/day.
Sucrose and other caloric sweeteners	Limit use; include based on ability to maintain blood glucose goals, nutritional adequacy of diet, and contribution to total meal plan.
Protein	The RDA for protein requirements during pregnancy is 1.1 g/kg/day or an additional 25 g/day. Protein intake may also increase due to decrease in carbohydrate intake.
Fat	Often increased due to increased protein intake; limit saturated fat.
Sodium	Not routinely restricted.
Fiber	The Adequate Intake (AI) for fiber during pregnancy is 28 g/day of total fiber. Fiber may be beneficial for relief of constipation.
Nonnutritive sweeteners	Generally safe in pregnancy.
Vitamins and minerals	Assess for specific individual needs; 400 µg of folic acid from foods or supplements; 30 mg/day (low-dose) iron supplementation during the second and third trimester; zinc supplements for women with low pregravid weight and low plasma zinc levels.
Alcohol	Avoid.
Caffeine	Limit to <300 mg/day (approximately 2 to 2½ 8-oz cups per day).[20,21]

Sources: American Dietetic Association[17] and Institute of Medicine.[19]

   c There is no agreement on the minimum caloric requirement for women with GDM.[3] A daily minimum of 1700 to 1800 kcals has been shown to prevent ketosis.[17] The use of hypocaloric diets in obese women has been suggested as a way to decrease blood glucose in GDM. However, energy restriction can lead to ketonemia and ketonuria, which can affect the fetus, and should be avoided during pregnancy.[22,23] In one study, a caloric reduction of 33% did not produce ketonuria but did improve glycemia.[24] However, at the present time, caloric restriction must be viewed with caution.[25]

9 Weight-gain goals are the same as for pregnant women without GDM and are based on prepregnancy body mass index (see Chapter 4, Pregnancy With Preexisting Diabetes, in Diabetes in the Life Cycle and Research).

   A Weight gain should be steady and progressive. Weight-gain charts can help in assessing appropriate weight gain.

   B Many women experience weight loss after the initiation of nutrition therapy for GDM. Women may find that making the recommended eating changes, consuming more nutrient-dense foods, and eating scheduled snacks reduces their appetite. They may eat fewer high-calorie and high-fat foods, resulting in a lower energy intake. Also, a shift from a high-carbohydrate diet to a diet moderate in carbohydrate and higher in protein may result in diuresis. Each case should be evaluated individually, the care plan adjusted as needed, and education provided to achieve appropriate weight gain (see Table 4.5 in Chapter 4, Pregnancy With Preexisting Diabetes, in Diabetes in the Life Cycle and Research, for recommended ranges of total weight gain for pregnant women).

10 Carbohydrate is the primary nutrient that affects postprandial blood glucose levels.

   A In practice, to adequately control postprandial blood glucose levels, carbohydrate generally accounts for 40% to 45% of total energy. Major et al[26] demonstrated that a carbohydrate intake of 42% reduced macrosomia and reduced the need for insulin therapy.

   B The Recommended Dietary Allowance (RDA) for carbohydrate for women in the nonpregnant state is 130 g/day.[19] This is the amount that should be sufficient to fuel central nervous system cells without having to rely on a partial replacement of glucose by ketoacids. However, in order to assure provision of the fetal brain with glucose (approximately 33 g/day) for fuel, as well as to supply the glucose fuel requirement for the mother's brain, plus the additional amount required during the last trimester of pregnancy, the RDA for carbohydrate during pregnancy is set at 175 g/day.

   C The amount and distribution of carbohydrate are based on clinical outcome measures (blood glucose levels, weight gain, appetite, and blood or urine ketone levels).[27,28] Evaluation guides changes in the food/meal plan or other management areas (eg, physical activity or insulin regimen).

   D Carbohydrate is generally less well tolerated at breakfast than at other meals. In pregnancy, increased levels of cortisol and growth hormone can contribute to morning glucose intolerance. Assessment, using blood glucose values, weight gain, and food records, should be used to determine the carbohydrate level at a particular time of day, including breakfast. A moderate restriction, usually no more than 30 to 45 g of carbohydrate, is generally recommended with the blood glucose response monitored closely.[17] Some clinicians recommend limiting breakfast carbohydrate to 15 to 30 g.[25,29]

   E During pregnancy, blood glucose monitoring is essential to determine the type and distribution of carbohydrate throughout the day to achieve desired outcomes and to avoid unnecessary food restrictions.[17]

   F Some carbohydrate-containing foods may produce an increased glycemic response resulting in elevated postprandial blood glucose levels. For example, this effect may be observed with the use of dry, processed cereal and instant and other highly refined food products. The use of whole grain and unrefined products, as well as nuts, legumes, and lentils, is encouraged because of their lower glycemic response. Clapp[30] reported lower postprandial blood glucose levels and blood glucose response to exercise with a low glycemic diet compared with a high glycemic diet in healthy non-pregnant and pregnant women. However, specific foods should not be labeled as acceptable or unacceptable for women with GDM. Each woman should be evaluated based on her glycemic response to particular foods and at different times of the day to determine what foods are appropriate for her.

G The value of dietary fibers in blood glucose control has been questioned; it is unknown if free-living individuals can consume amounts needed to demonstrate benefit.[18] A high-fiber meal (25 g/1000 kcal) slows gastric emptying time and reduces postprandial serum glucose and insulin levels;[31,32] this is considerably more than usual intake. The quantity of fiber rather than the proportion of soluble to insoluble fiber is reported to affect postprandial glucose metabolism.[33]
- All pregnant women are encouraged to eat a healthy diet that includes adequate fiber.
- The Dietary Reference Intakes[19] based on the amount of fiber that may help ameliorate constipation, attenuate blood glucose and lipid concentrations, and contribute to satiety, set an Adequate Intake (AI) for fiber for women in the nonpregnant state at 25 g/day of total fiber. Because of the increased energy requirement during pregnancy, the AI during pregnancy is set at 28 g/day.

H The distribution of carbohydrate throughout the day affects blood glucose levels. It is recommended that carbohydrate be distributed throughout the day into 3 meals and 2 to 4 snacks.[17] Snacks should have fewer grams of carbohydrate than meals. The results of SMBG guide the distribution of carbohydrate. If a woman has elevated blood glucose levels at a particular meal, some of the carbohydrate from that meal can be moved to a snack or to a meal at another time of day when her glucose tolerance is better. An evening snack is usually required to prevent starvation ketosis overnight. Lapses of more than 10 hours without food should be avoided.[34]

I If insulin therapy is added to nutrition therapy, it becomes necessary to maintain carbohydrate consistency at meals and snacks to facilitate making insulin adjustments. Without insulin therapy, consistency is still encouraged and prevents undereating. When using insulin therapy, a range of carbohydrate grams per meal or snack is given, with the emphasis on consistency. When a woman is not on insulin therapy, carbohydrate gram recommendations can be made based upon an upper limit per meal or snack.[17]

J There are currently no studies on the effect of sucrose ingestion during pregnancy. It is suggested that eliminating foods high in sucrose and other sugars helps in attaining blood glucose goals because elimination of these foods usually results in an overall reduction of carbohydrate intake.[17] Nonpregnant individuals with type 1 and type 2 diabetes can include sucrose and control blood glucose levels as long as the total carbohydrate content remains the same.[18] In pregnancy, the nutrient density of foods chosen is more important than the sucrose content.

K The Food and Drug Administration has approved 5 nonnutritive sweeteners for general use in the United States: aspartame, acesulfame potassium (acesulfame K), sucralose, saccharin, and neotame. Saccharin can cross the placenta and may remain in fetal tissue due to slow fetal clearance,[35] although there is no evidence that this is harmful. Nonnutritive sweeteners are rigorously tested to determine effects during pregnancy and lactation in animals. No adverse effects have been reported.[36] There is strong evidence that use of nonnutritive sweeteners is safe during pregnancy.[18] Use of these nonnutritive sweeteners can also help control carbohydrate intake.

L Sugar alcohols (polyols) are nutritive sweeteners approved by the Food and Drug Administration as safe for general use. The contain carbohydrate, but are only partially absorbed, so they have approximately half the calories as sucrose. Excessive ingestion of some sugar alcohols, such as sorbitol, can cause diarrhea.[18] Therefore in pregnancy moderation is advised.

11 Protein intake is increased during pregnancy.

A Peripheral glucose levels do not increase after protein ingestion.[37,38] Thus, food containing protein (meat and meat substitutes) can be included in meals and snacks in place of carbohydrate foods for additional calories and to increase satiety without affecting blood glucose levels.[19]

B The RDA for women in the nonpregnancy state is set at 0.80 g/kg/day or 56 g of protein.[19] The RDA for protein for pregnancy is in addition to the RDA of 0.8 g protein/kg/day for the nonpregnant woman and is the amount required for protein deposition during pregnancy. Thus, the RDA during pregnancy is 1.1 g/kg/day of protein or an additional 25 g/day of protein. This level is usually achieved in an eating plan for GDM because protein generally comprises 20% to 25% of energy.

12 The percentage of fat in the diet both in preexisting diabetes and pregnancy and for the management of GDM is generally higher than usually recommended for nonpregnant women. Decreasing the carbohydrate and increasing protein in the food/meal plan for GDM often increases the percentage of fat. Fat usually comprises 30% to 40% of calories.

A GDM is a short-term condition and the meals plans are not intended for long-term chronic disease prevention. Less that one third of the fat calories each day should be from saturated fat and less than one third from polyunsaturated fat; the balance should be from monounsaturated fats.[17]

B Pregnant women need adequate fat in their diet during pregnancy to provide essential fatty acids needed for fetal brain development.[39]

Management of Gestational Diabetes: Monitoring

1 A goal of managing GDM is to achieve normoglycemia. To do this, metabolic surveillance is critical.

2 Currently there is no consensus on the use of self-monitoring of capillary blood glucose versus venous laboratory samples in GDM.

A The Third International Conference-Workshop on Gestational Diabetes Mellitus reported that self-monitoring of capillary blood glucose has been useful in allowing the woman to participate in her own management, but its utility in mild GDM not requiring insulin, although reasonable and logical, has not been formally proved.[15] According to the Fourth International Conference-Workshop on Gestational Diabetes Mellitus[3] and the American Diabetes Association,[2] self-monitoring of blood glucose appears to be superior to less frequent glucose monitoring. The American College of Obstetricians and Gynecologists also support the use of SMBG in women with GDM.[40]

B There is evidence to support the role of SMBG in GDM.

- Wechter et al[41] concluded that a program of SMBG, intensive nutrition therapy, and institution of insulin therapy, when necessary, reduced the incidence of macrosomia in infants of women with GDM to that of the general population.
- Langer et al[42] compared an intensive schedule of monitoring capillary blood glucose (7 times per day) using memory reflectance meters with weekly venous glucose measurements supplemented by SMBG using visual strips (4 times per day) in women with GDM. Women in the intensified group had higher rates of insulin therapy but lower rates of macrosomia and other adverse pregnancy outcomes.

C The optimal timing of blood glucose testing has been controversial.

- In GDM it is recommended that glucose monitoring not be confined to fasting and preprandial testing, but also include postprandial blood glucose testing. Postmeal measurements at 1 or 2 hours are most commonly used.[3]
- DeVeciana et al[43] concluded that testing fasting and postprandial blood glucose levels improves glycemic control and infant outcomes.
- Sivan et al[44] compared the results of 1-hour postprandial glucose values with those obtained 2 hours postprandial. They found an increase in the percentages of abnormal values 1 hour after breakfast versus 2 hours after breakfast, but an increase in the percentage of abnormal values 2 hours after dinner versus 1 hour after dinner.
- Regardless of the method, it is the setting and achievement of blood glucose goals that produces positive outcomes.

D When SMBG is employed as a management tool, the woman should be taught how to use and care for her meter and supplies. The use of meters that electronically store results allow the healthcare team to compare stored results with a woman's written records.

E It is important that the accuracy of the meter results are verified by comparing a meter value with a laboratory reference on a routine basis. Any meter that varies from a laboratory value by more than 15% to 20% warrants investigation of the woman's technique, storage and care of supplies, and cleanliness of the meter. If no reason for the discrepancy can be found, the meter should be replaced.

F The results of SMBG can be used to help assess and guide nutrition and insulin therapies.

G It is important to note that both blood glucose goals and, thus, the criteria for initiation of insulin therapy, remain controversial in GDM.

- Blood glucose goals are listed in Table 5.4.[1]
- The American College of Obstetricians and Gynecology suggest the use of insulin therapy when fasting plasma glucose values exceed 95 mg/dL (5.3 mmol/L), 1-hour postprandial plasma values exceed 130 to 140 mg/dL (7.2 to 7.8 mmol/L) and 2-hour postprandial values exceed 120 mg/dL (6.7 mmol/L).[40]
- Other institutions and/or organizations may have alternative target plasma glucose goals. Research is needed as to when the optimum time is for insulin initiation.

H The frequency of testing is usually 4 times a day: in the fasting state and 1 or 2 hours after breakfast, lunch, and dinner. Once glucose goals have been achieved, the frequency of testing can be reduced. However, a more intensive testing schedule may need to be resumed as hormones antagonistic to insulin continue to rise as the pregnancy progresses.

I Postmeal testing provides information about the effects of the type and amount of food eaten. Women with GDM quickly learn the impact of food on their blood glucose levels. SMBG also may help identify women who are restricting foods excessively in order to maintain glucose control.

J Fasting or postprandial blood glucose levels that are out of range may warrant intensified management.

K Low average blood glucose levels in women with GDM have been associated with an increased incidence of small-for-gestational-age babies.[45]

Table 5.4. Glucose Goals During GDM

Insulin therapy is recommended when medical nutrition therapy fails to maintain self-monitored plasma glucose at the specified levels.

Time	
Fasting	Plasma glucose <105 mg/dL (5.8 mmol/L)
1-hour postprandial	Plasma glucose <155 mg/dL (8.6 mmol/L)
2-hour postprandial	Plasma glucose <130 mg/dL (7.2 mmol/L)

Source: American Diabetes Association.[1]

3 Urine or blood ketone testing can be used a management tool for women with GDM. However, the effectiveness of ketone testing in GDM to improve fetal outcomes has not been tested.[3]

A In the pregnant state, the body quickly reverts to fat storage for energy to spare glucose and amino acids for the fetus. The by-products of fat catabolism can produce ketones.

B Some studies suggest that high levels of ketones in the blood, or ketonemia, may cause lowered intelligence test scores and decreased psychomotor skills in the offspring of women with this alteration of metabolism.[22,23]

C The monitoring and frequency of urinary or blood ketone testing in GDM varies widely. It is currently recommended that prebreakfast urine ketone measurements be taken for women with GDM who follow hypocaloric or carbohydrate-restricted diets.[3]

D Reasons for insufficient food intake that might produce ketones include not following the appropriate food/meal plan, nausea, vomiting, or intentionally undereating to control blood glucose levels and/or to avoid the initiation of insulin therapy.

4 The use of measurements of glycated hemoglobin or other circulating proteins in GDM has not been established. This topic warrants further investigation.[3]

Management of Gestational Diabetes: Physical Activity

1 Physical activity can improve glucose tolerance in GDM and may be an alternative to insulin use. For women who are motivated to use this treatment, physical activity should be encouraged.[3]

  A The safety of physical activity/exercise in pregnancy is now well demonstrated,[46-48] but all pregnant women should receive medical clearance before beginning a physical activity/exercise program.

  B To achieve the effect of lowering blood glucose, the duration of activity may need to be 1 hour versus 30 minutes.[49]

2 The mechanisms that provide the metabolic benefits of exercise in GDM are not fully understood. It appears that the benefits are related, in part, to enhanced insulin sensitivity and decreased hepatic glucose output.[50]

3 There are some conditions that contraindicate exercise during pregnancy.[51] These include pregnancy-induced hypertension, premature rupture of membranes, intrauterine growth retardation, preterm labor or history of preterm labor, incompetent cervix/cerclage, and persistent bleeding in the second or third trimester.

Management of Gestational Diabetes: Insulin Therapy

1 Insulin therapy should be initiated if blood glucose goals are not consistently met with MNT.[3] Depending on the blood glucose goals, 20% to 50% of women with GDM require insulin therapy. Treatment with insulin reduces risk of fetal complications, especially macrosomia.[3]

2 Identifying women who would benefit from insulin therapy can be based on maternal blood glucose goals with or without assessment of fetal growth characteristics.[2]

3 Only human insulin is used in GDM, as in pregestational diabetes, to minimize the transplacental transport of anti-insulin antibodies and reduce the risk of future allergic reactions in women with GDM, who may go on to develop insulin-requiring diabetes later in life (see Chapter 4, Pregnancy With Preexisting Diabetes, in the Life Cycle and Research).

4 There is no one insulin regimen that has been shown to be most effective in managing women with GDM.[52] The insulin regimen should be individualized to achieve target blood glucose goals. Some centers may use initial doses based on body weight, while others may use a standard starting dose and make adjustments based on patterns of glucose elevations. Obese woman often require large amounts of insulin to overcome the combined insulin resistance of obesity and pregnancy.[53]

  A Insulin needs increase as the pregnancy progresses, and use of SMBG results to titrate the insulin dose is essential for maintaining tight control.

  B Insulin analogs have not yet been approved for use in GDM.[2] However, Jovanovic et al[54] demonstrated improved postprandial blood glucose levels in women with GDM treated with NPH/lispro insulin compared with women treated with

NPH/regular insulin. Pettitt et al[55] demonstrated that in women with GDM who required insulin, insulin aspart provided effective postprandial control. No studies using glargine during pregnancy have been published.

5 Many women are reluctant to take any medication during pregnancy, and insulin is no exception. Reassurance to the woman that commercial insulin is chemically identical to human insulin and will not harm her or her fetus is important. Also explain and assure her that the insulin is needed only until the baby is born.

Management of Gestational Diabetes: Oral Glucose-Lowering Agents

1 Oral glucose-lowering agents are not currently recommended during pregnancy by the American Diabetes Association or the American College of Obstetricians and Gynecologists. It has recently been suggested that oral agents be reconsidered as a therapy in GDM.

2 Langer et al[56] reported in a study of 404 women with GDM that glyburide, a second generation sulfonylurea, can be used to maintain glycemic control in women with GDM without any increase in incidence of maternal or fetal complications. Other researchers[57,58] have given women the option of using glyburide, instead of insulin, with varying degrees of success.

3 Several studies have been published recently regarding the use of metformin in women with polycystic ovary syndrome (PCOS). Vandermacher et al[59] and Kocak et al[60] demonstrated that metformin appears to improve the rate of ovulation and conception in women with PCOS. Glueck[61] and Jakubowicz[62] studied women who conceived on metformin and continued it during their pregnancy. Both showed a significantly lower rate of miscarriage with no increase in the rate of congenital anomalies. If metformin is shown to be safe to use in women with PCOS who become pregnant, metformin may then be considered for use in women with diabetes in pregnancy.

4 One case report with the use of acarbose in 6 women with GDM noted that all achieved adequate glycemic control and had normal newborns.[63] DeVeciana et al[64] compared acarbose to insulin therapy and achieved adequate glycemic control in both groups. However, insulin therapy was required in 6% of the acarbose group due to the inability to tolerate dosage increases, secondary to gastrointestinal side effects.

5 Although these studies are encouraging, there are no oral glucose-lowering agents approved by the FDA for use in the treatment of GDM.

Management of Gestational Diabetes: Fetal Surveillance

1 Fetal surveillance is an important part of managing the woman with GDM. The tests used for women with GDM are the same as those used for women with preexisting diabetes (see Chapter 4, Pregnancy With Preexisting Diabetes, in Diabetes in the Life Cycle and Research).

A Fetal ultrasound is a useful tool for assessing fetal growth.

B Determinations of fetal activity, such as teaching a woman to do kick counts or to note the amount of time elapsed between perceived fetal movement, can help identify the fetus at risk. When preset thresholds are not met, more sophisticated testing can be instituted.[3] Such tests include nonstress tests, contraction stress tests, biophysical profiles, or any combination of these tests.[65]

C Amniocentesis can be used to determine fetal lung maturity. This is not necessary after 38 weeks' gestational age in women who have good blood glucose control. The use of amniocentesis before 38 weeks' gestational age is individualized based on indications for preterm delivery.[3]

D Initiation and timing of these tests depend on the woman's glycemic status, fetal growth abnormalities, use of insulin therapy, whether the woman has any additional pregnancy complications, and what procedures have been established at the setting in which she receives her care.

2 Since the risk of hypertensive disorders in women with GDM is approximately twice that of pregnant women without GDM, maternal surveillance is also important. At each prenatal visit, measurement of body weight, blood pressure, and urinary protein is recommended. These tests can detect the presence of pregnancy-induced hypertension (preeclampsia). The treatment of hypertensive disorders in women with GDM is the same as for pregnant women who do not have GDM.[3] (See Chapter 4, Pregnancy With Preexisting Diabetes, in Diabetes in the Life Cycle and Research, for more information on hypertensive disorders.)

3 The diagnosis of GDM, in and of itself, is not an indication for cesarean delivery.[3,66] Women with GDM are generally allowed to begin labor spontaneously.

A Delivery past 38 weeks' gestational age can lead to an increase in large-for-gestational-age babies and no decrease in the rate of cesarean delivery, so some centers consider delivery at 38+ weeks' gestational age.[53]

B It is not known whether the morbidity and mortality risk is higher in infants of women with well-controlled GDM who are allowed to deliver past 40 weeks' gestational age. It seems prudent, however, to increase fetal surveillance.

C Once labor has begun, the management of women with GDM is the same as for women with pregestational diabetes (see Chapter 4, Pregnancy With Preexisting Diabetes, in Diabetes in the Life Cycle and Research). Blood glucose is checked on admission and plasma blood glucose levels should be maintained between 70 and 90 mg/dL (3.9-5.0 mmol/L).[66]

D Insulin can usually be discontinued after delivery. Postpartum evaluation can identify women who may develop or have undiagnosed type 2 diabetes in the nonpregnant state.

Postpartum Care

1 Most women return to normal glucose tolerance shortly after delivery. At this time, a period of improved insulin sensitivity occurs in GDM just as in women with preexisting diabetes (see Chapter 4, Pregnancy With Preexisting Diabetes, in Diabetes in the Life Cycle and Research). Glucose tolerance should be reevaluated at 6 to 12 weeks postpartum.[1,3]

A Use of the standard diagnostic criteria for diabetes is recommended.[1] Many practitioners prefer to use a 2-hour OGTT with 75 g of glucose. This test provides information useful for assessing the risk of future diabetes.[3]

B Even with normal glucose tolerance, women with previous GDM should be tested annually and receive preconception counseling before planning a subsequent pregnancy.[3]

C It is important to educate the woman with previous GDM to request annual testing for diabetes. She may change providers or be seen in a setting where testing would not be done routinely.

2 Contraception choices should be reviewed. Recommendations are the same for all women, regardless of whether they have had previous GDM.

A In women (n = 1940) in the Coronary Artery Risk Development in Young Adults (CARDIA) study, current use of oral contraceptives was associated with lower glucose levels in young African-American and white women and therefore may be associated with decreased risk of diabetes.[67]

B Low-dose combination oral contraceptives appear to be safe in women with previous GDM.

C The use of progestin-only oral contraceptives (the "mini pill") is safe but should not be used in breastfeeding women with GDM as it has been shown to triple the risk of developing type 2 diabetes.[68]

D Long-acting progestin-only methods and intramuscular depo-medroxyprogesterone acetate (DMPA) have not been studied in women with prior GDM. In healthy women, a deterioration of carbohydrate tolerance has been reported with the use of DMPA.[69,70] A long-acting progestin may be considered for women with a compliance problem, although this is not a first-line method.

E There are no apparent contraindications for use of the intrauterine device in women with previous GDM.

3 The postpartum period is a time when risk reduction for future development of diabetes should be addressed. The modifiable risk factors are obesity, future weight gain, and subsequent pregnancies. Other likely modifiable risk factors are eating habits, physical activity, and other lifestyle factors, such as smoking and avoidance of medications that adversely affect insulin resistance.[71]

A The woman with prior GDM should be counseled on a healthy eating style that is nutritionally balanced and low in fat. Energy intake should be adjusted to achieve desirable body weight.

B Many women with previous GDM have been sedentary. A program of regular physical activity should be encouraged after medical clearance.

C There is some evidence that the number of pregnancies has an impact on glucose tolerance in some high-risk populations.[71]

4 Breastfeeding should be strongly encouraged in women with previous GDM. As many as 50% of women with GDM are obese, and breastfeeding mobilizes fat stores. In addition, following a healthy eating plan may promote weight loss and reduce the risk of developing diabetes in the future.

A Many women with GDM believe that they cannot breastfeed because of the diagnosis of GDM. This misinformation should be corrected and other perceived barriers should be explored.

B If complications occur at delivery, women may be separated from their infants initially or maybe even for days. This possibility should be discussed before delivery so the woman is aware of the procedures at the institution where she will deliver. If initiation of breastfeeding is delayed for an extended period of time, pumping of breast milk is recommended to establish the milk supply.

C Women with previous GDM who continued to breastfeed were reported to have lower glucose levels at the postpartum OGTT and lower rates of diabetes compared with women who bottle-fed their infants.[72]

D Moderate weight loss does not negatively affect milk production. An overweight woman may lose up to 2 kg per month without adverse effects on her milk production. For Dietary Reference Intakes for energy, carbohydrate, and protein during lactation see Chapter 4, Pregnancy With Preexisting Diabetes, in Diabetes in the Life Cycle and Research.

E Moderate physical activity is also recommended and does not appear to affect lactation. The impact of more intense activity is not known.

Key Educational Considerations

1 Women can feel shock, guilt, fear, or denial about a diagnosis of GDM. This reaction is, in part, due to the fact that women with GDM are generally asymptomatic. Their pregnancy is almost at term and, in most cases, has been without complications.

A Educate the woman with GDM about the normal metabolic changes in the second half of pregnancy. Increased insulin requirements combined with the increase of hormones antagonistic to insulin produced by the placenta sets up an environment in which some women are unable to maintain their blood glucose levels within a normal range without intervention.

B Review the results of the OGTT and explain the implications of the various elevated values. Reinforce the fact that those numbers were in response to a glucose load, and a goal of therapy is to avoid exposing the woman to an excessive carbohydrate load throughout the rest of her pregnancy.

C Assure the woman that she did not do anything to cause this condition. Explain that now, however, her participation in a self-management program can help attain glucose control.

D Depending on the setting in which a woman with GDM receives care, the seriousness with which the diagnosis is treated may vary. Educate the woman about the importance of following self-management and medical recommendations.

2 Stress the importance of the diagnosis and treatment of GDM for both the mother and the baby. Discuss the potential fetal and neonatal complications of GDM and explain that high blood glucose levels increase these risks.

3 Review the desired outcome goals of GDM. Discuss blood glucose targets, weight gain goals, avoidance of ketones, and a healthy eating plan for pregnancy.

4 Stress that there are no bad foods, only foods that are more likely to raise blood glucose levels. Reinforce the importance of controlling carbohydrate intake and having frequent meals and snacks. Encourage the woman to keep food records.

5 Ensure that the woman is taught self-monitoring of blood glucose (SMBG) and how to use the results in self-management. If a woman had GDM in a previous pregnancy, be sure that she is not using outdated strips and that the accuracy of her meter is verified.

6 Discuss the implications of ketones. Teach the woman to check daily fasting ketones if she is on a hypocaloric or carbohydrate-restricted diet. Increased frequency of ketone testing may be indicated in illness, severe stress, continuous weight loss, in women who go for prolonged periods without eating, or in periods of increased activity or exercise.

7 Review blood glucose goals. Explain that if target goals cannot be met by meal planning and exercise, insulin therapy will be instituted.
   A Reassure her that insulin does not cross the placenta and does not harm the baby. Explain that insulin therapy helps the baby by lowering maternal blood glucose levels.
   B Explain that insulin therapy is used for the duration of the pregnancy and that it is likely that she will not have diabetes after the baby is born.
   C Educate the woman to recognize the signs and symptoms of a hypoglycemic reaction and how to treat it. Explain that the risk of low blood glucose levels decreases if she follows her food/meal plan. Also reassure her that she will not experience severe reactions, which she may have observed in other women who have type 1 diabetes.
   D Explain that oral glucose-lowering agents are not recommended for use during pregnancy.

8 Provide written guidelines outlining when it is necessary for the woman to contact a member of the healthcare team. Suggest she make contact if any of the following occurs: elevated blood glucose levels, hypoglycemia (if using insulin), moderate or large ketones, a decrease in fetal movement (in the second half of pregnancy), fever, vaginal bleeding, severe headache, blurred vision, uterine contractions, or other pregnancy complications.

9 Stress the importance of reevaluating her glycemic status postpartum. Advise her to have this done 6 to 8 weeks postpartum by means of a 75-g OGTT. If this test is normal, encourage her to be evaluated routinely thereafter. If testing is not offered to her, advise her to request it. Stress the importance of evaluating her glycemic status before planning another pregnancy.
   A Discuss the importance of risk reduction for type 2 diabetes because the incidence is higher in women with previous GDM. Emphasize the importance of becoming lean and fit after pregnancy.
   B Encourage the entire family to have healthy eating patterns and active lifestyles to reduce the risk of type 2 diabetes. The offspring of women with previous GDM are more likely to be obese and to develop type 2 diabetes during childhood through adolescence.

Self-Review Questions

1 Define gestational diabetes.

2 What are the normal metabolic changes that occur in the second half of pregnancy that can lead to GDM?

3 What are 2 potential fetal or neonatal complications of GDM?

4 What are the long-term implications of GDM on the mother and the baby?

5 What are the testing options for diagnosing GDM?

6 What are the various carbohydrate recommendations in nutrition therapy for GDM?

7 What is the recommended testing schedule and target glucose goals for GDM?

8 What is the criteria for insulin initiation?

9 What are 2 fetal surveillance tests used with GDM?

10 What are the postpartum concerns for women with GDM?

11 What are 2 modifiable risk factors to reduce the risk of type 2 diabetes in women with previous GDM?

Learning Assessment: Case Study 1

JS is a 27-year-old Hispanic woman with 2 previous pregnancies and a BMI of 36. She speaks only Spanish. She is married and both she and her husband work in a jewelry factory. She plans to breastfeed. At 30 weeks' gestational age she was transferred to the Diabetes in Pregnancy Program from her neighborhood health center due to an abnormal 3-hour OGTT. The results were as follows:

3-hour OGTT	
Time (h)	Plasma Glucose (mg/dL)
FPG	94
1	202
2	189
3	131

Her previous deliveries were in Guatemala, and JS reports that the birth weights of her 2 children were 8 lb 8 oz (3.86 kg) and 9 lb 10 oz (4.38 kg), respectively. She reports no complications with her previous deliveries, except that her youngest child has had problems with his left arm since birth. She was never tested for diabetes but believes that her mother and aunt in Guatemala have "sugar."

JS met with the dietitian and was given an individualized and culturally appropriate meal plan in Spanish. JS only attended school for 6 years but was able to demonstrate her ability to read. She was taught how to self-monitor her blood glucose levels 4 times a day. She was instructed to keep blood glucose and food records and to bring the glucose meter and her records to her next appointment. Her decision to breastfeed was reinforced.

At her appointment 1 week later, JS had gained 3/4 lb and had negative urine ketones. She provided the following sample of her plasma glucose values:

FPG	2 h after breakfast	2 h after lunch	2 h after dinner
89 mg/dL	101 mg/dL	108 mg/dL	135 mg/dL
91 mg/dL	112 mg/dL	115 mg/dL	141 mg/dL
87 mg/dL	94 mg/dL	110 mg/dL	145 mg/dL

Her monitoring technique was observed, and her meter was checked for accuracy. When she met with the dietitian to evaluate her eating plan, it was discovered that JS had been skipping her afternoon snack and eating excessive quantities of rice and beans at dinner. The meal plan was reinforced, and JS thought she would be able to make the suggested adjustments. Her plasma glucose levels remained within her target range for the duration of her pregnancy. She was instructed to monitor fetal movement and contact the medical team immediately if she noticed any decrease in movement. Nonstress tests were instituted at 36 weeks' gestation. At 40 weeks JS had a vaginal delivery of a healthy 7 lb 15 oz infant.

Questions for Discussion

1 Why is JS's past obstetrical history pertinent to her current management?
2 When would be the optimal time to screen JS for GDM?
3 What cultural and lifestyle factors should be addressed in educating JS?
4 How is JS feeling about the current and future pregnancies?
5 What type of postpartum education should be instituted?

Discussion

1 JS's second child was large for gestational age (LGA). There are no records available from Guatemala, but it is likely that the infant was macrosomic and the arm injury could be due to shoulder dystocia at delivery. JS was not tested for diabetes either during or after this pregnancy. There also may be a family history of diabetes, as reflected in her response to medical history questions.

2 A risk assessment should be done at her first prenatal visit. JS falls into the high risk category due to her ethnicity and her markedly elevated BMI prepregnancy. Subsequently, she should have a glucose screening as early in pregnancy as possible. If this screening is normal, and she has not been diagnosed with GDM prior to 24 weeks' gestation, she should be screened again at 24 to 28 weeks gestation.

3 Her culture and lifestyle may impact JS's care of her diabetes and her pregnancy. She should be questioned about her knowledge and beliefs about diabetes and pregnancy. She should be asked if she uses any alternative therapies, such as herbal medicines or dietary supplements, and counseled appropriately. JS's food/meal plan should reflect her usual food preferences. Modified portions of her familiar foods may increase adherence. Follow-up with blood glucose and food records is crucial. Adjustments in her food/meal plan and continued education made it possible for JR to control her GDM with nutrition therapy.
  A Because she has a young family, it is important to inquire if JS and her family have applied for the Special Supplemental Food Program for Women, Infants and

Children (WIC). The food assistance may be needed due to the extra expenses of having GDM (eg, testing equipment, time lost from work due to frequent appointments, etc). Refer if appropriate.

B Her work environment should be discussed. Will she be allowed time for SMBG and to eat her scheduled meals and snacks? Documentation of medical necessity can be provided to her, if needed.

4 Sometimes women with GDM feel overwhelmed by the unexpected diagnosis and the demands of learning self-management skills so quickly. Psychosocial support as well as education should be provided. It is also important to discuss family planning and the possibility of future pregnancies. Methods of contraception should be discussed. JS's religious, personal, and cultural concerns should be addressed. She should be encouraged to be tested for diabetes prior to planning any future pregnancies.

5 JS needs to be educated regarding her high risk of developing type 2 diabetes over her lifetime. Reinforce the need for a postpartum 2-hour OGTT to rule out type 2 diabetes. If this test is normal she should be advised to have her blood glucose tested on a yearly basis. She should also be aware of the signs and symptoms of hyperglycemia and told to contact her healthcare provider if these occur. Risk reduction strategies to prevent development of future type 2 diabetes should be encouraged. These include weight loss and a low-fat diet, a plan of physical activity, and supportive education.

Learning Assessment: Case Study 2

CG is a 38-year-old Caucasian woman with 1 previous pregnancy and a BMI of 23. She had a history of GDM with her first pregnancy, 2 years ago, which was controlled successfully by nutrition therapy. CG delivered an 8 lb 2 oz (4.2 kg) healthy infant vaginally. Her postpartum 2-hour OGTT was within normal limits. She reports that her grandmother developed diabetes in her 60s, but there was no other significant family history of diabetes. CG is married and works part-time as an accountant. She plans to bottle-feed her baby. A private obstetrician screened her for GDM early in her pregnancy with normal results. She was rescreened at 25 weeks' gestational age. Results of the glucose challenge test were 161 mg/dL. Results of the 3-hour oral glucose tolerance test were as follows:

Time (h)	3-hour OGTT Plasma Glucose (mg/dL)
FPG	92
1	181
2	179
3	135

CG was subsequently transferred to the Diabetes in Pregnancy Program. She remembered the basic principles of a food/meal plan for GDM and just wanted to follow the meal plan she was on during her first pregnancy, to save time. She was encouraged to see the dietitian for reassessment of the plan because her lifestyle had changed dramatically since the birth of her first child. CG was given an updated food/meal plan. Self-monitoring of blood glucose was reviewed. She was instructed to test blood glucose 4 times a day and keep food and blood glucose records. Instructions for assessing fetal movement were reviewed. CG was medically cleared and started a physical activity program of walking on the treadmill 30 minutes per day, beginning gradually. Activity guidelines were provided. Breastfeeding was encouraged, but she adamantly refused.

At 29 weeks, CG's plasma glucose levels remained within her target range, with appropriate weight gain and negative ketones. By 33 weeks' gestational age, her plasma glucose levels began to rise. A sample of her plasma glucose values were as follows:

FPG	2 h after breakfast	2 h after lunch	2 h after dinner
106 mg/dL	112 mg/dL	130 mg/dL	119 mg/dL
108 mg/dL	110 mg/dL	117 mg/dL	105 mg/dL
112 mg/dL	114 mg/dL	99 mg/dL	102 mg/dL

At that time she reported that she was too fatigued to continue her activity program. A review of her eating plan showed that she was doing well adhering to the plan. She was eating an appropriate bedtime snack and was not getting up to eat or drink during the night. The length of the time between her bedtime snack and breakfast was 10 hours. Due to her increasing fatigue, CG did not want to eat her bedtime snack later. CG was then started on bedtime NPH insulin therapy to control her fasting plasma glucose levels. CG was upset and felt that she had "failed" because her plasma glucose levels were above target range.

At 36 weeks' gestational age, CG had lost 4 pounds and had moderate urinary ketones. The following is a sample of her plasma glucose records:

FPG	2 h after breakfast	2 h after lunch	2 h after dinner
91 mg/dL	135 mg/dL	139 mg/dL	140 mg/dL
101 mg/dL	128 mg/dL	145 mg/dL	131 mg/dL
89 mg/dL	133 mg/dL	137 mg/dL	139 mg/dL

Her eating plan was reviewed, and it was determined that CG had not been consuming all of the recommended calories. CG stated that she had been intentionally restricting food to avoid additional insulin injections. After discussion regarding the health of her baby, CG agreed to increase insulin therapy to 2 daily injections of NPH and regular insulin, 1 before breakfast and 1 before dinner. She also agreed to eat the recommended amount of food in her plan. Her insulin doses were adjusted as needed throughout the rest of the pregnancy. Weight gain was appropriate at ½ to 1 lb per week. Nonstress tests were started at 36 weeks' gestational age. She had a vaginal delivery at 39 weeks' gestational age of a healthy 8 lb 5 oz (3.8 kg) baby. She bottle-fed her baby as she had previously planned.

Questions for Discussion

1 When was the appropriate time to screen CG for GDM?

2 Should CG just find her old meal plan and follow it?

3 What factors need to be considered when CG expresses the desire to use her meter from her previous pregnancy?

4 What information might reassure CG when target glucose goals are not maintained, and it is recommended that insulin therapy be instituted or intensified?

Discussion

1 Screening CG as early in the pregnancy as possible, for the existence of GDM, was appropriate because having had a previous pregnancy with GDM places a woman at high risk for developing GDM in subsequent pregnancies. The follow-up screening and OGTT diagnosed her GDM at the usual gestational age.

2 A thorough nutrition assessment should be completed for each pregnancy. GG's prepregnancy weight status may be different in this pregnancy. Lifestyle changes often occur after the birth of a child. Her daily activity at home, as well as the timing of her meals and snacks, may be very different than it was 2 years ago; perhaps her employment status has changed. Every pregnancy can also be different in terms of food cravings, aversions, and intolerances. Pregnancy symptoms can affect food choices. CG's familiarity with the principles of nutrition management may make the education process easier the second time. Often the addition of caring for a child, as well as oneself can make adherence to the plan of care more of a challenge. Though CG was not open to discussion of breastfeeding, initially, a diabetes team member should attempt to gently bring up discussion of breastfeeding, and possible perceived barriers, at a follow-up visit. Breastfeeding is recommended in women with GDM.

3 If CG uses her meter from 2 years ago, the meter should be verified against a laboratory reference; any outdated strips should be discarded and replaced with new strips. If the strips are not outdated, they should be checked with new control solution for accuracy. Her technique should be observed and corrected, if necessary. Target plasma glucose goals and the testing schedule should be reviewed.

4 Most pregnant women feel an increased responsibility for the health of their unborn baby after the diagnosis of GDM. It is sometimes viewed as a personal failure when nutrition therapy alone does not maintain recommended blood glucose levels. Women may also intentionally undereat to avoid insulin use, an increase in dosage, or an increase in the number of injections. It is important to explain that due to the hormones of pregnancy and the demands of the fetus, it is not unusual for a woman with GDM to require insulin therapy, even if she is following her food/meal plan carefully. As the pregnancy progresses insulin resistance continues to increase and insulin requirements are expected to increase. Sometimes intensified insulin therapy is necessary. These changes are not due to any failure of CG's adherence to the self-management plan. Remind her that insulin will only help, not hurt, the baby and that she must continue to provide adequate nourishment for herself and her baby.

References

1 Coustan DR. Gestational diabetes. In: National Diabetes Data Group. Diabetes in America. 2nd ed. Bethesda, Md: National Institutes of Health, National Institute of Diabetes and Digestive and Kidney Disorders; 1995. NIH publication 95-1468:197-201.

2 American Diabetes Association. Gestational diabetes mellitus (position statement). Diabetes Care. 2003;26(suppl 1):S103-S105.

3 Metzger BE, Coustan DR, eds. Proceedings of the Fourth International Workshop-Conference on Gestational Diabetes Mellitus. Diabetes Care. 1998;21(suppl 2).

4 American Diabetes Association. Report of the Expert Committee on the Diagnosis and Classification of Diabetes Mellitus. Diabetes Care. 2003;26(suppl 1):S5-S20.

5 Homko CJ, Jorsney D. Pregnancy: preconception to postpartum. In: Franz MJ, Kulkarni K, Polonsky WH, Yarborough P, Zamudio V, eds. A Core Curriculum for Diabetes Education. 4th ed. Diabetes in the Life Cycle and Research. Chicago: American Association of Diabetes Educators; 2001:33-69.

6 Kjos SL. Postpartum care of the woman with diabetes. Clin Obstet Gynecol. 2000;43:75-86.

7 Phelps RL, Metzger BE, Freinkel N. Carbohydrate metabolism in pregnancy. XVII. Diurnal profiles of plasma glucose, insulin, free fatty acids, triglycerides, cholesterol, and individual amino acids in late normal pregnancy. Am J Obstet Gynecol. 1981;140:730-736.

8 Coustan DR. Management of gestational diabetes. In: Reece EA, Coustan DR, eds. Diabetes Mellitus in Pregnancy. New York: Churchill-Livingston; 1995:59-64.

9 Catalano PM, Tyzbir ED, Wolfe RR, et al. Carbohydrate metabolism during pregnancy in control subjects and women with gestational diabetes. Am J Physiol. 1993;264:E60-E67.

10 Hod M, Rabinersin D, Peled Y. Gestational diabetes mellitus: is it a clinical entity? Diabetes Reviews. 1995;3:602-613.

11 Schaefer UM, Songster G, Xiang A, et al. Congenital malformations in offspring of women with hyperglycemia first detected in pregnancy. Am J Obstst Gynecol. 1997;177:1165-1171.

12 Shand JL, Tapsell LC. The recurrence of gestational diabetes: could dietary differences in fat intake be an explanation? Diabetes Care. 1997;20:1647-1650.

13 Plagemann A, Harder I, Kohlhoff R, Rohde W, Dorner G. Overweight and obesity in infants of mothers with long-term insulin-dependent or gestational diabetes. Int J Obes Related Metab Disord. 1997;21:451-456.

14 Freinkel N. Summary and recommendations of the Second International Workshop-Conference on Gestational Diabetes Mellitus. Diabetes. 1985;34(suppl 1):123-126.

15 Metzger BE and the Organizing Committee. Summary and recommendations of the Third International Workshop-Conference on Gestational Diabetes Mellitus. Diabetes. 1991;40(suppl 2):197-201.

16 World Health Organization. WHO Expert Committee on Diabetes Mellitus: Second Report. Geneva, Switzerland: World Health Organization; 1980. Tech Rep Ser 646.

17 American Dietetic Association Medical Nutrition Therapy Evidence-Based Guides for Practice. Nutrition practice guidelines for GDM [CD-ROM]. Chicago: American Dietetic Association; 2001.

18 American Diabetes Association. Evidence-based nutrition principles and recommendations for the treatment and prevention of diabetes and related complications (position statement). Diabetes Care. 2003;26(suppl 1):S51-S61.

19 Institute of Medicine of the National Academies. Dietary Reference Intakes: Energy, Carbohydrate, Fiber, Fat, Fatty Acids, Cholesterol, Protein, and Amino Acids. Washington, DC: The National Academies Press; 2002.

20 Nawrot P, Jordan S, Eastwood J, et al. Effects of caffeine on human health. Food Addit Contam. 2003;20:1-30.

21 March of Dimes. During your pregnancy: what you need to know: caffeine Available at: http://www.modimes.org. Accessed January 7, 2003.

22 Rizzo T, Metzger B, Burns W, Burns K. Correlations between antepartum maternal metabolism and intelligence of offsprings. N Eng J Med. 1990;325:911-916.

23 Silverman BL, Rizzo TA, Cho NH, Metzger BE. Long-term effects of the intrauterine environment, birth weight, and breast-feeding in Pima Indians. Diabetes Care. 1998;21(suppl 2):B142-B149.

24 Knopp RH, Magee MS, Raisys V, et al. Hypocaloric diets and ketogenesis in the management of obese gestational diabetic women. J Am Coll Nutr. 1991;10:649-667.

25 Gunderson E. Intensive nutrition therapy for gestational diabetes. Diabetes Care. 1997;20:221-226.

26 Major CA, Henry MJ, DeVeciana M, Morgan MA. The effects of carbohydrate restriction in patients with diet-controlled gestational diabetes. Obstet Gynecol. 1998;91:600-604.

27 Peterson CM, Jovanovic-Peterson L. Percentages of carbohydrate and glycemic response to breakfast, lunch and dinner in women with gestational diabetes. Diabetes. 1991;40:172-194.

28 Mahaffey PJ, Podell SK. Euglycemic control of gestational diabetes mellitus by specific dietary manipulation, a case study presentation. Diabetes. 1991;17:460-465.

29 Fagan C, Kling J, Erick M. Nutrition management in women with gestational diabetes mellitus: a review by the American Dietetic Association Diabetes Care and Education Dietetic Practice Group. J Am Diet Assoc. 1995;95:460-467.

30 Clapp JF. Effect of dietary carbohydrate on the glucose and insulin response to mixed caloric intake and exercise in both nonpregnant and pregnant women. Diabetes Care. 1998;21(suppl 2):B107-B112.

31 Benini L, Castellani G, Brighenti F, et al. Gastric emptying of a solid meal is accelerated by the removal of dietary fibre naturally present in food. Gut. 1995;36: 825-830.

32 Anderson JW, O'Neal DS, Riddell-Mason S, Floore TL, Dillon DW, Oeltgen PR. Postprandial serum glucose, insulin, and lipoprotein responses to high- and low-fiber diets. Metab. 1995;44:848-854.

33 Guevin N, Jacques H, Nadeau A, Galibois I. Postprandial glucose, insulin, and lipid responses to four meals containing unpurified dietary fiber in non-insulin-dependent diabetes mellitus (NIDDM), hypertriglyceridemic subjects. J Am Coll Nutr. 1996; 15:389-396.

34 Metzger B. Pregnancy in diabetes. In: Powers MA, ed. Handbook of Diabetes Medical Nutrition Therapy. 2nd ed. Gaithersburg, Md: Aspen Publishers; 1996:503-526.

35 Pitkin RM, Reynolds W, Filer LJ, et al. Placental transmission and fetal distribution of saccharin. Am J Obstet Gynecol. 1971;111:280-286.

36 World Health Organization Expert Committee on Food Additives. Toxicological Evaluation of Certain Food Additives and Food Contaminants. Geneva, Switzerland: World Health Organization; 1981;16:11-27, 1983;18:12-14.

37 Nuttall FQ, Gannon MC. Plasma glucose and insulin response to macronutrients in non-diabetic and NIDDM subjects. Diabetes Care. 1991;14:814-838.

38 Nuttall FQ, Mooradian AD, Gannon MC, Billington CJ, Krezowski PA. Effect of protein ingestion on glucose and insulin response to a standardized oral glucose load. Diabetes Care. 1998;21:16-22.

39 Duque A. The role of lipids in fetal brain development. In: The Perinatal Nutrition Report: a quarterly publication of the Perinatal Nutrition Dietetic Practice Group of the American Dietetic Association; 1997;(Spring):4-5.

40 American College of Obstetricians and Gynecologists. Practice Bulletin: Gestational Diabetes. Washington, DC: American College of Obstetricians and Gynecologists; 2001.

41 Wechter DJ, Kaufman RC, Amankwah KS, et al. Prevention of neonatal macrosomia in gestational diabetes by the use of intensive dietary therapy and home glucose monitoring. Am J Perinatol. 1991;8:131-134.

42 Langer O, Rodriquez DA, Xenakis MJ, McFarland MB, Berkus MD, Arredondo F. Intensified versus conventional management of gestational diabetes. Am J Obstet Gynecol. 1994;170:1036-1047.

43 DeVeciana M, Major CA, Morgan MA, et al. Postprandial versus preprandial blood glucose monitoring in women with gestational diabetes mellitus requiring insulin therapy. N Engl J Med. 1995;333:1237-1241.

44 Sivan E, Weisz B, Homko CJ, et al. One or two hour postprandial glucose measurements: are they the same? Am J Obstet Gynecol. 2001;185:604-607.

45 Langer O, Levy J, Brustman L, Anayaegbunan A, Meskatz R, Divon M. Glycemic control in gestational diabetes mellitus: how tight is tight enough: small for gestational age? Obstet Gynecol. 1989;161:646-653.

46 Avery MD, Leon AS, Kopher RA. Effects of a partially home-based exercise program for women with gestational diabetes. Obstet Gynecol. 1997;89:10-15.

47 Paolone AM, Shangold M. Artifact in the recording of fetal heart rates during maternal exercise. J Appl Physiol. 1987;62:848-849.

48 Clapp JF, Capeless EL. Neonatal morphometrics after endurance exercise during pregnancy. Am J Obstet Gynecol. 1999;163:1805-1811.

49 Soultanakis HN, Artal R, Wiswell RA. Prolonged exercise in pregnancy: glucose homeostasis, ventilatory and cardiovascular responses. Semin Perinatol. 1996;20:315-317.

50 Langer O, Hod M. Management of gestational diabetes mellitus. Obstet Gynecol Clin North Am. 1996;21:137-159.

51 Exercise during pregnancy and the postpartum period. ACOG Tech Bull 189. February 1994.

52 Jovanovic-Peterson L, Peterson CM. Nutritional management of the obese gestational diabetic woman. J Am Coll Nutr. 1992;71:921-927.

53 Jovanovic-Peterson L, Peterson CM. Rationale for prevention and treatment of glucose-mediated macrosomia. A protocol for gestational diabetes. Endocr Pract. 1996;2:118-129.

54 Jovanovic-Peterson L, Ilic S, Pettitt D, et al. The metabolic and immunology effects of insulin lispro. Diabetes Care. 1999;22:1422-1427.

55 Pettitt DJ, Ospina P, Kolaczynski JW, Jovanovic L. Comparison of an insulin analog, insulin aspart, and regular human insulin with no insulin in gestational diabetes mellitus. Diabetes Care. 2003;26:183-186.

56 Langer O, Conway D, Berkus MD, Henakis EMJ, Gonzalez O. A comparison of glyburide and insulin in women with gestational diabetes. N Engl J Med. 2000;343:1134-1138.

57 Kitzmiller J. Limited efficacy of glyburide for glycemic control. Am J Obstet Gynecol. 2001;185:S198.

58 Chmait R, Dinise T, Daneshmand S, Kim M, Moore T. Prospect cohort study to establish glyburide success in gestational diabetes mellitus. Am J Obstet Gynecol. 2001;185:S197.

59 Vandermolan DT, Ratts VS, Evans WS, Stovall DW, Kauma SW, Nestler JE. Metformin increases the ovulatory rate and pregnancy rate from clomiphene citrate in patients with polycystic ovary syndrome who are resistant to clomiphene citrate alone. Fertil Steril. 2001;2:310-315.

60 Kocak M, Caliskan E, Simsir C, Haberal A. Metformin therapy improves ovulatory rates, cervical scores, and pregnancy rates in clomiphene citrate-resistant women with polycystic ovary syndrome. Fertil Steril. 2002;77:101-106.

61 Glueck CJ, Phillips H, Caneron D, Sieve-Smith L, Wang P. Continuing metformin throughout pregnancy in women with polycystic ovary syndrome appears to safely reduce first trimester spontaneous abortion: a pilot study. Fertil Steril. 2001;75:46-52.

62 Jakubowicz DJ, Iurono MJ, Jackubowicz S, Roberts KA, Nestler JE. Effects of metformin on early pregnancy loss in the polycystic ovarian syndrome. J Clin Endocrinol Metab. 2002;87:524-529.

63 Zorate A, Ochoa R, Hernandez M, Basurto L. Effectiveness of acarbose in the control of glucose tolerance worsening in pregnancy. Ginecol Obstet Mex. 2002;87:524-529.

64 DeVeciana M, Trail PA, Evans AT, Dulaney K. A comparison of oral acarbose and insulin in women with gestational diabetes. Obstet Gynecol. 2002;99(suppl 4):5S.

65 Coustan DR. Management of gestational diabetes. In: Reece EA, Coustan DR, eds. Diabetes Mellitus in Pregnancy. New York: Churchill-Livingston; 1995:283-284.

66 Jovanovic L, ed. Medical Management of Pregnancy Complicated by Diabetes. 3rd ed. Alexandria, Va: American Diabetes Association; 2000.

67 Kim C, Siscovick DS, Sidney S, Lewis CE, Kiefe CI, Koepsell TD. Oral contraceptive use and association with glucose, insulin, and diabetes in young adult women. The CARDIA study. Diabetes Care. 2002; 25:1027-1032.

68 Kjos SL, Peters RK, Xiang A, Thomas D, Schaefer V, Buchanan TA. Contraception and the risk of type 2 diabetes mellitus in Latina women with prior gestational diabetes mellitus. JAMA. 1998;280:533-538.

69 Fahmy K, Abdel-Razik M, Shaaraway M, et al. Effect of long-acting progestagen-only injectable contraceptives on carbohydrate metabolism and its hormonal profile. Contraception. 1991;44:419-429.

70 Konje JC, Otolorin EO, Ladipo AO. The effect of continuous subdermal levonorgestrel (Norplant) on carbohydrate metabolism. Am J Obstet Gynecol. 1992:166:15-19.

71 Dornhorst A, Rossi M. Risk and prevention of type 2 diabetes in women with gestational diabetes. Diabetes Care. 1998;21(suppl 2):B43-B49.

72 Kjos SL, Henry O, Lee R, Buchanan TA, Mishell DR Jr. The effect of lactation on glucose and lipid metabolism in women with recent gestational diabetes. Obstet Gynecol. 1992;82:451-455.

Suggested Readings

American College of Obstetricians and Gynecologists. ACOG Practice Bulletin No. 30. Gestational Diabetes. Obstetrics & Gynecology. 98:525-538, 2001.

American Diabetes Association. Gestational diabetes mellitus (position statement). Diabetes Care. 2003;26(suppl 1):S103-S105.

American Dietetic Association Medical Nutrition Therapy Evidence-Based Guides for Practice. Nutrition practice guidelines for GDM [CD-ROM]. Chicago: American Dietetic Association; 2001.

California Diabetes and Pregnancy Program. Sweet Success: Guidelines for Care. Campbell, Ca: Education Program Associates; 2002.

Fagan C. Nutrition therapy for pregnancy and lactation. In: Franz MJ, Bantle JP, eds. American Diabetes Association Guide to Medical Nutrition Therapy for Diabetes. Alexandria, Va: American Diabetes Association; 1999:229-248.

Franz MJ, Bantle JP, Beebe CA, et al. Evidence-based nutrition principles and recommendations for the treatment and prevention of diabetes and related complications. (Technical review). Diabetes Care. 2002;25:148-198.

Jovanovic L, ed. Medical Management of Pregnancy Complicated by Diabetes. 3rd ed. Alexandria, Va: American Diabetes Association; 2000.

Metzger BE, Coustan DR, eds. Proceedings of the Fourth International Workshop-Conference on Gestational Diabetes Mellitus. Diabetes Care. 1998;21(suppl 2).

Slocum JM, Burke Sosa ME. Use of antidiabetes agents in pregnancy: current practices and controversies. J Perinat Neonat Nurs. 2002;16:40-53.

Learning Assessment: Post-Test Questions

Gestational Diabetes

5

1 Which of the following is not true regarding gestational diabetes?

  A Gestational diabetes occurs only in high-risk women who are obese

  B Approximately 1% to 14% of all pregnancies are complicated by gestational diabetes

  C Gestational diabetes places a woman at increased risk of developing type 2 diabetes later in life

  D Some medications can increase the risk of a pregnant woman developing gestational diabetes

2 Which of the following metabolic changes does not occur in the second half of pregnancy?

  A Insulin resistance results in higher and more prolonged postprandial blood glucose concentration than in the nonpregnant state

  B Basal insulin levels decrease in relation to placental growth

  C Insulin resistance appears to be related to placental hormones (eg, human placental lactogen, prolactin, estrogen, and cortisol)

  D Women are prone to the condition of accelerated starvation, which can result in elevated plasma and urinary ketone levels

3 The current testing recommendations for diagnosing gestational diabetes include all of the following except:

  A Every pregnant woman should have a risk assessment for the development of gestational diabetes at 24 to 28 weeks' gestational age

  B A fasting plasma glucose of >126 mg/dL (7.0 mmol/L) or a casual plasma glucose of >200 mg/dL (11.1 mmol/L) is suggestive of diabetes and warrants immediate follow-up

  C Having 2 or more glucose levels out of target range on the oral glucose tolerance test warrants the diagnosis of gestational diabetes

  D The diagnosis of gestational diabetes can be made with either a 1-step 75-g oral glucose tolerance test or the 2-step process using a 50-g glucose screen and, if abnormal, a 100-g oral glucose tolerance test

4 Which of the following is currently not approved as a management method for gestational diabetes?

  A An individualized pregnancy eating plan, provided by a registered dietitian

  B Institution of individualized insulin therapy when target plasma glucose goals are not met

  C A program of moderate physical activity for women with gestational diabetes without medical or obstetrical complications

  D The use of oral glucose-lowering agents in place of insulin in women with gestational diabetes who are not able to meet target glucose goals

5 KG has gestational diabetes and has received nutrition therapy from a registered dietitian. She is self-monitoring her blood glucose and keeping food records at home. She has a history of preterm labor and is not medically cleared for exercise. Her blood glucose levels after lunch are elevated. What would be the initial recommendation for management?

A Start insulin therapy immediately, due to elevated postprandial blood glucose values

B Evaluate her food choices at lunch and change either the carbohydrate type or amount for a trial period

C Have her start a regimen of brisk walking after lunch to decrease postprandial blood glucose values

D Increase the amount of carbohydrate at lunch to counterbalance the protein choices

6 With the diagnosis of gestational diabetes there are associated possible neonatal complications. Which of the following complications is not usually associated with gestational diabetes?

A Macrosomia and hypoglycemia

B Shoulder dystocia and polycythemia

C Small-for-gestational-age infants and birth defects

D Hyperbilirubinemia and macrosomia

7 In gestational diabetes, self-monitoring of blood glucose values guides management. Which of the following is not a concern?

A Age of the meter and strips

B Type of lancet device used

C Whether meter and laboratory reference use whole blood or plasma values

D Verification of the meter accuracy against a laboratory reference

8 According to the American Diabetes Association, which of the following are target blood glucose goals for pregnancy complicated by GDM?

A Fasting whole blood glucose <105 mg/dL, 1-hour postprandial whole blood glucose <155 mg/dL, 2-hour postprandial whole blood glucose <130 mg/dL

B Fasting plasma blood glucose <105 mg/dL, 1-hour postprandial plasma blood glucose <155 mg/dL, 2-hour postprandial plasma blood glucose <130 mg/dL

C Fasting plasma blood glucose <105 mg/dL, 1-hour postprandial plasma blood glucose <135 mg/dL, 2-hour postprandial plasma blood glucose <140 mg/dL

D Fasting whole blood glucose <100mg/dL, 1-hour postprandial whole blood glucose <130 mg/dL, 2-hour postprandial whole blood glucose <115 mg/dL

9 Which of the following may not be a concern in the postpartum care of women with previous gestational diabetes?

A Achieving a normal body mass index (BMI)

B Remaining lean and fit throughout life

C Staying on insulin postpartum if insulin was required during pregnancy

D Having a follow-up oral glucose tolerance test 6 to 12 weeks postpartum

10 Which of the following is true when recommending infant feeding options to women with previous gestational diabetes?

A Breastfeeding is encouraged unless the woman required insulin therapy

B Breastfeeding is not recommended if the woman continues to have elevated blood glucose levels and is diagnosed with type 2 diabetes

C Breastfeeding mobilizes fat stores and may aid in weight reduction

D Breastfeeding a macrosomic infant may increase the risk of obesity later in life

See next page for answer key.

Post-Test Answer Key

Gestational Diabetes   5

1	A		**6**	C
2	B		**7**	B
3	A		**8**	B
4	D		**9**	C
5	B		**10**	C

A Core Curriculum for Diabetes Education

Diabetes in the Life Cycle and Research

Diabetes in Older Adults

6

Anne T. Nettles, RN, MS, CDE
Diabetes CareWorks
Minneapolis, Minnesota

Introduction

1 Diabetes mellitus has been underdiagnosed and undertreated in the United States, particularly among people in the oldest age groups.

2 In 2001, the prevalence of those diagnosed with diabetes among US adults increased to 7.9% from 7.3% in 2000 and 4.9% in 1990.[1] However, of US adults aged 60 years or older, 15.1% had diagnosed diabetes. More individuals may be affected by hyperglycemia after the age of 75 years because of rising glucose intolerance with age.[2] However, glucose intolerance is not inevitable, even in 100 year olds.[3]

3 Because the classical symptoms of diabetes often are absent in older adults, diagnosis is more often made when the long-term effects of poor glucose control result in a crisis or complication.[4] Harris et al[5] estimate that the diagnosis is made an average of 6.5 years after the onset of the disease.

4 Because of the magnitude of underdiagnosis, the American Diabetes Association, in cooperation with worldwide health organizations, modified the recommendations for diagnosis in 1997. If the recommendations are put into practice, elderly individuals will be diagnosed and treated sooner.

5 Diabetes educators need to understand the atypical manifestations of diabetes in older adults to properly educate and care for them.

6 Better understanding aged patients' needs, priorities, and the developmental tasks of aging may assist in more effective interventions. Educators must appreciate the vast differences in those 65 years to those 95 years of age.

Objectives

Upon completion of this chapter, the learner will be able to
1 Describe the pertinent changes that occur with aging.
2 Identify the unique risks of poor glucose control in the elderly.
3 Explain adaptations in treatment approaches for older individuals.
4 List potential barriers and strategies for teaching older adults about diabetes management.

Changes of Aging

1 Aging is more than a matter of physiological changes. Psychosocial factors play a significant role in how aging is expressed.

2 When aging is addressed from a developmental perspective, providers can anticipate and offer expected adaptations. Change is inevitable, but can be accommodated.

3 Developmental tasks include retirement, marital changes, widowhood, grandparenting, dying, and death. Loss and dependence are common. But having time to enjoy children and grandchildren, not worrying about the opinions of others, and pursuing interests are positive counterbalances.

4 Patient concerns about functional abilities, health, quality of life, and health care become prominent. Maintaining independence is often a priority.

5 Many of the physiological changes of aging resemble those of diabetes and include impaired hormone regulation, decreased vision, decreased glomerular filtration, bone loss, muscle wasting, and loss of skin tone. The changes of aging are accelerated and compounded by having diabetes (Table 6.1).

6 Careful individual assessment is needed to differentiate between changes of normal aging, diseases of older adults, and effects of hyperglycemia or diabetes with each individual.

7 Intrinsic and extrinsic factors contributing to hyperglycemia in the elderly are shown in Figure 6.1.[3]

Diagnosis and Treatment

1 Undiagnosed and untreated diabetes is more common in older adults. The prevalence of diabetes is higher among elderly African Americans, Hispanics, Pima Indians, Micronesians, Scandinavians, and male Japanese.[6] Elderly Hispanics have twice the rate of diabetes as non-Hispanic whites.[7]

2 The same diagnostic criteria used for all adults are used for older adults. Recent changes in diagnostic criteria, especially the use of fasting glucoses, may reveal more older adults in need of treatment for diabetes. Yet some believe fasting glucoses miss another portion of the undiagnosed population.[8]

3 Because consensus has not been established regarding target glucose levels for older adults, diabetes management should be individualized with initial priority given to eliminating glycemic symptoms. Longevity and potential risks for acute and long-term effects of poor glucose control also should be considered. Personal glucose goals are as important for this age group as for younger people with diabetes.

4 Uncontrolled diabetes causes symptoms and acute illnesses that, at the least, impair quality of life; some complications such as hyperosmolar hyperglycemic state (HHS) may be fatal[9] (see Chapter 2, Hyperglycemia, in Diabetes and Complications).

5 The lifespan of people in the US is increasing (Table 6.2); therefore, people over age 65 may live long enough to develop the long-term complications of diabetes.[10] Do not assume that an elderly person has a short life expectancy or that glucose control is not important.

Table 6.1. Aging and Disease of the Elderly That Influence Diabetes Care

Ophthalmic
- Decreased acuity
- Slowed light/dark adaptation
- Decreased color perception
- Increased blinding diseases (senile cataracts, macular degeneration)

Cardiovascular
- Conduction defects
- Systolic hypertension (disease)
- Decreased cardiac output
- Increased vascular resistance
- Increase in cerebral vascular accidents
- Increase in myocardial infarction
- Peripheral vascular diseases

Gastrointestinal
- Decreased secretion, absorption, motility
- Changes in appetite

Dental Diseases
- Tooth loss
- Gum/periodontal disease

Musculoskeletal
- Arthritis, joint diseases
- Decreased muscle mass and strength
- Foot deformities

Neurological
- Slower learning, processing time
- Slower reactions
- Decreased taste, smell, and thirst
- Peripheral and autonomic neuropathic diseases
- Increase in organic brain diseases

Renal
- Decreased glomerular filtration rate (GFR)
- Altered ability to concentrate or dilute urine
- Decreased active renin production
- Decreased antidiuretic hormone (ADH) responsiveness

Figure 6.1. Nondietary Factors Contributing to Hyperglycemia in the Elderly

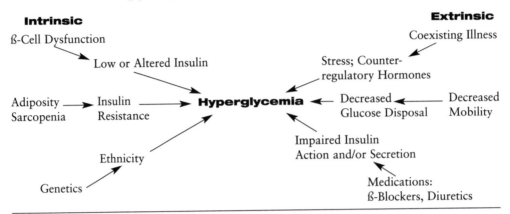

Source: Adapted with permission from Samos and Roos.[3]

Table 6.2. Life Span of Older Adults in the United States

Age, years	Additional Years of Life Expectancy
60	21.4
65	17.7
70	14.3
75	11.2
80	8.5
85	6.3
90	4.5
95	3.3
100	2.5

Source: Adapted from National Vital Statistics Report.[10]

Management Issues

1 Older adults primarily have type 2 diabetes resulting from impaired insulin release. Insulin resistance is prominent in obese older persons.[6,11]

2 Cardiovascular risk reduction strategies such as smoking cessation, lipid and hypertension control, and aspirin are equally important with aging.

3 Dementia, certain cognitive disorders, energy level, quality of life, and memory have been shown to improve with glucose control.[12,13]

4 Improved functional health has been shown to be associated with physical activity, body mass index (BMI), and positive mood in older patients.[14]

5 Among obese people, modest weight loss and mildly increased physical activity can improve glucose control.[15] However, in weight loss, physical activity, and educational programs, drop out is more common in older age groups. It therefore becomes important to incorporate strategies to remove barriers to attendance such as timing, cost, or accessibility.[14,16]

Medical Nutrition Therapy

1 Failure to thrive among older people is generally due to a combination of malnutrition, decreased physical function, depression, and cognitive impairment.[17] Elderly people with diabetes are at additional risk because of high rates of depression.

2 Glycemic control, nutritional status, and other risk factors for malnutrition should be assessed. Age-related physiological changes that affect nutritional status include lower energy needs (10% to 20%), changes in body composition, changes in the mouth, increased carbohydrate intolerance, and decline in renal function.[18]

3 Protein needs for the aged are the same or slightly higher than other adults. Protein-dense foods that cost less and are easily eaten include beans, legumes, milk, eggs, and cheese. Adequate nutrition is the primary goal of meal planning.

4 Nutrient intake may be limited due to financial constraints, cultural and eating habits, depression, cognitive or functional impairment, or simply not being aware of new food products.

5 Fluid intake may be inadequate because of changes in thirst perception and access to fluids, predisposing people to dehydration. Those with renal changes or taking diuretics have additional risk.

6 Malnutrition can result from poor dentition, changes in taste, lack of transportation, physical disabilities, medications, alcohol use, or social isolation. Patients who are dependent or have low functional ability should be assessed regularly for signs of malnutrition. Detailed criteria for nutritional screening are available.[19]

7 Implementing dietary changes may have adverse financial effects. When working with older adults, anticipate costs and routinely provide alternative low-cost strategies (see Table 6.3).[18]

Table 6.3. Nutritional Support Resources for Elderly Persons[18]

• Community nutrition sites	• Meals on Wheels
• Food stamps	• Commodity foods
• Adult day care centers	• In-home personal aides
• County extension agents	• Centers on aging
• Social services	• Geriatric specialists

8 Retirement, widowhood, or needing to live with others for the first time can require a number of lifestyle changes that can affect nutrition. Individuals may need to adjust household responsibilities. Loneliness, boredom, or depression can sometimes cause irregular eating habits in older adults.

9 Mobility and transportation limitations can make obtaining food difficult for some older adults. Emergency food supplies might include frozen meals, no-cook options (tuna, dried fruit, evaporated or dried milk, soup, peanut butter, or crackers).

10 Approximately 40% of those over 65 are edentulous, which can lead to avoidance of coarse fiber and protein-containing foods.
  A Dental problems may cause a decrease in mastication which contributes to digestive disturbances. This, in turn, may lead to a decline in intake or omission of certain foods or food groups, with resultant malnutrition.
  B Educators can provide information on the ongoing value of routine dental exams and ways to avoid constipation.[20]

11 Clinicians need to be alert for rapid weight loss or other coexisting problems in underweight older people and refer these individuals for diagnosis and treatment.

12 Meal planning for weight maintenance or weight gain includes the following considerations:
  A Preference
  B Palatability
  C Food consistency
  D Lifelong eating habits
  E Purchasing and preparing food
  F Financial considerations
  G Cultural preferences and/or religious practices

13 The need for weight loss in overweight older adults should be carefully evaluated. If the benefits outweigh the risks, the following weight reduction strategies are suggested:
  A Use a gradual approach.
  B Incorporate and prioritize other restrictions such as sodium.
  C Provide adequate protein, calcium, vitamin D.
  D Reduce overall fat content.

14 Evidence of benefits from light-to-moderate alcohol use in the general adult population is growing. However, alcohol and drug abuse is high among the elderly and further compounds nutrition and metabolic control problems.[18] The use of alcohol and controlled substances (including prescribed) should be assessed and information incorporated into educational opportunities.

Physical Activity

1 Physical activity plans are based on the patient's preferences, functional capacity, and coexisting illnesses such as cardiovascular, neurological, or eye diseases. Physical activity has been shown to prevent and reverse some microvascular/muscle changes in older people.[14,15]

2 Starting at 50% to 60% maximum heart rate is a reasonable goal for older adults beginning a physical activity program. The goal can be increased very gradually, resulting in significant improvement in oxygen-carrying power and decreased body fat.[21]

3 Physical limitations can be accommodated through a variety of activities such as stationary bicycling, swimming, water aerobics, walking, or chair exercises.

4 Exercising with others provides additional safety as well as opportunities for socialization.

5 Education is needed about risks and benefits, hypoglycemia avoidance, and timing of exercise with older adults as it is with younger people. (See Chapter 2, Physical Activity/Exercise, in Diabetes Management Therapies.)

Medications

1 Including a pharmacist in the diabetes management team can improve detection of duplicate therapies, improve detection of drug-drug, drug-disease, and drug-food interactions and identify ways to simplify medication programs for those with comorbidities.

2 The number of new drugs on the market increased the management options for older adults. However, the lack of long-term experience administering these drugs to elderly patients and the small number of studies on previously administered ones makes selection a challenge. No specific guidelines for prescribing oral glucose-lowering medications in the elderly are available and diabetes specialists often have conflicting recommendations. To date, however, most of the recently developed oral agents have been used safely in elderly populations when carefully monitored and individualized.[6,22-30] Table 6.4 lists glucose-lowering medications and cautions for their use. (For additional information on glucose-lowering medications see Chapter 3, Pharmacologic Therapies for Glucose Management, in Diabetes Management Therapies.)

3 Oral glucose-lowering agents are started at the lowest possible doses and titrated slowly to minimize the risk of adverse effects.

4 Key considerations for selection of oral diabetes agents include the following:
  A Simplified regimens (eg, less frequent dosing)
  B Other drugs may interfere with effectiveness
  C Comorbidities may create contraindications
  D Side effects may complicate management of other existing diseases
  E Safety profile, including risk of hypoglycemia
  F Costs may be prohibitive for some agents
  G Effects on weight or lipids

5 The appropriateness of all drug therapy should be assessed at each visit especially when patients have renal, liver, or cardiac impairment.

Table 6.4. Oral Glucose-Lowering Agents

Oral Agent	Use With Caution in Persons With:
Sulfonylureas • Glyburide • Glipizide • Glimepiride	• Renal impairment, impaired liver function
Non-sulfonylurea secretagogues • Repaglinide • Nataglinide	• Impaired liver function
Biguanidines • Metformin	• Renal impairment
Thiozolidinediones (TZDs) • Rosiglitizone • Pioglitazone	• Impaired liver function • Heart failure
Alpha-glucosidase inhibitors • Acarbose • Miglitol	• Gastrointestinal disease

6 Polypharmacy or multiple medication use is common in older adults with diabetes.[31] Older adults often take 5 or more medications.

   A This may be appropriate since adequate treatment of hypertension, coronary artery disease, and renal disease rely on aggressive pharmacotherapy. However, many of these comorbid complications often go undiagnosed or are undertreated.

   B On the other hand, use of more medications than are appropriate is also common. In one report, modest interventions making caregivers aware of agents in use has lead to significant reductions. Careful withdrawal of unnecessary drugs is needed as untoward effects may be seen in the elderly.[31] Table 6.5 lists general suggestions for appropriate prescribing of medications for the elderly.

7 The effectiveness of therapy increases when medications are taken at recommended times. The following approaches may increase the likelihood of patients taking their medications as prescribed:

   A Address costs and complexity of the existing medication regimen, simplify when possible.

   B Incorporate medication schedule into daily routines.

   C Teach patients to understand their prescription labels.

   D Devise or procure memory aids such as calendars, pill boxes, or timers.

   E Recommend pill-splitting aids or magnifiers as needed.[32]

Table 6.5. General Suggestions for Appropriate Prescribing for the Elderly

- Attempt nonpharmacological measure when feasible.
- Before starting a new drug, consider that the patient's symptoms may be from an adverse drug reaction.
- When starting a new drug, educate about indications, how to administer, common side effects, potential serious adverse effects, and what to do if these occur.
- Regularly review all medications; include OTC products, herbals, vitamin/mineral supplements. Help patients maintain a current medication list.
- Coordinate care with all providers to eliminate prescription duplication.
- Identify indications for each medication prescribed. Discontinue those not indicated.
- Regularly assess therapeutic responses to medications. Discontinue those that have not achieved goal.
- Avoid medications with high incidence of adverse effects in the elderly. [33]
- When possible, combine indications with a single drug.
- Regularly assess patient adherence, especially before changing doses or adding a new drug.
- Choose drugs with wide therapeutic windows when possible.
- Maintain your knowledge of potential drug interactions; commercial software is available.
- Consider age and comorbidities when weighing benefits of pharmacotherapy for prevention.

Source: Adapted from Good.[31]

8 Provide brief, easy-to-read written, visual, and verbal information about the specific oral agent that is being used. Inquire about side effects (and appropriate lab tests for monitoring), timing, costs, and complexity at each visit. Table 6.6 is a list of cost-saving suggestions that can be given to older adults.

9 Insulin is frequently initiated when maximum doses of single or combined oral agents fail to control glucose levels. Patients should be informed that diabetes is a progressive disease and they have not personally "failed."

A Physician and educator attitudes have been shown to be the most important factors in acceptance of insulin therapy. Discussing the benefits and potential challenges of insulin therapy may help patients make a decision about whether to take insulin or not.[34] The need for insulin can be presented as the treatment for the patient's particular stage of diabetes. Some patients appreciate the cost savings and view insulin as a more "natural" product.

B Time for supervised practice for those with motor or visual problems should be provided and can improve the accuracy of insulin administration. Consider newer injection devices available that simplify administration.

C The patient's insulin administration technique should be observed on a regular basis to detect a need for adaptive strategies, such as additional lighting, magnification, and alternative delivery devices. Family members, home care nurses, and visiting nurses can assist with implementing these techniques in the home.

Table 6.6 Cost Saving Suggestions That May be Offered to Older Adults

General	• Consider generic over the-counter medication. • Keep and submit receipts for insurance and tax benefits. • Shop drug stores for coupons and pricing. • Consider mail order. • Limit supplements and herbs.
Provider Assistance	• Implement lifestyle changes that would replace the need for medication. • Do not pressure your provider for highly advertised drugs • Ask about new medications that are less expensive than those you use, ask for samples. • Discuss generic substitution. • Make sure your provider has your insurance list of preferred product with lower copays. • Review all medications annually, deleting those not needed.
Low Income	• Ask about pharmacy or grocery senior discount cards. • Explore the AARP pharmacy service. • Ask about low income programs of drug companies. • Ask about free clinics. • Ask about state programs for low income elderly or disabled individuals.

Source: Adapted from Good.[31]

D Patients who require insulin may benefit from using a rapid-acting insulin because it may reduce the likelihood of hypoglycemia for those with variable food intake or unpredictable digestion/absorption.[35]

10 When appropriate, family members who are involved in day-to-day care should be included in educational and clinical sessions. These caregivers often are older spouses for whom educational adaptation will also be needed.[36]

11 Collaborative goals for management should be established by discussing with the patient existing diabetes complications, comorbidities, abilities, and willingness to carry out the treatment plan.[37]

Monitoring

1 Monitoring frequency and method will depend on the stability and level of glucose control as well as self-testing skills, desire, and willingness. Older people can learn to monitor as accurately as younger people.[38]

    A Determining whether problems exist with manual dexterity, vision, or memory of the procedure is important.

B Providing information about meters that accommodate their needs is helpful.

2 Urine ketone testing for those with known type 1 diabetes and those with type 2 diabetes who are lean and take insulin (since the latter may actually have ketosis-prone diabetes) should be included in educational sessions.

3 A1C test accuracy is affected by hemoglobinopathies such as anemia. Some providers advocate use of fructosamine in older adults.[3,39]

Self-Management Education

1 Older patients may or may not have had previous diabetes education. Therefore, it is important to evaluate their current level of knowledge about diabetes, correct existing misconceptions, and provide updated information.

2 Positive attitudes of educators can have a positive effect on patient behavior. Assume that mental or physical capacities are intact unless your assessment indicates otherwise.

3 Cultural or social barriers may exist between older people and the educator in part because of age differences. Create a comfortable, accepting environment to overcome these barriers.

4 Provide meaningful and practical information. Avoid medical jargon and unnecessary detail.

5 Assess the social and financial support available as well as the patient's expectations about the relationship with healthcare providers.

6 Because hyperglycemia impairs learning and retention,[13,40] simplify instruction and include significant others. Provide written reinforcement and access to the educator for clarification especially when hyperglycemia is present.

7 When glucose is under control, assess residual mental changes using standardized instruments, such as the Mini Mental State, Short Portable Mental Status, or Neurobehavioral Cognitive Status Examination.[41]

8 The following approach can be effective for accommodating persistent sensory or neurological limitations:
  A Slow the pace of teaching; focus on 1 or 2 points and make the learning sessions brief.
  B Use printed materials that are easy to read; assess color vision (use red, orange, or yellow instead of green or blue if color perception changes exist), and use fonts that are simple, bold, and large size. Magnifiers are often needed.[42]
  C Present audio information clearly, speak slowly and distinctly, augment spoken information with visual aids, avoid shouting, and prevent distracting noises or activity. Patients who have decreased hearing may appear confused.
  D Include frequent practice opportunities, telephone follow-up, or home care for those with limited mobility.

E Enhance memory by using cues such as calendars or pillboxes, repeating key learning points, and using familiar concrete examples.

9 Consider group education that includes coping skills. This approach may significantly improve glycemic control as well as enhance learning over time.[43] Interaction, group-driven objectives, and structured question-and-answer times are also possible strategies.[16]

Psychosocial Issues

1 Erickson calls this phase of the life cycle "integrity versus despair." During this phase, individuals review their lives for meaningfulness and develop a sense of acceptance or rejection.[44]

2 Retirement is often viewed as the start of this phase of the life cycle. Retirement can be viewed positively or negatively. Creating new relationships with adult children, grandparenting, adjusting to changes in health of self and spouse, divorce, widowhood, remarriage, changes in financial status, changes in residence, and recognition of the inevitability of death are also issues common to older adults.

3 The developmental tasks of aging represent many changes, adjustments, and losses. It is one of the most stressful periods of the life span.[45] Limited income, isolation, loss of a spouse, or limited mobility can lead to inadequate self-care or a sense of hopelessness.

4 Depression is common among members of this age group. Although 15% to 20% of people with diabetes in this age group have depression, it is often unrecognized by healthcare providers.
  A Depression may be masked among older adults with multiple physical symptoms and other mental changes associated with medication or the aging process.[46] A common myth is that depression is inevitable or natural in the aged. Hearing loss and other sensory or functional impairments that contribute to social isolation can exacerbate depression.
  B Depression may be accompanied by alcohol and drug abuse. It has also been correlated with mortality in older people with diabetes.[47]
  C Older adults who are members of minority ethnic groups appear to be at the greatest risk for negative impacts on income, health, and other measures of quality of life.[48]
  D Assess for signs and symptoms of depression at each visit. Because diagnosis may be difficult in the presence of dementia or cognitive impairment, refer patients to mental health professionals for evaluation when you suspect depression. (See Chapter 2, Psychosocial Assessment, in Diabetes Education and Program Management.)

5 Advocate for assistance with transportation, shopping, social contact, or negotiation with healthcare systems when patients appear to need this type of support.[49]

6 The ability to make the adjustments needed during this stage of life is a function of whether tasks of previous stages were successfully completed and of previous coping skills and abilities. Many adults are able to review their lives, place events in perspective, and resolve lifelong issues and conflicts.[48]

7 Older adults can experience strong feelings when confronted with an illness such as diabetes. The experiences of others in their families and social groups may influence their beliefs about diabetes and its seriousness. It is particularly important among cultural groups who are taught not to express emotions to carefully assess patients' perceptions of diabetes and their feelings about it.

Hyperosmolar Hyperglycemic State (HHS)

1 HHS is most often seen in the elderly with untreated (20%) or undertreated type 2 diabetes and especially those in long-term care facilities. Mortality is highest in the oldest patients (see Chapter 2, Hyperglycemia, in Diabetes and Complications, for more information).

2 Both patient and provider-related causes can increase the risk of HHS:
A The most common cause is infection.[9] Other causes are stroke, alcohol abuse, pancreatitis, myocardial infarction, trauma, and drugs. Inadequate fluid intake in people with hyperglycemia is also a cause.
B Provider-related causes include reluctance to aggressively treat elderly people and inadequate monitoring, especially in settings where patients are dependent or during concurrent illness (see Chapter 9, Illness and Surgery, in Diabetes Management Therapies, for more information).

Hypoglycemia

1 Older adults are at higher risk for medication-induced hypoglycemia due to the following conditions:
A Renal changes
B Slowed hormonal counterregulation
C Inadequate hydration
D Polypharmacy
E Inadequate or erratic food intake
F Slowed intestinal absorption

2 Hypoglycemia can cause cardiac arrhythmias.

3 Review individual signs and symptoms of hypoglycemia regularly with patients and caregivers. Be aware that their first symptoms may be unsteadiness, lightheadedness, poor concentration, trembling, or sweating.[50] Caregivers may attribute neurological changes to cardiac or cerebrovascular causes. Patients may attribute hypoglycemic symptoms to comorbidities, drug side effects, or normal aging.

4 Appropriate bedtime snacks for people on diabetes medication can prevent nocturnal hypoglycemia. Keeping a carbohydrate source at the bedside may help prevent related ataxia and subsequent falls.

5 Avoid reliance on symptoms because they may be absent or confused with other disease symptoms. Blood glucose monitoring can be used to detect asymptomatic hypoglycemia.

6 Oral agents without hypoglycemic effects should be used when feasible.

7 Higher blood glucose targets may be appropriate for people with a history of severe hypoglycemia.

8 A "check-in" system can be helpful for those at high risk of developing hypoglycemia. Individuals who live alone can call a relative at a preappointed time; emergency pager devices also may be useful.

Other Related Acute Problems

1 Older adults with diabetes have higher rates of anxiety and forgetfulness. They have increased susceptibility to hypothermia, absence of fever with infection, and tuberculosis. Unique syndromes include painful shoulder periarthritis, amyotrophy, neuropathic cachexia, or bullae of the feet (the last resolve spontaneously).[3]

2 Older women with diabetes have an increased risk of fractures. These occur most often in the hip, humerus, and foot.[51]

Long-Term Complications of Diabetes

1 Older adults have a higher incidence and accelerated development of long-term complications. Some complications (especially retinal, peripheral vascular, and lower extremity neuropathies) often are present at diagnosis.[52,53]

2 Amputation is twice as common in patients over age 65. Peripheral neuropathy and decreased vision can compromise self-detection of lower extremity problems (see Chapter 4, Diabetes Foot Care and Education, in Diabetes and Complications, for more information).
  A Stress the importance of frequent foot inspection, incorporating assistance from others (family, friends, and home health nurses) as needed.
  B Create teaching opportunities by observing foot care and inspecting footwear during clinical visits.
  C Assist patients to obtain footwear that accommodates the shape of their feet and specific sensation problems. Refer to a podiatrist or orthotic specialist as necessary.

3 Hypertension, a diabetes-related complication, contributes to stroke, renal failure, and myocardial infarction.
  A Screen blood pressure regularly.
  B Evaluate sodium intake and teach patients ways to decrease if appropriate.
  C Alternative seasonings can be suggested for those with decreased taste sensation.
  D Advocate for early treatment.
  E Monitor closely for drug side effects (eg, orthostatic hypotension, decreased cardiac output).

F Consider potential drug-drug interactions each time a new medication is started. (See Chapter 3, Pharmacologic Therapies for Hypertension and Dyslipdemia, in Diabetes Management Therapies, for more information.)

4 Myocardial infarction and cerebrovascular incidents are more prevalent in elderly persons with diabetes. In addition to the usual preventive care and education, the elderly person has special needs to consider.

   A Weigh preventive strategies against needed treatments for comorbidities and expected benefits.

   B Stroke prevention efforts for the elderly are focused on glucose control, treating atrial fibrillation, and control of hypertension.[54]

   C Routine EKGs should be performed. Monitor and educate patients about the signs/symptoms of congestive heart failure if there is evidence of earlier cardiac damage.[55]

5 Vision loss is more likely to occur in the elderly.

   A Eye diseases, in general, are more common with aging. This fact, coupled with changes from diabetes, makes older people more susceptible to vision loss.

   B Cataract surgery is 95% effective. Macular edema can be detected with a simple in-office Amsler grid.[42]

   C The risk of new retinopathy is also present in the aged.[56] Annual screening and treatment of retinopathy and maculopathy for older patients can save vision.[57]

   D Glucose control affects the progression of retinopathy in the elderly.[58]

   E Emphasize the importance of annual screening because yearly eye exams are not ordered routinely.[59]

   F Limited vision can seriously impact self-care for diabetes.

   G Assess functional vision regularly and during educational sessions to determine its impact on self-monitoring, medication administration, and foot care. (See Chapter 7, Eye Disease and Adaptive Diabetes Education for Visually Impaired Persons, in Diabetes and Complications, for more information on eye disease and vision loss.)

6 Diabetic nephropathy coupled with the renal changes associated with aging and other causes of renal insufficiency (eg, arteriosclerosis, hypertension, congestive heart failure, drugs, infection, and cancer) can precipitate kidney failure.

   A Routine screening for kidney disease is needed for early detection and treatment (see Chapter 8, Nephropathy, in Diabetes and Complications, for more information).

   B Warn patients about the dangers of nephrotoxic contrast media and selected drugs.

   C Teach signs/symptoms of urinary tract infections to foster early treatment.

   D Carefully evaluate the need for a low-protein diet.

7 The effect of dental diseases on eating and nutrition can be significant. Dental disease is also linked to coronary heart disease.[20]

   A Assess whether mobility or financial difficulties are limiting preventive care.

   B Assess and facilitate oral hygiene and dental care (see Chapter 5, Skin and Dental Care, in Diabetes and Complications).

   C Evaluate whether dry mouth symptoms have caused food intake problems.

8 Cognitive function declines with age.

A Changes in short-term memory, information processing speed, and attention span normally decline with age. Some changes occur more often in people with chronic hyperglycemia at all ages and specifically affect memory, sensorimotor (information processing) speed, cognitive flexibility (problem-solving), and fluency.[60]

B Cognitive testing can guide self-management and educational interventions.

Care of the Hospitalized Elderly

1 Elderly people are hospitalized more frequently than younger people. One third of those who are 75 years of age and have diabetes are hospitalized in the course of a year.[61,62]

2 Because 65% of elderly people who are hospitalized are undernourished at admission, assess the nutritional status of elderly diabetes patients on admission and provide follow-up as needed.[63] Use this opportunity to update previous nutrition recommendations that may now be obsolete.

3 The diagnosis of diabetes may not be included in the hospital records of patients with diabetes. Furthermore, undetected diabetes is common in hospital populations.[64] Hospitalization does not assure adequate screening or treatment of complications.[65]

4 Hospital-based diabetes educators have a unique opportunity to promote diagnosis and improve treatment of older people with diabetes. Changes in therapy requiring changes in self-care are often initiated in the hospital. Ageism should not prevent referral for educational programs. Ensure that outpatient medical and educational appointments are made before discharge.[66]

5 Earlier detection and treatment in the geriatric population may help reduce personal suffering and financial burden. Hospitalization expenses make up 40% of all costs of care for people with diabetes, and as with other populations 10% of individuals comprise 56% of expenditures.[67,68]

Nursing Facilities

1 Dependent individuals with diabetes comprise 18.3% of residents in nursing care facilities. Evidence suggests that standards of care and monitoring may not be in use.[69,70]

2 Priorities of care for residents with diabetes include the following:
   A Personal/family priorities
   B Eliminating glycemic symptoms
   C Achieving/maintaining optimal daily functioning
   D Balancing treatment with overall prognosis

3 A team approach is possible for residents with diabetes because the involvement of nurses, dietitians, pharmacists, physicians, and therapists is mandated by regulations for long-term care facilities. The nature of this environment in terms of consistency and team care can result in optimal control of diabetes without unnecessary burden. Staff education is necessary and has been shown to be effective.[71-73]

4 Selected common diseases of the elderly are

    A Eyes: senile cataract, senile macular degeneration, open angle glaucoma

    B Renal insufficiency caused by arteriosclerosis, hypertension, coronary heart failure, drug effects

    C Foot problems: arthritis, arteriopathy

Key Educational Considerations

1 Assess older adults as individuals but anticipate special needs related to sensory and other deficits related to aging.

2 Determine the patient's priorities. Limit instruction to content that matches the older adult's specific diabetes-related goals.

3 Modify instruction so that key information is presented in easily read or heard messages. Use groups and active learning methods.

4 Routinely teach at a slower pace, use memory aids, and incorporate significant others and caregivers in instruction.[5] Help patients organize information by defining the topic to be discussed at the beginning of the presentation and summarizing key points at the end.

5 Evaluate learning often, especially when hyperglycemia or sensory or cognitive deficits are present.

6 Evaluate care recommendations with consideration for cost, accessibility, safety, support systems, and the effect on perceived quality of life.

Learning Assessment: Case Study 1

FM is a 70-year-old Native American man who lives on the local reservation. He has been admitted to the hospital for hypoglycemia, and you have been asked to evaluate his treatment and educational needs. His A1C test value is 10.0%. Currently, FM is taking the following medications:

- Rosiglitizone, 8 mg daily; glipizide 10 mg bid
- 70/30 insulin: 45 units before breakfast, 25 units at 6 PM
- Aspirin, 1 daily
- Lasix, 40 mg daily
- Vasotec, 5 mg daily
- Albuterol, 2 puffs 4 times daily

FM has had diabetes for 15 years and is seen at the reservation clinic several times a year. Due to poor eyesight he is not using his blood glucose meter to test his blood glucose.

Questions for Discussion

1 What approach would you use for your first visit with this patient?

2 Are the patient's current medications appropriate for him?

3 What resource issues will need to be assessed?

Discussion

1 To prepare for FM's first visit:

  A Ask FM to bring a family member or friend with him.

  B Ask FM to bring all of his medications and monitoring supplies.

  C Make sure you have magnifiers and low-vision educational materials available for FM to use.

  D Contact his provider to confirm his medications and get his most recent lab results.

  E Determine if community health workers or home health care are available to him on the reservation.

2 The first visit will likely focus on assessing FM's concerns, his willingness and ability to do self-care, the cause of his current episode of hypoglycemia, food intake and nutritional needs, identification of support systems, and influence of his cultural beliefs and practices on his self-care (eg, food preparation and choices, use of alternative therapies). Basic information regarding meal planning can be provided. Provide time for him and his family to ask questions.

3 It is likely that FM's diabetes medication regimen can be simplified to assure accurate administration.

  A Sulfonylureas may not reduce glucose levels because FM is likely to have reduced insulin secretion at his age. However, if effective they may be the lowest cost option.

  B Combination regimens with 3 or more drugs are not usually recommended. A simplified regimen is more likely to result in increased accuracy in dosing, administration, and reduced costs.

  C Liver and renal function must be tested to determine safety of the oral agents.

4 FM has visual problems that will have to be accommodated.

5 Develop a teaching plan with FM so that other educational and management issues can be addressed at future visits. This plan also can be used to report back to FM's case manager or provider as needed.

6 It is likely that FM will benefit from ongoing brief educational sessions. Include a significant other to help with reinforcement or memory problems. Given the high incidence of diabetes among Native Americans, FM's family members or friends may personally benefit from receiving information about diabetes.

7 A community health worker or home health nurse can assist with instruction and evaluate his home environment.

Learning Assessment: Case Study 2

EK is an obese 76-year-old widow with type 2 diabetes. She is referred to you for instruction about blood glucose monitoring. EK lives alone in a high-rise apartment building in a large city. Her daughter lives nearby and drives her to medical appointments. Although she takes glyburide 5 mg twice daily, her blood glucose levels are consistently 300 mg/dL (16.7 mmol/L) when measured using the glucose meter in her provider's office.

EK does not report symptoms of high or low blood sugar but is concerned about having to get up during the night to urinate as a result of her "water pill." Other medical problems that she reports are arthritis (which limits her activity), cataract surgery 2 years earlier, and a mild heart problem for which she takes digoxin.

Questions for Discussion

1 What difficulties might EK have doing blood glucose monitoring?

2 What might be the causes of her persistent hyperglycemia?

3 In addition to her concerns, what other areas might you identify in your educational plan?

Discussion

1 In light of her previous cataract surgery, EK may have difficulty seeing adequately, and her manual dexterity may be affected by her arthritis.

2 She may benefit from (1) a meter with easy-to-use features, (2) being given supervised opportunities to practice using her meter, and (3) receiving brief written reminders on how to use the device. Demonstrate different meters that are available so she can understand her options in making a selection.

3 Until her blood glucose is in target range, EK may have difficulty learning and retaining information. Reinforce all verbal information with written materials. Her daughter can also be taught how to reinforce her mother's technique and recall, such as by posting the procedure where she tests and making sure there is good lighting.

4 EK is at risk for dehydration because of her hyperglycemia and polyuria; getting up at night increases her risk of falling since her mobility is limited.

5 Her glyburide is at maximum dose and improved glycemic control may be better achieved with an oral agent that does not cause hypoglycemia.

6 Another possible cause of her hyperglycemia is infection. The upper respiratory tract is a common site of infection in people with diabetes. If signs or symptoms are present, follow-up medical evaluation can be recommended.

7 Information on meal planning, weight, blood pressure, recent A1C test, serum and urine creatinine, and EKG may need to be provided. Offer chair exercises, stretching, or mild calisthenics to maintain range of motion in light of her arthritis. Include a foot exam at every office visit, provide a referral to an ophthalmologist, and emphasize regular eye care during educational sessions.

8 Financial and access issues must be discussed early so that appropriate resources can be provided.

9 Determine whether the cause of her hyperglycemia has been addressed and follow up on treatment progress in future visits. Other issues to assess include activity level and other medications.

References

1 Mokdad AH, Ford ES, Bowman BA, et al. Prevalence of obesity, diabetes, and obesity-related health risk factors, 2001. JAMA. 2003;289:76-79.

2 Kenny SJ, Aubert RE, Geiss LS. Prevalence and incidence of non-insulin-dependent diabetes. In: National Diabetes Data Group. Diabetes in America. 2nd ed. Bethesda, Md: National Institutes of Health; 1995. NIH publication 95-1468:49-54.

3 Samos LF, Roos BA. Diabetes mellitus in older persons. Med Clin North Am. 1998;82:791-803.

4 Croxson SCM, Burden AC. Polyuria and polydipsia in an elderly population: its relationship to previously undiagnosed diabetes. Practical Diabetes International. 1998:15:170-172.

5 Harris MI, Klein R, Welborn TA, Knuiman MW. Onset of NIDDM occurs at least 4-7 yr before clinical diagnosis. Diabetes Care. 1992;15:815-819.

6 Meneilly GS, Tessier D. Diabetes in the elderly. Diabetic Med. 1995;12:949-960.

7 Lindeman RD, Romero LJ, Hundley R, et al. Prevalences of type 2 diabetes, the insulin resistance syndrome, and coronary heart disease in an elderly, biethnic population. Diabetes Care. 1998;21:959-966.

8 Chau MD, Edelman SV. Clinical management of diabetes in the elderly. Clinical Diabetes. 2001;19:172-175.

9 Kitabchi AE, Umpierrez GE, Murphy MB, et al. Management of hyperglycemia crises in patients with diabetes. Diabetes Care. 2001;24:131-153.

10 National Vital Statistics Report. 47(28). December 1999:6-7.

11 Sacks DB, McDonald JM. The pathogenesis of type II diabetes mellitus. A polygenic disease. Am J Clin Pathol. 1996;105:149-156.

12 Gradman TJ, Laws A, Thompson LW, Reaven GM. Verbal learning and/or memory improves with glycemic control in older subjects with non-insulin-dependent diabetes mellitus. J Am Geriatr Soc. 1993;41:1305-1312.

13 Testa MA, Simonson DC. Health economic benefits and quality of life during improved glycemic control in patients with type 2 diabetes mellitus: a randomized, controlled, double-blind trial. JAMA. 1998;280:1490-1496.

14 Caruso L, Silliman R, Demissie S, Greenfield S, Wagner E. What can we do to improve physical function in older persons with type 2 diabetes? J Gerontol. 2000;55A: M372-M377.

15 Williamson JR, Hoffmann PL, Kohrt WM. Endurance exercise training decreases capillary basement membrane width in older nondiabetic and diabetic adults. J Appl Physiol. 1996;80:747-753.

16 Funnell M, Arnold M, Fogler J, Merritt J, Anderson L. Participation in a diabetes education and care program: experience from the Diabetes Care for Older Adults Project. Diabetes Educ. 1997;23:163-167.

17 Markson EW. Functional, social, and psychological disability as causes of loss of weight and independence in older community-living people. Clin Geriatr Med. 1997;13:639-652.

18 Stanley K. Assessing the nutritional needs of the geriatric patient with diabetes. Diabetes Educ. 1998;24:29-36.

19 Nutrition Screening Initiative. Nutrition Interventions Manual for Professionals Caring for Older Americans. Washington DC; 1992.

20 Loesche WJ, Schork A, Terpenning MS, Chen YM, Dominguez BL, Grossman N. Assessing the relationship between dental disease and coronary heart disease in elderly US veterans. J Am Dent Assoc. 1998; 129:301-311.

21 Pratley RE, Hagberg JM, Dengel DR, Rogues EM, Muller DC, Goldberg AP. Aerobic exercise training-induced reductions in abdominal fat and glucose-stimulated insulin responses in middle-aged and older men. J Am Geriatr Soc. 2000;48:1055-1061.

22 Bressler R, Johnson DG. Oral antidiabetic drug use in the elderly. Drugs Aging. 1996;9:418-437.

23 Mooradian AD. Drug therapy of non-insulin dependent diabetes mellitus in the elderly. Drugs. 1996;51:931-941.

24 Oki JC, Isley WL. Rethinking new and old diabetes drugs for type 2 disease. Practical Diabetol. 1997;16(3):27-40.

25 Umeda F. Potential role of thiazolidine-diones in older diabetic patients. Drugs Aging. 1995;7:331-337.

26 White JR. Combination oral agent/insulin therapy in patients with type 2 diabetes mellitus. Clinical Diabetes. 1997;152:102-112.

27 Shorr RI, Ray WA, Daugherty JR, Griffin MN. Incidence and risk factors for serious hypoglycemia in older persons using insulin or sulfonylureas. Arch Intern Med. 1997;157:1681-1686.

28 Gregorio F, Ambrosi F, Filipponi P, Manfrini S, Testa I. Is metformin safe enough for aging type 2 diabetic patients? Diabetes Metab. 1996;22:43-50.

29 Jennings PE. Oral antihyperglycemics. Considerations in older patients with non-insulin-dependent diabetes mellitus. Drugs Aging. 1997;10:323-331.

30 Johnson P, Lebovitz H, Coniff R, Simonson C, Raskin P, Munera C. Advantages of alpha-glucosidase inhibition as monotherapy in elderly type 2 diabetic patients. J Clin Endocrinol Metab. 1998;83:1515-1522.

31 Good. CB. Polypharmacy in elderly patients with diabetes. Diabetes Spectrum. 2002; 15:240-248.

32 Wallsten SM, Sullivan RJ Jr, Hanlon JT, Blazer DG, Tyrey MJ, Westlund R. Medication-taking behaviors in the high- and low-functioning elderly: MacArthur field studies of successful aging. Ann Pharmaco Ther. 1995;29:359-364.

33 Beers MH. Explicit criteria for determining potentially inappropriate medication by the elderly. Arch Intern Med. 1997;157:1531-1536.

34 Wolffenbuttel BH, Drossaert CH, Visser AP. Determinants of injecting insulin in elderly patients with type II diabetes mellitus. Patient Educ Couns. 1993;22:117-125.

35 Hoogwerf BJ, Mehta A, Reddy S. Advances in the treatment of diabetes mellitus in the elderly. Development of insulin analogues. Drugs Aging. 1996;9:438-448.

36 Silliman RA, Bhatti S, Khan A, Dukes KA, Sullivan LM. The care of older persons with diabetes mellitus: families and primary care physicians. J Am Geriatr Soc. 1996;44:1314-1321.

37 Halter J. Geriatric patients. In: Lebovitz HE, ed. Therapy for Diabetes Mellitus and Related Disorders. 3rd ed. Alexandria, Va: American Diabetes Association, 1998:234-240.

38 Bernbaum M, Albert SG, McGinnis J, Brusca S, Mooradian AD. The reliability of self-blood glucose monitoring in elderly diabetic patients. J Am Geriatr Soc. 1994;42:779-781.

39 Morley JE. An overview of diabetes mellitus in older persons. Advances in the care of older people with diabetes. Clin Geriatr Med. 1999;15:211-224.

40 Meneilly GS, Cheung E, Tessier D, Yakura C, Tuokko H. The effect of improved glycemic control on cognitive functions in the elderly patient with diabetes. J Gerontol. 1993;48:M117-M121.

41 Chenitz WC, Stone JT, Salisbury SA. Clinical Gerontological Nursing. Philadelphia: WB Saunders; 1991.

42 Butler F, Faye EE, Guazzo E, Kupfer C. Keeping an eye on vision: new tools to preserve sight and quality of life. Geriatrics. 1997;52:48-56.

43 Garcia R, Suarez R. Diabetes education in the elderly: a 5-year follow-up of an interactive approach. Patient Educ and Couns. 1996;29:87-97.

44 Erickson E. Childhood and Society. New York: Norton; 1963.

45 Woodruff-Pak DS. The Neuropsychology of Aging. Malden, Ma: Blackwell; 1997.

46 Lustman PJ, Griffith LS, Clouse RE. Recognizing and managing depression in patients with diabetes. In: Anderson BA, Rubin RR, eds. Practical Psychology for Diabetes Clinicians. Alexandria, Va: American Diabetes Association; 1996:143-152.

47 Ganzini L, Smith DM, Fenn DS, Lee MA. Depression and mortality in medically ill older adults. J Am Geriatr Soc. 1997; 45:307-312.

48 Kart CS, ed. The Realities of Aging: An Introduction to Gerontology. 3rd ed. Boston: Allyn and Bacon; 1990.

49 Zrebiec JF. Caring for elderly patients with diabetes. In: Anderson BA, Rubin RR, eds. Practical Psychology for Diabetes Clinicians. Alexandria, Va: American Diabetes Association; 1996:35-42.

50 Jaap A, Jones G, McCrimmon R, Deary I, Fruer B. Perceived symptoms of hypoglycaemia in elderly type 2 diabetic patients treated with insulin. Diabetic Med. 1998; 15:398-401.

51 Schwartz A, Sellmeyer DE, Ensrud KE, et al. Older women with diabetes have an increased risk of fracture: a prospective study. J Clin Endocrinol & Metab. 2001; 86:32-38.

52 Abraira C, Colwell J, Nuttall F, Sawin CT, Henderson W, Comstock JP. Cardiovascular events and correlates in the Veterans Affairs Diabetes Feasibility Trial. Arch Intern Med. 1997;157:181-188.

53 Turner RC, Holman RR. Lessons from UK prospective diabetes study. Diabetes Res Clin Pract. 1995;28:S151-S157.

54 Kuusisto J, Mykkanen L, Pyorala K, Laakso M. Non-insulin-dependent diabetes and its metabolic control are important predictors of stroke in elderly subjects. Stroke. 1994;25:1157-1164.

55 Azzarelli A, Dini FL, Cristofani R, et al. NIDDM as unfavorable factor to the postinfarctual ventricular function in the elderly: echocardiography study. Coronary Artery Dis. 1995;6:629-634.

56 Cohen O, Norymberg K, Neumann E, Dekel H. Complication-free duration and the risk of development of retinopathy in elderly diabetic patients. Arch Intern Med. 1998;158:641-644.

57 Agardh E, Agardh CD, Hansson-Lundblad C, Cavallin-Sjoberg U. The importance of early diagnosis of treatable diabetic retinopathy for the four-year visual outcome in older-onset diabetes mellitus. Acta Ophthalmol Scand. 1996;74:166-170.

58 Morisaki N, Watanabe S, Kobayashi J, Kanzaki T, Takahashi K, Yokote K. Diabetic control and progression of retinopathy in elderly patients: five year follow-up study. J Am Geriatr Soc. 1994;42:142-145.

59 Pagano G, Bargero G, Vuolo A, Bruno G. Prevalence and clinical features of known type 2 diabetes in the elderly: a population based study. Diabetic Med. 1994;11:475-479.

60 Van Boxtel M, Buntinx F, Houx P, Melsemakers J, Knottnerus A, Jolles J. The relation between morbidity and cognitive performance in a normal aging population. J Gerontol. 1998;53A:M147-M154.

61 Aubert RE, Geiss LS, Ballard DJ, Cocanougher B, Herman WH. Diabetes-related hospitalization and hospital utilization. In: National Diabetes Data Group. Diabetes in America. 2nd ed. Bethesda, Md: National Institutes of Health, 1995; NIH publication 95-1468:559.

62 Rosenthal MJ, Fajardo M, Gilmore S, Morley JE, Naliboff B. Hospitalization and mortality of diabetes in older adults. Diabetes Care. 1998;21:231-235.

63 Sullivan D, Lipschitz D. Evaluating and treating nutritional problems in older patients. Clin Geriatr Med. 1997;13:753-768.

64 Levetan CS, Passaro M, Jablonski K, Kass M, Ratner RE. Unrecognized diabetes among hospitalized patients. Diabetes Care. 1998;21:246-249.

65 McClellen W, Knight D, Karp H, Brown W. Early detection and treatment of renal disease in hospitalized diabetic and hypertensive patients: important differences between practice and published guidelines. Am J Kidney Dis. 1997;29:368-375.

66 Davis E. A quality improvement project in diabetes patient education during hospitalization. Diabetes Spectrum. 2000;13:228-231.

67 American Diabetes Association. Diabetes 1996 Vital Statistics. Alexandria, Va: American Diabetes Association; 1997:67.

68 Krop JS, Powe NR, Weller WE, Shaffer TJ, Saudek CD, Anderson GF. Patterns of expenditures and use of services among older adults with diabetes: implications for the transition to capitated managed care. Diabetes Care. 1998;21:747-752.

69 Mayfield JA, Deb P, Potter DEB. Diabetes and long term care. In: National Diabetes Data Group. Diabetes in America. 2nd ed. Bethesda, Md: National Institutes of Health, 1995; NIH publication 95-1468:571-586.

70 Mooradian AD. Caring for the elderly nursing home patient with diabetes. Diabetes Spectrum. 1992;5:318-322.

71 Sherriff P, Allison J, Large DM, Quinn C, Routledge A, Hall E, Broughton DL, Kelly WF. Out of sight, out of mind? Elderly patients with diabetes in nursing homes. Practical Diabetes International. 2000; 17:73-76.

72 Tonino R. Diabetes education: what should health-care providers in long-term nursing care facilities know about diabetes? Diabetes Care. 1990;13:55-59.

73 Wylie-Rosett J, Villeneuve M, Mazze R. Professional education in a long term care facility: program development in diabetes. Diabetes Care. 1985;8:481-485.

Suggested Readings

Amato L, Paolisso G, Cacciatore F, Ferrara N, Canonico S, Rengo F. Non-insulin-dependent diabetes mellitus is associated with a greater prevalence of depression in the elderly. Diabetes Metab. 1996;22:314-318.

American Association of Diabetes Educators. Special considerations for the education and management of older adults with diabetes [position statement]. Diabetes Educ. 2003;29: 93-96.

Atiea JA, Moses JL, Sinclair AJ. Neuropsychological function in older subjects with non-insulin-dependent diabetes mellitus. Diabetic Med. 1995;12:679-685.

Belmin J, Valensi P. Diabetic neuropathy in elderly patients. What can be done? Drugs Aging. 1996;8:416-429.

Funnell M. Care of the nursing home resident with diabetes. Clin Geriatr Med. 1999; 15:413-422.

Funnell M, Merritt JH. Impact of diabetes mellitus on the aging population. In: Haire-Joshu D, ed. Management of Diabetes Mellitis: Perspectives of Care Across the Life Span. 2nd ed. St. Louis. Mosby; 1996:755-834.

Funnell M, Merritt JH. The older adult with diabetes. Nurse Practitioner Forum. 1998;9:98-107.

Gurwitz JH, Field TS, Glynn RJ, et al. Risk factors for non-insulin-dependent diabetes mellitus requiring treatment in the elderly. J Am Geriatr Soc. 1994;42:1235-1240.

Helkala EL, Niskanen L, Viinamaki H, Partanen J, Uusitupa M. Short-term and long-term memory in elderly patients with NIDDM. Diabetes Care. 1995;18:681-685.

Leibson CL, Rocca WA, Hanson VA, et al. Risk of dementia among persons with diabetes mellitus: a population-based cohort study. Am J Epidemiol. 1997;145:301-308.

McLaughlin S. Nutrition therapy for the older adult with diabetes. In: Franz MJ, Bantle JP, eds. American Diabetes Association Guide to Medical Nutrition Therapy for Diabetes. Alexandria, Va: American Diabetes Association. 1999;249-273.

Niskanen L, Rauramaa R, Miettinen H, Haffner SM, Mercuri M, Uusitupa M. Carotid artery intima-media thickness in elderly patients with NIDDM and in nondiabetic subjects. Stroke. 1996;27:1986-1992.

Learning Assessment: Post-Test Questions

Diabetes in Older Adults   6

1 The physiological changes of aging include all of the following except:
A Increased GFR
B Slower reaction time
C Decreased muscle mass and strength
D Increased vascular resistance

2 When counseling a 65-year-old man with type 2 diabetes who has never exercised in the past, it would be important to first:
A Assess his functional capacity and existing comorbidities
B Caution him against participating in strenuous activity
C Advise him to join an aerobic class
D Advise him to swim for 45 minutes every other day

3 Failure to thrive in older people:
A Occurs in patients who have 1 or more changes in functional ability
B Occurs in patients who experience recent weight loss
C Usually results from a combination of changes in physical and cognitive function
D Is seldom related to rates of depression

4 When considering blood glucose monitoring for an older adult, it is important to take into account all of the following, but the least critical is:
A Finances
B Manual dexterity
C Blood glucose goals
D Age of patient

5 When providing education to older adults an appropriate strategy is to:
A Be technical and complete
B Direct your message only to the individual with diabetes
C Be meaningful and practical
D Be directed by agency policies and protocols

6 In your teaching with an elderly patient you note markedly poor short-term memory. You should do all of the following except:
A Reassess mental status after glycemic control is achieved
B Provide supplemental sources of information
C Limit time for practice
D Slow the pace of teaching

7 Hypoglycemia is more problematic in older adults due to:
A Greater sensitivity to glucagon
B Different symptomatology
C Greater total body fat
D Subsequent rebound hyperglycemia

8 Which of the following statements about older people is true?
A Depression is uncommon in persons with diabetes
B Depression may be masked in the elderly by physical symptoms
C Assessment of signs and symptoms of depression should only be done by mental health professionals
D Aside from feeling sad, depression has no serious effects

9 All of the following actions are routinely appropriate in reducing the risk of hypoglycemia in older people except:
A A regular review of their signs and symptoms of hypoglycemia
B The use of appropriate bedtime snacks to avoid nocturnal hypoglycemia
C Use of blood glucose monitoring
D Lowering target blood glucose goals to avoid risk of complications of hypoglycemia

10 One of the most serious complications of type 2 diabetes in the older adult is:
A Hyperosmolar hyperglycemic state (HHS)
B Diabetic ketoacidosis (DKA)
C Nocturnal hyperglycemia
D Cataracts

See next page for answer key.

Post-Test Answer Key

Diabetes in Older Adults

6

1	A	**6**	C
2	A	**7**	B
3	C	**8**	B
4	D	**9**	D
5	C	**10**	A

A Core Curriculum for Diabetes Education
Diabetes in the Life Cycle and Research

Biological Complementary Therapies in Diabetes

7

Laura Shane-McWhorter, PharmD, BCPS, FASCP, BC-ADM, CDE
College of Pharmacy
University of Utah
Salt Lake City, Utah

Introduction

1 Because of the growing demand for alternative therapies in the United States and to promote research on the use of these agents, the US Senate created the Office of Alternative Medicine (OAM) in 1992 at the National Institutes of Health (NIH). In 1998, Congress changed the name of the OAM to the National Center for Complementary and Alternative Medicine (NCCAM).[1]

2 In 1993, Eisenberg et al[2] published a landmark survey that indicated a high prevalence of the use of alternative medicine.
  A Eisenberg's definition of "alternative medicine" included such modalities as acupuncture, relaxation techniques, massage, chiropractic, and spiritual healing as well as herbal medicine and megavitamins.
  B Examples of other alternative medicine practices include aromatherapy, Qigong, reflexology, curanderismo, and meditation relaxation techniques.[3]

3 The NCCAM has provided a definition of complementary and alternative medicine. According to the NCCAM, complementary and alternative medicine (CAM) covers a broad range of healing philosophies, approaches, and therapies. It is generally defined as treatments and healthcare practices not widely taught in medical schools, not generally used in hospitals, and not usually reimbursed by insurance companies. In many therapies, the healthcare practitioner considers the whole person, including physical, mental, emotional, and spiritual aspects, hence the term holistic. Some of these therapies are used alone and referred to as alternative, while some are used in combination with other alternative or conventional therapies and referred to as complementary.

4 This chapter focuses on biological complementary therapies, which include botanical, vitamin, and mineral products.

5 Diabetes educators need to have a clear understanding of biological complementary therapies in diabetes to be able to
  A Provide unbiased, nonjudgmental information to patients about these therapies.
  B Understand the proposed mechanism of action of these agents.
  C Provide information regarding potential side effects of these therapies.
  D Provide information regarding potential drug interactions between biological complementary therapies and concurrently used diabetes medications.
  E Understand that there is insufficient evidence to recommend routine use of the biological complementary therapies discussed in this chapter by people with diabetes.

Objectives

Upon completion of this chapter, the learner will be able to
1 State the epidemiology of use of complementary and alternative medicine (CAM).
2 State reasons why persons with diabetes use CAM.
3 Describe reasons for concern with the use of CAM.
4 Describe the main components of the Dietary Supplement Health and Education Act (DSHEA) of 1994.
5 Describe how to evaluate claims from manufacturers of dietary supplements.

6 List biological complementary therapies commonly used in diabetes.

7 Explain the proposed mechanism of action of biological complementary therapies in diabetes.

8 Describe side effects and drug interactions that may occur with use of biological complementary therapies.

9 Provide information and recommendations to persons with diabetes regarding the use of biological complementary therapies.

10 Describe how to talk with individuals in a nonjudgmental manner about the use of biological complementary therapies.

11 List references that may be used to answer questions about CAM products and resources.

Key Definitions

1 *Ayurveda.* An ancient healing system practiced in such countries as India and Sri Lanka that employs diet, yoga, meditation, massage, and botanical remedies for treatment of medical diseases. The word is a Sanskrit term from 2 root words: Ayus meaning life and Vid meaning knowledge.

2 *Adaptogen.* An agent that may increase resistance against physical or mental stress or noxious stimuli without impairing physiologic functions.

3 *Biological complementary therapies.* A subset of CAM that includes vitamin, mineral, and botanical products.

4 *Decoction.* A botanical product prepared by boiling the herb directly in water and then straining it to remove the solid plant material.

5 *Dietary Supplement Health and Education Act* (DSHEA). Legislation established in 1994 that defined dietary supplements as orally ingested foods that include botanical products (such as herbs and different plant products), nonbotanical substances (such as vitamins and minerals), and traditional cultural remedies (such as Asian herbal prescription medicines). Under DSHEA, these products are not required to undergo the same approval process that is required for drugs. These products do not require proof that they are safe and effective to be marketed.

6 *Glycerite.* A botanical preparation made by using glycerin as a solvent. It is less stable than an alcoholic extract.

7 *Infusion.* A tea made by pouring boiling water over a botanical product and letting it steep.

Epidemiology of Complementary and Alternative Medicine Use

1 A landmark study in 1990 indicated that 33.8% of Americans were using alternative medicine.[2] The study was repeated in 1997 and found that use had increased to 42.1%.[4]

    A According to the 1997 survey, 15 million adults had taken alternative agents concurrently with prescription drugs.

B Results from this survey also showed that 12.1% of patients were taking herbals and 5.5% were taking megavitamins. From 1990 to 1997, herbal product use increased 380% and megavitamin use increased 130%.[3]

C A report published in 2002 of medication use in the United States indicated that herbals or supplements were used by 14% of the population surveyed.[5]

D There is no currently available large survey that thoroughly evaluates how many patients with diabetes are using CAM, although more information is becoming available.

E CAM treatments that have been used by patients with diabetes include faith healing, macrobiosis (eating a macrobiotic diet), membership in religious sects, clinical ecology (using chromium and nicotinic acid treatment), astrotherapy (tying pieces of coral around the arms), reflexology (massaging areas on the foot that are said to represent internal organs), pearl therapy (boiling oyster pearls in milk and drinking the liquid), cellular nutrition (ingesting a liquid replacement feed), gnosis (practicing a subconscious healing technique), herbal treatment, meditation, and homeopathy.[6]

F Recent publications have addressed CAM use by patients with diabetes. One study used 1996 Medical Expenditure Panel Survey data and reported that patients with diabetes are 1.6 times more likely than patients without diabetes to use CAM (8% vs. 5%, $P<.0001$).[7] The most commonly used therapies were nutritional advice and lifestyle diets (Ayurvedic diets, naturopathic or homeopathic nutrition diets, as well as orthomolecular therapies such as melatonin, vitamin megadoses, or magnesium) administered by CAM practitioners, spiritual healing, herbal remedies, massage therapy, and meditation training.

G Other recent surveys of diabetes clinic patients indicate that 17% to 57% use CAM.[8-10]

- In one study 17% used CAM therapies. Acupuncture, homeopathy, and herbal therapy were used most often.[8]
- In another study, 31% of patients used supplements. The most commonly used biological therapies included garlic, echinacea, herbal mixtures, glucosamine, chromium, Ginkgo biloba, fish oil, cayenne, and St John's wort.[9]
- Data from a national survey of CAM use found that in persons with diabetes 57% had used these products in the past year. Reported most often were prayer and spiritual practices, herbal remedies, commercial diets, and folk remedies.[10] A smaller percentage, 35%, reported use specifically for diabetes.

H The use of CAM therapies in specific ethnic groups with diabetes has also been reported. In Navajos with diabetes 39% used CAM therapies,[11] in Hispanics with diabetes in South Texas 49% used CAM,[12] and in a Vietnamese population with diabetes two thirds used CAM.[13]

2 Several surveys have reviewed patients' reasons for using complementary and alternative medicine.[14-16]

A According to a national survey, individuals were not dissatisfied with conventional medicine but felt that using alternative medicine was more consistent with their health care beliefs and philosophy concerning health and life.[14]

B Another survey found that the major reason for using alternative medicine was the belief that it would work.[15] Other reasons for use included prevention of illness or injuries, wellness beliefs, and treatment of specific health problems such as back pain, headache, anxiety/emotional problems, neck pain, musculoskeletal problems, and infections. Patients who used alternative medicine in combination with conventional care believed that complementary medicine may "work and achieve faster resolution of symptoms."[15]

C Reasons for use reported in another survey included the belief of added benefits, lower cost, and perceived fewer side effects of alternative agents.[16] In this survey, the converse belief was expressed that prescription medications may cause more side effects or that natural medicines are better.

D Reasons for use have also included "health or good for you" as well as "diet supplement." A frequently cited reason was for prophylaxis, most often for osteoporosis and "colds or influenza."[5]

E Patients with diabetes have felt that complementary therapies were useful but less so than their pharmaceuticals.[9]

Reasons for Concern Regarding Use of Complementary Therapies

1 As with conventional medicines, 2 issues arise with use of complementary therapies—potential side effects and/or drug interactions. Other concerns include variability of products, problems with standardization, contamination, or misidentification. Furthermore, there are additional costs with using complementary and alternative medicines and potential delays in initiation of more effective interventions.

A Since less than 40% of patients tell their healthcare provider they are using these treatments,[2,4] a patient may experience a side effect that the provider may attribute to another medication. Many serious side effects have been experienced by patients taking complementary therapies.[17,18]

B Another concern is potential drug interactions.[19,20] Since patients with diabetes often take other medications, concomitant use of complementary therapies may result in toxicity secondary to exaggerated or subtherapeutic effects from their medications.

2 The variability of products is another issue of concern.

A Products are available as capsules and tablets as well as other forms including water extracts (also called decoctions or infusions), tinctures (hydroalcoholic extracts), and glycerides (glycerin-extracted preparations that are alcohol-free).

B The quality of botanical products may depend on what part of the plant was used, how it was grown and stored, length of storage, the processing technique, and how the extract was prepared.[18] Contamination of CAM products used to treat diabetes has been reported.[21,22]

C Some products are available in a form that is standardized for pharmacologic activity. Standardization should guarantee consistency from batch to batch and stability of the active ingredients. However, standardization is not a simple process because the active constituents are unknown for many botanicals. A product that is standardized for 1 or more markers may show consistency, but the marker may not be the active ingredient. Pharmacologic action may be due to additive or synergistic effects of several ingredients, none of which separately has the same activity as the whole plant.[23]

D Active constituents in extracts or dried botanicals may vary secondary to differences in geographic location and/or soil, exposure to sunlight and/or rainfall, harvest time, and methods of drying, storage, and processing. These variables may affect pharmacologic activity.[24]

E Other factors involve potential misidentification, mislabeling, and possibly the addition of unnatural toxic substances, such as adulteration with heavy metals or steroids and contamination with microbes, pesticides, fumigants, and radioactive products.[24] A recent example is the inadvertent substitution of Aristolochia serpentaria for Stephania tetranda in a weight-loss product that resulted in Chinese herb nephropathy.[25]

3 Another concern is the potential increased indirect cost of diabetes care because patients may substitute ineffective complementary therapies or delay treatment with proven therapeutic agents. These costs may include increased hospitalizations, acute complications such as ketoacidosis, acute hyperglycemia, or chronic complications such as retinopathy.[6] Other potential costs include decreased work productivity and diminished ability to function in a social or occupational setting.

Dietary Supplement Health and Education Act of 1994

1 Biological complementary therapies are classified as dietary supplements. Prior to 1994, these products were classified as foods or drugs, depending on their intended use. In 1994, Congress passed the Dietary Supplement Health and Education Act (DSHEA). This legislation created a separate category for botanicals and other products that classifies them as dietary supplements.[26]

A Under this legislation, these products are not required to undergo the same stringent approval process that is required for drugs and hence do not require proof of safety and effectiveness to be marketed.

B The reclassification has resulted in a serious dilemma. Sometimes contaminants or substitutes have been found in the products. For instance, diabetes products have been contaminated with lead [21,22] and plantain contaminated with digitalis produced bradycardia and heart block.[27]

C A possible solution would be the use of standardized products. Standardization guarantees that each dose provides a consistent level of the active ingredient. However, proponents of biological complementary therapies argue that standardized extracts may not always contain all of the therapeutic ingredients found in the natural product.

2 The DSHEA allows manufacturers of biological complementary therapies to make claims regarding the ability to maintain "structure and function" of the body, but not regarding diagnosis, treatment, cure, or prevention of disease.[26]

A If a manufacturer makes a claim stating the product affects body structure or function, the label must include the following statement: "This statement has not been evaluated by the Food and Drug Administration (FDA). This product is not intended to diagnose, treat, cure, or prevent any disease."

B The manufacturer must also notify the FDA within 30 days after a product is on the market if it bears such a label.

3 In January 2000, the FDA implemented new regulations that banned implied as well as expressed disease claims.[26] For example, any claims made by a manufacturer that a patient could misconstrue easily as a treatment or prevention of a disease are no longer allowed.

A The definition of disease was also changed so that symptoms associated with different life stages are no longer considered diseases. Some examples include hot flashes associated with menopause or wrinkles associated with aging.

B In the new regulations, a product may make health maintenance claims but not disease claims ("maintains a healthy prostate" is allowed but not "treats benign prostatic hyperplasia").

4 The FDA has published a Dietary Supplement Strategy (Ten Year Plan).[28] This plan sets the year 2010 as the goal for the FDA to have a "science-based regulatory program that fully implements DSHEA, in an effort to provide consumers with a high level of confidence in the safety, composition, and labeling of dietary supplement products." This program will assist diabetes educators in providing better information to persons with diabetes who use complementary therapies.

5 Testing of dietary supplements is now possible to verify accuracy and purity of the product ingredients listed on the label. However, efficacy is not evaluated. Two independent organizations have established certification programs of dietary supplements. These entities include the US Pharmacopeia (USP) and NSF International (formerly known as National Sanitation Foundation).

A The USP program is called the Dietary Supplement Verification Program.[29] A product containing the DSVP mark on the label indicates the label product ingredients are accurate, the product is pure, and the product has been manufactured using good manufacturing practices (GMPs).

B NSF International also verifies products for label and content accuracy, checks purity and contaminants, and audits the manufacturing process for GMP compliance.[30]

C Consumer Lab is also testing supplements.[31] It tests certain classes for accuracy of ingredient content and purity. All 3 entities require manufacturers to pay for testing.[32]

D Consumer Reports also tests different groups of products and reports findings in their publication.[33]

E Another group, the National Nutritional Foods Association (NNFA), has also launched a GMP program. More information may be obtained at the following Web site: http://www.nnfa.org/services/science/gmp.htm.

Evaluating Claims From Manufacturers of Dietary Supplements

1 Diabetes educators should be aware of deceptive marketing tactics that manufacturers may use to promote their products. The National Council for Reliable Health Information identified certain claims that may be questionable, such as claims made using "borrowed" science (information taken from other sources that is adopted as one's own), misrepresenting data (partially accurate information but with the truth "bent"), stating that research is underway, using testimonials, providing poorly designed research (available only in abstract form), promoting a patent (a patent only means that a product is unique; it has no safety or efficacy claims), or stating that research is unavailable. Even products that do have research supporting their use are often not the same forms commonly available in the United States.

2 The FDA Center for Food Safety and Applied Nutrition has established a Web site for consumers to evaluate information about dietary supplements. The Web site is Tips for the Savvy Supplement User: Making Informed Decisions and Evaluating Information. It is available at: http://www.cfsan.fda.gov/~dms/ds-savvy.html. The Web site includes basic points to consider such as checking with a healthcare provider before using a supplement, broaching the issue that some supplements may interact with prescription or over-the-counter medicines, unwanted effects during surgery, how to report adverse effects of dietary supplements. Furthermore, tips are given on searching the web for information on dietary supplements, such as finding out who operates the site, the purpose of the site, information source and references, or whether the information is current.

3 Diabetes educators may obtain information about specific products through a literature review. The following information published in The Health Professional's Guide to Popular Dietary Supplements[34] also may be helpful:

A Review the product label for clarity or unrealistic claims. If such claims appear, the manufacturer may not be following DSHEA rules.

B The United States Pharmacopeia (USP) symbol on supplements ensures standards for disintegration, dissolution, purity, strength, packaging, labeling, and weight variation.

C Other products may have the National Formulary (NF) designation alone or in addition to USP. This indicates the product complies with NF standards. Neither USP nor NF labeling indicates efficacy.

D Some brands provide information about standardization, which ensures that supplements contain the same amount of the product's active ingredient from bottle to bottle and pill to pill.

E Check the manufacturer name. Nationally known companies are more likely to have strict quality control and good manufacturing practices (GMPs).

F Some companies import products tested in Europe. A list of these is included in The Complete German Commission E Monographs: Therapeutic Guide to Herbal Medicines.[35]

G When contacting the manufacturer, the following questions from The Health Professional's Guide to Popular Dietary Supplements[34] can serve as a guide:

- Has the product been evaluated in clinical studies published in peer-reviewed journals? If so, can the company share these studies?
- Can the manufacturer explain the pharmacologic mechanism? Is there research to support this mechanism?
- Does the company complete an analysis on the active and inert ingredients?
- Does the company complete an analysis on the final product to insure that contents in the package match what is on the label?
- Does the product meet bioavailability standards for disintegration dissolution?
- Are there any storage/stability issues?
- What are product use contraindications?

Biological Complementary Therapies Used for Diabetes and Its Complications

1 Botanical biological complementary therapies used to lower blood glucose include *Gymnema sylvestre* R.Br., fenugreek (*Trigonella foenum-graecum*), bitter melon (*Momordica charantia*), ginseng (*Panax ginseng*), and nopal (*Opuntia streptacantha*). Claims have been made for aloe, bilberry, and milk thistle (*Silybum marianum*) but there is less evidence for these and other products.

2 Nonbotanical biological complementary therapies thought to lower blood glucose include chromium, vanadium, coenzyme Q10, and nicotinamide.

3 Biological complementary products thought to decrease the complications of diabetes include the vitamin-like substance alpha-lipoic acid, vitamin E, and magnesium as well as the botanical products gamma linolenic acid, Ginkgo biloba, and garlic. (See Chapter 1, Medical Nutrition Therapy for Diabetes, in Diabetes Management Therapies, for information on vitamin E and magnesium.)

4 Another biological complementary product frequently used is St John's wort, which is used to treat depression rather than diabetes or its complications.

Botanical Products That May Lower Blood Glucose Levels

1 *Gymnema sylvestre* R.Br., a member of the milkweed family, is a woody climbing plant that is found in the tropical forests of India and also in Africa.[36,37] Gymnema leaf has been used for centuries to treat diabetes and as a digestive system stimulant, anti-malarial, laxative, and diuretic. Its chemical constituents include the gymnemic acids (gymnemosides), saponins, stigmasterol, quercitol, and the amino acid derivatives betaine, choline, and trimethylamine.[38]

A Although the exact mechanism of action of gymnema is unknown, there are a variety of theorized mechanisms.
- Besides impairing the ability to discriminate sweet taste,[36] gymnema may increase the enzyme activity responsible for glucose uptake and utilization.[39]
- Other research has shown that gymnema may stimulate beta cell function, increase beta cell number, and/or increase insulin release by increasing cell permeability to insulin.[40]
- In pancreatectomized animals, no hypoglycemic effect is seen with gymnema use, indicating that residual beta cell function may be necessary to exert this effect.[41]

B No side effects of gymnema use have been reported. Gymnema may produce hypoglycemia and may have additive hypoglycemic effects with either insulin or insulin secretagogues. Doses of existing drug therapy may have to be adjusted if gymnema is used.

C There are only a few human studies but no randomized controlled trials studying gymnema. There is limited evidence of efficacy of gymnema in humans. Uncontrolled trials conducted in persons with type 1 and type 2 diabetes reported decreases in levels of A1C, fasting blood glucose, and lipids.[42,43] However, these studies did not report important details of study design, such as blinding and randomization.

D Typical doses are 400 mg/day, standardized to contain 24% gymnemic acids. The product should not be used without medical supervision.

2 Fenugreek (*Trigonella foenum-graecum*) is a member of the *Leguminosae* family along with other plants such as chickpeas, peanuts, and green peas.[36,37] The plant grows in India, Egypt, and other parts of the Middle East. It has been used as a cooking spice and flavoring agent for centuries.[37]

A The seed extracts are used to flavor imitation maple syrup. It has also been used as a medicinal agent to treat diabetes, constipation, and hyperlipidemia.

B Topically it has been used to treat inflammation, and it has been used postpartum with a substance called jaggery to promote lactation. Since the taste and odor resemble maple syrup, it has been used to mask the taste of medicines.

C Due to high fiber content, fenugreek is thought to delay gastric emptying, slow carbohydrate absorption, and inhibit glucose transport.[44] It has been shown to increase erythrocyte insulin receptors and improve peripheral glucose utilization, thus showing potential pancreatic as well as extra-pancreatic effects.[45] One potential active constituent, 4-hydroxy-isoleucine, may directly stimulate insulin secretion.[37]

D The main side effects of fenugreek are flatulence and diarrhea, which subside after a few days. It also has uterotonic properties.[37]

- Hypersensitivity reactions have occurred, including rhinorrhea, wheezing, and fainting after inhalation of the seed powder. Wheezing and facial angioedema was reported in a patient with chronic asthma after application of a topical fenugreek paste for dandruff.[46]

- Because of the coumarin constituents, fenugreek may potentially increase the risk of bleeding if combined with drugs or herbs with anticoagulant activity.[37] There is now a case report of an interaction between warfarin and and a product containing the digestive agent, boldo, in combination with fenugreek. The result was an increase in international normalized ratio (INR).[47]

- It may inhibit corticosteroid drug activity, interfere with hormone therapy, and potentiate MAO inhibitor activity.[37]

E There are few human studies on fenugreek; most are short term involving few patients, and details of the study design are not well reported. Most studies have used unusual forms of fenugreek, such as defatted seed powder in "chapati" (unleavened bread) or powdered fenugreek seed. Although clinical studies have been done in both type 1 and type 2 diabetes, details of the study design are often sketchy or missing.[48-50] A recent study indicated that in 25 newly diagnosed patients with type 2 diabetes, fenugreek improved glycemic control, decreased insulin resistance, and improved hypertriglyceridemia.[51]

F In the United States, fenugreek has been categorized as Generally Recognized as Safe (GRAS). The recommended dose has varied. One author recommended a dose of 1 to 2 g of the seed or the equivalent 3 times daily, or 1 cup of the tea several times a day, prepared by steeping 500 mg of seed in 150 mL of cold water.[37] These doses are lower than those used in the clinical studies, which ranged from 15 g to 50 g twice daily.

3 Bitter melon (*Momordica charantia*) is also known by other names such as bitter gourd, bitter apple, bitter cucumber, karolla, and karela. It is a vegetable cultivated in tropical areas, including India, Asia, South America, and Africa. The vegetable is yellow-orange, resembles a gherkin, and is bitter but edible. It has been used as an ingredient in certain curries.[36,37] Bitter melon has been used to treat diabetes, for HIV supportive therapy and psoriasis, and has been studied as a potential contraceptive agent.[36,37]

A The bitter melon fruit and fruit extracts are thought to contain the active ingredients and seem to have hypoglycemic effects in human and diabetes animal models.[37] However, hypoglycemic activity may be dependent on viable beta cell function.[52]

B Certain adverse events including severe hypoglycemia, favism, and potential uterine bleeding and contractions may occur.[37] It has also been shown to have additive hypoglycemic properties when combined with chlorpropamide.[53]

- It should not be used by children, and in pregnant women there is a potential for miscarriage.[37]
- Other cautions include the potential for additive hypokalemia when combined with other medications or herbs that lower serum potassium, such as stimulant laxatives, diuretics, or botanicals such as licorice rhizome. Bitter melon may produce gastrointestinal discomfort.
- Hypoglycemic coma from a tea containing bitter melon has been reported in 2 children as well as favism, which is characterized by headache, fever, abdominal pain, and coma.[36,37]
- The red arils around the seeds have produced toxicity; vomiting, diarrhea, and death occurred in a child.[36]

C Most studies of bitter melon in humans involve few patients, are of short duration, and provide only vague details of the study design, including blinding and randomization. Studies have been done primarily in type 2 diabetes,[54-56] although a small study using injectable polypeptide-P, an insulin-like polypeptide, included patients with type 1 diabetes.[55] Results from these various studies have shown that there are responders as well as nonresponders. Long-term studies have not been done, but 1 trial in a small number of patients demonstrated a decline in A1C levels after 7 weeks.[57]

D There is insufficient information to recommend a reliable dose of bitter melon.[37] Various forms have been used in research, including powdered, extract, juice, and the cooked vegetable. Some sources recommended eating 1 small unripe melon daily or drinking 50 mL of fresh juice daily with food.[36] Tinctures and oral forms are starting to become available. Medical supervision is always necessary when using bitter melon.

4 Different products are called ginseng. The 3 most commonly used are *Panax ginseng* CA Meyer (Asian or Korean ginseng), *Panax quinquefolius L* (American ginseng), or *Eleutherococcus senticosus Maximum* (Russian or Siberian ginseng). The root of the plant is used.[36] Korean and American ginseng belong to the plant family *Araliaceae* and the genus *Panax*. They contain saponins or ginsenosides. Siberian ginseng belongs to a separate genus, *Eleutherococcus*, and contains eleutherosides, including lignans and other phenylpropanoid glycosides such as coumarins.[37]

A Ginseng has been described as an adaptogen, which is a drug that may increase resistance to adverse influences such as infection and stress.[58] Individuals use ginseng to enhance physical or psychomotor performance and cognitive function and for immunomodulation, infections, and diabetes.[59]

B *Panax ginseng* contains a family of steroid-like compounds called ginsenosides. Although there are many ginsenoside subtypes, they are tetracyclic triterpenoid saponin glycosides thought to have various, often opposing, hormonal and central nervous system (CNS) effects.

C Some individual compounds show contradictory effects. For example, ginsenoside Rg1 has hypertensive and CNS stimulant effects while ginsenoside Rb1 has hypotensive and CNS depressant effects.[36,58]

D Ginseng has also been used to treat diabetes. However, only Korean and American ginseng has been studied in diabetes.

- In diabetes, the mechanism of beneficial effect of ginseng is unknown. Animal research has indicated that ginseng may lower blood glucose by decreasing the rate of carbohydrate absorption into the portal hepatic circulation and possibly increasing glucose transport and uptake. Another potential mechanism may involve modulation of insulin secretion. Some ginseng fractions have increased the serum insulin level and glucose-stimulated insulin secretion in mice.[60]

E Side effects of ginseng include hypertension, estrogenic effects, hepatitis, insomnia, nervousness, neurologic effects, and possibly other psychiatric effects. The most commonly reported side effects of ginseng are nervousness and excitation.[36,37]

- The ginseng abuse syndrome is a controversial adverse effect reported in 14 of 133 long-term users of high daily doses.[61] The syndrome consisted of hypertension, nervousness, sleeplessness, skin eruptions, increased libido, and morning diarrhea.

- Drug interactions may occur with diuretics, estrogens, warfarin, and phenelzine (an MAO inhibitor) and potentially with steroids, hormones, and diabetes medications.[37] Preliminary evidence indicates ginseng may inhibit medications metabolized by the Cytochrome P450 (CYP450) 2D6 isoenzyme system, resulting in approximately a 6% increase in serum drug concentrations.[37] Consequently this may increase the effect of many medications such as beta blockers and certain antidepressants or neuroleptics as well as certain pain medications including codeine and other opiates.

- Ginseng products have been found to be adulterated with other substances, including mandrake root or phenylbutazone; 1 case even led to a positive doping test in an athlete.[62] Furthermore, there has been inconsistency between the actual amount of active ginsenosides contained in ginseng products and the amount stated on the label.[63]

- Concomitant use of ginseng with diabetes agents may cause hypoglycemia. Furthermore, patients may lose hypertension control due to possible increases in blood pressure.

F Ginseng has been studied extensively. A recent meta-analysis evaluated the effects of ginseng on physical or psychomotor performance, cognitive function, immunomodulation, and other miscellaneous uses.[59] This analysis, which comprised only randomized, placebo-controlled studies, showed suboptimal efficacy of ginseng.

- Ginseng 100 mg or 200 mg daily was compared to placebo in patients with newly diagnosed type 2 diabetes. Although baseline values for glucose and A1C levels were not given, lowered A1C values were reported.[64] However, the A1C level in the 200-mg ginseng group was 6% and 6.5% in the 100-mg and placebo groups, which may be considered an irrelevant difference by many clinicians.

- In two other studies American ginseng was reported to acutely lower postprandial glucose levels.[60,65]

- In a double-blind crossover trial, Korean red ginseng has been shown to improve erectile dysfunction, which may be of importance to patients with diabetes.[66]

G Typical doses of ginseng are 200 to 600 mg/day.[37] These doses are lower than in the study using American ginseng (capsules), which used 3 g/day, but higher than the tablets used in the study of newly diagnosed patients with diabetes, 100 and 200 mg per day. Other forms of ginseng that have been used range from fresh and dried roots to extracts, solutions, sodas, teas, and cosmetics. The root contains at least 1.5% ginsenosides. Length of use should be limited to 3 months, due to concerns about hormone-like effects.[35]

5 Nopal (*Opuntia streptacantha*), also known as prickly pear, is a member of the cactus family.[36] Multiple species are known as *Opuntia*, including *Opuntia megacantha*, *Opuntia ficus indica*, and *Opuntia fuliginosa*. Research has focused on *Opuntia streptacantha Lemaire* to lower blood glucose. Nopal stems are used as a food source in Mexico. Leaves and stems are also used for other reasons, such as for treating diabetes and hyperlipidemia. Nopal contains mucopolysaccharide soluble fibers and phytochemicals.[37]

    A The mechanism of nopal action is unknown. Animal research has shown that activity does not depend on the presence of insulin since hypoglycemic activity is seen in pancreatectomized animals.[67] The fiber content of nopal may help decrease intestinal glucose absorption. Another theorized mechanism is increased insulin sensitivity.[68]

    B Reported adverse effects include increased stool volume, frequency, abdominal fullness, and dermatitis.[37] The potential for additive hypoglycemia with insulin secretagogues is a theoretical concern.

      - There are no known risks with nopal use, but long-term studies with good study design have not been done.

    C Most trials with nopal have been small and published in Spanish only, although abstracts are available in English. In 2 small trials in persons with type 2 diabetes, the acute glucose response of nopal, water, and zucchini were compared.[68,69] A decrease in the postprandial glucose response from nopal was noted.

    D The dose used is 100 to 500 g of broiled or fresh nopal stems taken with meals.[37] However, ideal doses and the optimal preparation have not been established.

6 Aloe is a desert plant with a cactus-like appearance that belongs to the family *Liliaceae*.[36] There are over 500 species, but the most familiar form is aloe vera. There are 2 forms: dried juice from the leaf and aloe gel.[36]

    A The dried aloe juice is latex from pericyclic cells obtained beneath the skin of leaves that has evaporated to form a sticky substance known as drug aloes or aloe.

    B Aloe gel is obtained from the inner portion of the leaves and contains a polysaccharide, glucomannan, that is similar to guar gum.

    C Aloe gel is used topically for burns, sunburn, wound healing, moisturizing, and other skin problems, including psoriasis and seborrhea. Orally it has also been used to enhance the immune system and treat asthma and diabetes.

    D The mechanism of action of aloe is not well documented.

    E In laxative form, aloe may cause abdominal cramps and pain with subsequent fluid and electrolyte disturbances. No problems have been reported with topical use. The laxative form may deplete potassium, predisposing persons to cardiac abnormalities and may potentially interact with glycosides because of the hypokalemic effects.[37]

Additive cathartic effects may also occur when different laxatives are combined, and additive hypokalemia may occur when aloe is coadministered with other drugs that deplete potassium, such as diuretics and corticosteroids.

- It is important to stress to patients that one of the oral forms of aloe could potentially produce a laxative effect that results in diarrhea and electrolyte disturbances. An aloe gel product could potentially be contaminated with the cathartic form that contains anthraquinones. As of November 5, 2002, the FDA is requiring the removal of aloe laxatives from the market.[37]
- Aloe gel taken internally may exacerbate Crohn disease and ulcerative colitis.[37]

F In a small, uncontrolled study that was conducted in persons with type 2 diabetes, improvements in fasting blood glucose and A1C levels were reported with aloe use.[70]

G Doses of aloe are variable, ranging from 50 to 200 mg/day of aloe gel.[37] There is insufficient evidence for use of aloe in diabetes. Supplementation is not recommended.

7 Bilberry is a plant related to the American blueberry, cranberry, and huckleberry.[36] Two forms of bilberry are used: the dried fruit and the leaf.

A The dried fruit is used to treat diarrhea and improve night vision, cataracts, and varicose veins.[35-37]

B The leaf is used for diabetes, arthritis, and circulatory disorders.[35,36] In folk medicine, bilberry is used as a blood-sugar-reducing drug and is therefore a common constituent in antidiabetic teas. However, there are no trials in humans to document efficacy.

C Anthocyanosides are bioflavonoids, the chemical constituents in bilberry fruit that are thought to decrease vascular permeability and redistribute microvascular blood flow.[37] These substances are similar to some of the agents found in grape seed and are proposed as the active ingredients in vision and vascular-related claims.

- The mechanism of action of bilberry in diabetes may be related to the high chromium content in the bilberry leaf (9 ppm). However, further research is required to determine whether this proposed mechanism of action in diabetes is valid.

D Most of the reported adverse effects of bilberry have been benign, such as mild digestive distress, skin rashes, and drowsiness. There are no known drug interactions.

E During World War II, bilberry preserves were speculated to improve night vision in Royal Air Force pilots.[36] However, this effect has not been demonstrated in controlled trials.[71]

F Standard doses of the dried ripe berries are 20 to 60 g daily. Decoctions have also been prepared by placing 5 to 10 g of mashed berries in cold water, simmering the mixture for 10 minutes, and then straining and drinking the liquid. The leaf is prepared as a tea using 1 g of finely chopped dried leaf in 150 mL of boiling water and steeping it for 5 to 10 minutes. Overall, bilberry leaves have been constituents in antidiabetic teas, but research has not been done in humans to verify the effectiveness.[37]

8 Milk thistle (*Silybum marianum*) is a member of the aster family (*Asteraceae* or *Compositae*), which also includes daisies and thistles.[72] Milk thistle has been used extensively for various hepatic disorders. It is used for uterine complaints and stimulating menstrual flow. In Europe it is also used as a vegetable. Recently, its use has been proposed in diabetes to diminish insulin resistance.[73] Chemical constituents are found in the fruit, seeds, and leaves of the plant.

A There are several proposed mechanisms of action of milk thistle in hepatic disease or impairment.[72] One mechanism is inhibition of hepatotoxin binding to hepatocyte membrane receptor sites. Another mechanism is decreased glutathione oxidation, which may replenish diminished glutathione levels in the liver and intestines.

- Lipoperoxidation may adversely affect patients with diabetes and replenishment of antioxidants may improve diabetes.[73]

B Side effects of milk thistle include diarrhea, weakness, sweating, and possible allergic reactions in persons who have sensitivity to ragweed, chrysanthemums, marigolds, and daisies.[37,72]

- No known adverse interactions have been reported with milk thistle. Beneficial interactions, however, have included attenuation of hepatotoxicity associated with acetaminophen, antipsychotics, halothane, and alcohol.[72]

C The studies that have been done evaluating milk thistle have had serious problems with study design.

- Several studies have evaluated effects of milk thistle on hepatic disease with inconclusive results.[74]
- Milk thistle was evaluated in a randomized, open-label trial in a small number of type 2 diabetes patients with cirrhosis.[73] Improvements in glycemia and liver function were reported.

D The typical dose of milk thistle for liver disease is 200 mg 3 times daily. Milk thistle extract should be standardized to contain 70% silymarin (140 mg of silymarin). Since phosphatidylcholine enhances oral absorption, preparations containing this ingredient may be dosed at 100 mg/day.[72] These doses differ from doses used in clinical studies, which ranged from 280 to 800 mg/day.

Nonbotanical Biological Complementary Products That May Lower Blood Glucose

1 Chromium is a trace element found as a trivalent or hexavalent form. The hexavalent form is a carcinogen with toxicity occurring only in industrial exposure. It is not found in chromium-containing foods such as brewer's yeast, oysters, mushrooms, liver, potatoes, beef, cheese, and fresh vegetables.[36,37]

A Chromium deficiency may occur if a patient is on total parenteral nutrition (TPN), during pregnancy, or if a patient has a poor diet, high glucose intake, or poor glucose control. There is currently no evidence to show that chromium deficiency rates are different in persons with diabetes versus the general population.

B Chromium has been used for weight loss, for its ergogenic properties, and to improve lipid and glycemic control.[36,37] Since increased chromium excretion may occur with steroid use, chromium supplementation has been used to reverse corticosteroid-induced diabetes.[75]

C The Food and Nutrition Board of the Institute of Medicine determined there was not sufficient evidence to set an estimated average requirement for chromium.[76] An adequate intake (AI) was set based on estimated mean intakes. The AI for young men is 35 µg/day and 25 µg/day for young women. Because few serious adverse effects are reported from excess intake of chromium from food, no tolerable upper level was established.

D Since there is no accurate assay for body chromium stores, it is difficult to determine when an individual has chromium deficiency and how supplementation may affect the deficiency.

E The specific mechanism by which chromium impacts glucose metabolism is unknown. It is known that chromium is an essential mineral for glucose metabolism. Supplementation is likely beneficial in deficiency states. Current knowledge is based on the effects of chromium deprivation and supplementation. The trivalent form is believed to play a role in potentiating the cellular effects of insulin. It may increase insulin receptor number, insulin binding, and/or insulin activation. The proposed overall effect of chromium may be to increase insulin or beta cell sensitivity.[77]

F Reported side effects of chromium are renal toxicity, including acute renal failure caused by severe interstitial nephritis; severe systemic illness, including hemolysis; thrombocytopenia; hepatic dysfunction; and renal failure.[36,37] Studies have demonstrated the safety of large doses of chromium III;[78] however, additive hypoglycemia with insulin or insulin secretagogues may occur.[37]

G Positive effects of chromium have been shown in persons with type 1 and type 2 diabetes.[78-80] Studies have shown variable benefits for diabetes and hyperlipidemia. Trials with negative results used less bioavailable forms of chromium, such as chromium chloride or chromium-rich yeast.

- In a randomized, double-blind placebo-controlled trial in 180 Chinese persons, fasting blood glucose and A1C levels decreased significantly in the group taking 1000 μg/day of chromium picolinate compared with the 500 μg/day group and placebo group.[78] However, these individuals may have significantly different dietary chromium intake compared with the US population and may be leaner than many obese persons with type 2 diabetes in the United States. Effects were dose-dependent and were seen within 2 months and 4 months.

- Two other controlled trials evaluating chromium chloride[81] or chromium-rich yeast[82] for lipids have shown no benefit for blood glucose and variable benefits for lipids.

- A recent meta-analysis of randomized controlled trials that evaluated the effects of chromium use on insulin and glucose reported that data are inconclusive and more studies are needed to evaluate the role of chromium supplementation in diabetes.[83]

H Although higher doses of chromium have been studied and shown to be more effective, a typical dose is 200 μg/day.[37] Dose-related responses have been shown, but the safety of higher doses is not known. Results from chromium research are not conclusive, particularly in light of lack of information regarding the most appropriate biomarkers for chromium or the most appropriate formulation. The FDA does not allow claims on chromium supplement labels regarding hypoglycemic effects.

2 Vanadium is a trace element found in several foods, including breakfast cereals, sunflower seeds, certain vegetables, grains, wine, and beer.[37] Vanadium has been used for diabetes and for bodybuilding, although it has not been found effective for bodybuilding[84] and it has limited evidence of efficacy in diabetes.

A Vanadium intake is reported to range from 6.5 to 11 μg/day for infants, children, and adolescents and from 6 to 18 μg/day for adults and the elderly.[76] Indicators for establishing an adequate intake for vanadium are not currently available. The estimate of tolerable upper level for vanadium for adults is 1.8 mg/day.

B It has been administered to humans as the sodium metavanadate and vanadyl sulfate salts.[76]

C Vanadium may function in various parts of the insulin signaling pathway.[85] It is also thought to have direct insulin-mimetic activity and may increase tissue sensitivity to insulin.[86]

D Side effects of vanadium include diarrhea, abdominal cramping, nausea, and flatulence that may last a few days.[37] Serious safety issues have been raised from animal research, such as the potential for accumulation until toxicity occurs.[87] Vanadium may potentiate the anticoagulant effects of antiplatelets and enhance therapeutic and/or adverse effects of digoxin.[37]

E Vanadium use in humans has only been evaluated in small studies. It has been studied in type 1 and type 2 diabetes. Improvements included decreased fasting plasma glucose and A1C levels, and decreased insulin requirements in patients with type 1 diabetes and enhanced insulin sensitivity in patients with type 2 diabetes.[86,88,89]

F Vanadium has not yet been shown to be essential in the diet. There is no established recommended daily allowance. The estimate of tolerable upper level for adults is 1.8 mg/day, and studies used doses far exceeding this amount (100 to 125 mg/day). Studies have been done only in small numbers of patients, and vanadium supplementation is therefore not recommended.

3 Coenzyme Q10 (CoQ10) is a vitamin-like substance that serves as a cofactor in the mitochondrial electron transport chain, necessary for ATP production. It has various antioxidant activities and may improve glucose-stimulated insulin secretion.[36,37]

A CoQ10 has been used as adjunctive therapy for various cardiac diseases, including congestive heart failure, cardiomyopathy, hypertension, angina, and certain arrhythmias. CoQ10 has also been used to treat cancer, muscular dystrophy, and periodontal disease.[90]

B In diabetes, suboptimal CoQ10 activity is thought to occur in beta cells. By increasing the activity of glycerol-3-phosphate dehydrogenase (G3PD) and improving ATP production, CoQ10 may improve glucose-stimulated insulin secretion.[91] Some patients with diabetes may take CoQ10 to replenish endogenous levels that may be lowered with the use of certain medications including beta blockers, statins, or sulfonylureas.[37] However, need for CoQ10 supplementation as a result of use of these medications has not been studied.

C Less than 1% of patients taking CoQ10 experience gastric upset, including diarrhea, nausea, anorexia, and epigastric distress. Dose-related adverse effects have included mild insomnia and slight increases in serum transaminases without hepatotoxicity.[36]

- Since CoQ10 is a structural analog of vitamin K, it has decreased international normalized ratio (INR), a measure of anticoagulant activity, when used with warfarin.[37] Diabetes educators should inform their patients that drug interactions include decreased INR with warfarin use, and CoQ10 may also interact with other medications that persons with diabetes may take.

D CoQ10 is a much-studied agent for cardiovascular disease, but the study designs have had many flaws. Endpoints have not always been acceptable or well defined. For example, although a significant decline in systolic and diastolic pressures have been reported with CoQ10 use, endpoint values are still much higher than advocated for persons with diabetes.[37,90]

E In studies of persons with type 1 and type 2 diabetes, CoQ10 supplementation has shown variable effects on diabetes endpoints, with decreases in fasting glucose and A1C, but not different than placebo.[92,93]

F Doses of CoQ10 have varied in different studies. In diabetes, the typical dose is 150 mg/day.[37] Lower doses have been studied.[93] Further studies are needed to determine the role of CoQ10 in diabetes therapy since there is insufficient evidence to warrant its use.

4 Nicotinamide is one form of vitamin B_3,[37] which is necessary for appropriate functioning of over 50 enzymes in the body. Dietary sources of nicotinamide include yeast, bran, almonds, peanuts, wild/brown rice, whole wheat, barley, and peas.[37]

A Nicotinamide is being studied in diabetes prevention[94] and has been used to improve blood glucose control.[95,96]

B The vitamin is available in 2 major forms, nicotinic acid (niacin) and nicotinamide (niacinamide). Both forms have similar effects in low doses. In high doses, they have differing effects: nicotinic acid is used as a treatment for dyslipidemia and nicotinamide for diabetes and diabetes prevention.[37]

C Nicotinamide may preserve, improve, and protect beta cell function by improving resistance to autoimmune destruction. At the intracellular level, nicotinamide may inhibit the enzyme poly (ADP-ribose) polymerase (PARP), thereby preventing depletion of NAD+. Low intracellular NAD+ levels may contribute to islet cell destruction via apoptosis.[97]

D Potential side effects of nicotinamide are varied and include headache, skin reactions, allergies, and other gastrointestinal disturbances. Nicotinamide use warrants monitoring of liver enzymes, platelet function, and blood glucose.[37] Use is contraindicated in patients with active liver disease. Nicotinamide may exacerbate gallbladder disease, gout, peptic ulcer disease, and allergies. There is a potential for decreased insulin sensitivity and decreased first phase insulin release. Nicotinamide may increase serum drug concentrations of certain anticonvulsants.[37]

E Nicotinamide trials in diabetes have focused on treatment and prevention. A meta-analysis of 10 randomized trials in recently diagnosed persons with type 1 diabetes reported higher C-peptide levels in nicotinamide-treated patients but no differences in insulin doses and A1C levels after 1 year.[95] A small single-blind trial in persons with type 2 diabetes reported improved C-peptide levels in the groups receiving nicotinamide.[96] A large nonrandomized population-based trial in high-risk children in New Zealand showed promise of decreasing the incidence of type 1 diabetes by administering nicotinamide.[94] Other trials have not shown promising results, including preliminary results from a German trial that found no effect.[37] A long-term trial, the European Nicotinamide Diabetes Intervention Trial (ENDIT), is underway to evaluate whether regular use of nicotinamide can prevent diabetes.[98] Data presented at the American Diabetes Association 2003 Scientific Sessions indicated that results from ENDIT demonstrated a lack of benefit from nicotinamide.

F A variety of doses of nicotinamide have been used, but studies have generally used a dose of 500 mg 2 or 3 times daily.[37] Although nicotinamide use may have potential merit in diabetes, caution should be exercised until long-term trial results and more information are obtained.

Biological Complementary Therapies That May Treat Complications of Diabetes

1 Alpha-lipoic acid (ALA), also known as thioctic acid, is a disulfide compound that is synthesized in the liver. ALA functions as a cofactor in enzyme complexes such as pyruvate dehydrogenase and assists in the conversion of pyruvic acid to acetyl-coenzyme A in oxidative glucose metabolism.[99] ALA may increase insulin sensitivity.[100] ALA has been widely used in Germany to treat peripheral neuropathy.[37]

   A Alpha-lipoic acid is readily converted to the reduced form, dihydrolipoic acid (DHLA). ALA and DHLA are both potent antioxidants.[101] In vitro and animal research has shown that elevated glucose may increase free radical–mediated oxidation, which in turn is implicated in the pathogenesis of diabetic neuropathy.[102] Since ALA may decrease oxidative stress (caused by increased blood glucose), it may potentially help to minimize symptoms of neuropathy.[37] Decreases in A1C levels have not been significant.[103-105]

   B To date, no serious side effects from ALA have been reported, even though it has been used in IV doses and in long-term trials.[103-105] However, ALA may produce gastrointestinal side effects and possible allergic skin conditions. Potential hypoglycemia when combined with secretagogues may occur.[101]

   C Alpha-lipoic acid has been studied in a series of Alpha-Lipoic Acid in Diabetic Neuropathy (ALADIN) trials.
   - The first trial in type 2 diabetes patients with symptomatic peripheral neuropathy reported improvements in symptoms of neuropathy after 3 weeks of intravenous (IV) ALA.[103]
   - ALADIN II was a trial in patients with type 1 or type 2 diabetes with polyneuropathy symptoms.[104] ALA was administered IV for 5 days and then orally for 2 years. Improvements were again noted in symptoms of neuropathy.
   - ALADIN III was a trial in patients with type 2 diabetes.[105] Both IV and oral ALA were studied and improvements in symptoms were noted.
   - The NATHAN I (Neurological Assessment of Thioctic Acid in Neuropathy) trial is a long-term, multicenter trial in North America and Europe that is assessing the role of oral alpha-lipoic acid in prevention and treatment of diabetes neuropathy.[106] NATHAN II will address the use of an intravenous agent for relief of painful neuropathy symptoms.

   D Typical doses of ALA are 600 to 800 mg/day.[37] Long-term trials are necessary to determine whether ALA slows the progression of neuropathy versus only improving the neuropathy symptoms. The American Diabetes Association does not recommend use of ALA.

2 Gamma linolenic acid (GLA) is an omega-6 fatty acid. The main source used in nutritional supplements is evening primrose oil,[36,37] which is extracted from the small seeds of the plant.

   A GLA is used as a nutritional supplement or as an ingredient in food products in many countries. GLA has been used to treat diabetic neuropathy, hyperlipidemia, mastitis, premenstrual syndrome (PMS), eczema, rheumatoid arthritis, and multiple sclerosis.[36]
   - Linolenic acid conversion to GLA is thought to be impaired in neuropathy, potentially leading to problems with nerve function. Supplementation with GLA may alleviate these problems.[107]

- Since A1C levels do not improve with GLA, the beneficial effects on symptoms of neuropathy are not secondary to blood glucose control.[107,108]

B Most adverse effects of GLA are mild and include headache and gastrointestinal effects such as bloating and loose stools.[37] There are reports of prolonged bleeding time and a case report of seizures.[37] If GLA is combined with phenothiazines, seizures may potentially occur because these drugs may lower the seizure threshold.[37]

C Two main clinical trials have evaluated GLA in peripheral neuropathy. A small trial in patients with type 1 and type 2 diabetes reported improvements in neuropathy scores.[107] In a 1-year, multicenter trial in patients with type 1 and type 2 diabetes who were given 480 mg of GLA, significant improvements were reported in 13 of 16 parameters of neuropathy.[108]

D Doses of GLA used to treat neuropathy are 360 to 480 mg/day.[37] For maximal absorption, it should be taken with food. The role of GLA in treating neuropathic complications is unknown at this time.

3 *Gingko biloba* is one of the world's oldest living tree species, dating back over 200 million years.[36] Extracts from dried leaves of younger trees are used in complementary therapies. Gingko biloba is one of the most widely used drugs in Germany, where it is used for cerebrovascular insufficiency and dementia.[109]

A In diabetes, Gingko biloba may be useful for peripheral circulatory problems such as intermittent claudication.[37] A recent meta-analysis evaluated the effect of Gingko biloba on intermittent claudication and reported an increase in pain-free walking distance.[110]

B There is some evidence that Gingko biloba may help with sexual dysfunction.[111,112]

C Gingko biloba has been found to be effective in patients with dementia,[113] although it has not been compared with prescription medications for Alzheimer's disease.

D In a recent report, Gingko biloba use for 3 months in type 2 hyperlinsulinemic patients (who were taking secretagogues) resulted in elevated blood glucose.[114]

E A reported side effect of gingko biloba is transient headache for the first 2 to 3 days of use. Another recently reported side effect is seizures.[115] The main drug interaction is the potential for additive antiplatelet activity when combined with antiplatelet drugs such as warfarin, aspirin, Cox-2 inhibitors such as celecoxib or rofecoxib, or with botanical products that also have antiplatelet activity, such as ginger, garlic, and feverfew.[37] Recently a case report indicated that concomitant use with a widely used antidepressant, trazodone, resulted in coma in a patient with dementia.[116]

F Doses of Gingko biloba are variable: 120 to 240 mg/day for dementia and 120 to 160 mg/day for peripheral vascular disease.[37] Gingko biloba is administered in divided doses, usually 2 to 3 times daily. Administration for 6 to 8 weeks is required to determine the benefit. The role of Gingko biloba in diabetes is still unknown.

4 Garlic, a member of the lily family, has been used in cooking for thousands of years.[36] Garlic is used for hyperlipidemia, hypertension, cancer prevention, and antibacterial activity. Garlic has been reported to reduce blood glucose in animals and humans.[117]

A Garlic contains the sulfur-based chemical constituent alliin, which must be converted to the active form, allicin, by the enzyme alliinase. This reaction occurs when the garlic bulb is chewed or crushed.[36]

B Commercial preparations of garlic usually contain alliin, not allicin or ajoene. Conversion requires alliinase, which is unstable in stomach acids. Dried garlic preparations may be effective only if the product is enteric coated to prevent gastric acid breakdown and permit release in the small intestine. Fresh garlic is effective.[36,37]

C Allicin has antibacterial and antioxidant activity. Ajoene is formed by the acid-catalyzed reaction of 2 allicin molecules. It decreases the activity of factors needed for lipid synthesis by reducing the thiol group in coenzyme A and HMG CoA reductase and by oxidizing NADPH. Ajoene has antiplatelet activity and interferes with thromboxane synthesis.[36] Another constituent, allylpropyl disulfide, may reduce blood glucose and increase insulin.[37] Researchers have noted that garlic use may be associated with increased serum insulin and improved liver glycogen storage.[118]

D Side effects of garlic include breath odor, mouth and gastrointestinal burning or irritation, heartburn, flatulence, and rare topical reactions. There are cases of spontaneous spinal epidural hematoma[119] and excessive bleeding.[120,121]

E A recently published meta-analysis of garlic reported that garlic reduced total cholesterol modestly (15.7 mg/dL).[122] Therefore, patients should be told that garlic may be of benefit only in mild hyperlipidemia. Persons with diabetes generally need more aggressive lipid-lowering agents to insure that LDL cholesterol is less than 100 mg/dL.
  - A meta-analysis of the effect of garlic on mild hypertension indicated a modest decrease in systolic blood pressure (7.7 mm Hg) and diastolic blood pressure (5 mm Hg) compared with placebo.[123] Persons with diabetes may need more aggressive antihypertensive effects than garlic can provide.
  - A review of trials that have evaluated garlic use for cardiovascular risk factors has indicated a small, short-term benefit on lipids, an insignificant effect on blood pressure, and no effect on glucose levels.[124]

F For fresh garlic, the dose is 1 clove taken 1 to 2 times daily.[37] Dried garlic powder preparations standardized to 1.3% allicin content have been used in studies. Dried garlic preparations should be enteric coated to prevent breakdown by stomach acids. The dose for garlic supplements is 600 to 900 mg/day in divided doses. More studies are needed to determine if garlic can be of any significant value in diabetes treatment.

Biological Complementary Product That May Treat Depression

1 St John's wort (*hypericum perforatum*) is a perennial that grows throughout the United States, Canada, and Europe. Its bright flowers bloom in late June, and the flowering top is used in the product.[36] It has been used to treat depression, anxiety, and insomnia.

A Side effects of St John's wort include phototoxicity,[125] as well as sleep difficulties, gastrointestinal upset, anxiety, and withdrawal-like symptoms when discontinued abruptly.[126] Patients should be counseled to wear sunscreen when using St John's wort and to gradually taper when discontinuing this product. St John's wort may also increase thyroid stimulating hormone.[127,128]

B St John's wort had been found to produce serotonin syndrome when combined with serotonergic agents such as fluoxetine (Prozac).[129] St John's wort may decrease serum concentrations of drugs that a patient with diabetes may be taking including digoxin, oral contraceptives, cyclosporine, warfarin, theophylline, certain statins, protease inhibitors, and possibly other medications.

C St John's wort has been compared with placebo and traditional antidepressants.

- The Cochrane Review assessed randomized controlled studies.[130] In about half of the studies, more patients responded to St John's wort than placebo, and fewer side effects were reported.
- Another study reported greater efficacy of St John's wort than placebo but equal efficacy when compared to the tricyclic antidepressant, imipramine.[131] St John's wort has been found equal in efficacy to the antidepressants fluoxetine,[132] and sertraline.[133] A recent study, however, reported no benefits for major depression.[134]
- Numerous studies continue to be published – some confirm the efficacy of St John's wort in mild to moderate depression. Other trials do not corroborate this effect, particularly for severe depression.[135]

D Doses of St John's wort are 300 to 600 mg 3 times daily.[37] Standardized extracts used in studies include 0.3% hypericin and the hyperforin-stabilized version of this extract. Patients should always inform their healthcare providers if they are taking St John's wort, particularly because of the potential for drug interactions with medications that diabetes patients may be using.

Other Biological Complementary Products

1 A recent systematic review by Yeh et al of herbs and dietary supplements for glycemic control is the most comprehensive review to date.[136] Most of the products included in this chapter were discussed in that publication, but the review also included other products such as *Coccinia indica*, *Bauhinia forficata*, and *Myrcia uniflora*, magnesium, vitamin E, L-Carnitine, and certain combination products. The reader may find this publication by Yeh et al a valuable resource. Quality of evidence for products reviewed was assessed using the US Preventive Services Task Force criteria[137] and the American Diabetes Association evidence grading system[138] for clinical practice recommendations.

2 Furthermore, the reader is also directed to the statement by the American Diabetes Association on unproven therapies that acknowledges the widespread use of alternative therapies and the need for cautious evaluation of these products.[139]

Key Educational Considerations

1 Because of the increasing popularity of complementary alternative medicines, diabetes educators may find themselves serving as a resource for individuals with diabetes who are interested in using such therapies. Diabetes educators should strive to familiarize themselves with current research in this area.

A An open-minded, yet evidence-based approach is important. Many individuals are reluctant to inform their healthcare providers of complementary therapy use.

B Individuals with diabetes who are considering use of these therapies are likely to be very actively involved in their own health care and should be congratulated for their initiative and interest.

C Diabetes educators should work in partnership with their patients to encourage open communication about complementary therapy use, provide safety and efficacy information about supplements, and discourage the use of dangerous or ineffective products or those for which there is little evidence.

2 Encourage patients to keep the healthcare providers informed about any dietary supplements they may be taking. Complementary therapies are not benign; they have side effects and may interact with concomitant diseases, drugs, nutrients, or other complementary therapies. Healthcare providers should know the entire spectrum of products the patient is using to provide the best possible care.

3 Advise patients that if these supplements are used, it should be in addition to the essential elements of the diabetes care regimen, such as meal planning, physical activity, and medications. They should not be used as replacements for prescribed modalities.

4 Inform patients that natural products are not necessarily safer than other products. Because most natural agents are not subject to rigorous government safety and efficacy testing, they may be potentially more dangerous than conventional forms of medication.

5 Suggest that patients do background research on a product before they begin taking it, particularly since many products are very expensive and may provide questionable health benefits. There is less published evidence for use of complementary therapies than for conventional diabetes medications. There is insufficient information to support universal use of these products by patients with diabetes and again the reader is referred to the American Diabetes Association's statement on unproven therapies.[139]

6 Teach patients to read labels carefully, look for telephone numbers and addresses on the labels of products, and ask questions of the manufacturers.

7 Tell patients to purchase products that are standardized whenever possible. Encourage patients to buy products from companies that invest in research and meet good manufacturing practice (GMP) guidelines, as noted on the product label, to ensure product purity and safety. Recent problems have included contamination of products with ingredients that were not listed on the label. Tell patients to obtain products that have been evaluated through DSVP by the USP or NSF International.

8 Tell patients about the FDA Web site that provides information for supplement users. (Tips for the Savvy Supplement User: Available at http://www.cfsan.fda.gov/~dms/ds-savvy.html).

9 Inform patients that it is usually better to start with single-ingredient products than multiple-ingredient products because if there is an adverse effect or a worsening of blood glucose, it is easier to determine which ingredient is responsible. Many healthcare providers suggest beginning with a small dose of a product and working up to the recommended dose to determine whether the supplement has any effect on blood glucose levels. For some products it may take several weeks to determine whether there is efficacy or any effect on blood glucose.

10 Advise patients to monitor their blood glucose levels frequently when taking any type of nutritional supplement and share any concerns about changes in blood glucose with their healthcare team. Remind patients that taking a pill does not make up for an unhealthy lifestyle or unhealthy behaviors.

11 Advise patients to keep records to assess progress toward desired effects such as improvements in blood glucose, lipid profile, blood pressure, weight, neuropathy symptoms, and other aspects of diabetes care.

12 Ask patients to look for expiration dates on the bottle, look for telephone numbers, or Web sites to contact the manufacturer of the product. The patient may wish to save a few pills in the bottle should the need arise to perform an assay of the product (in case of adverse effects).

13 Ask patients to consider using the product for a limited time to evaluate the effect. If there is no benefit, then discontinue use of the product.

14 A key role of educators is to help patients identify what they hope to achieve when using a biological complementary therapy, keep records of the effects, and evaluate the impact on diabetes care.

Self-Review Questions
1 What is the official FDA classification of complementary therapies?
2 Which complementary products are reported to lower blood glucose?
3 Which complementary therapies are used to treat complications of diabetes?
4 What are some side effects that may occur when complementary therapies are used?
5 What are some drug interactions that may occur when complementary therapies are used with other drugs commonly used by patients with diabetes?
6 Which complementary therapies may interact with insulin secretagogues?
7 Which complementary therapies may interact with antiplatelet agents?
8 What practical advice may be provided to patients who want to take complementary therapies?

Learning Assessment: Case Study 1
A man with type 2 diabetes and a history of deep venous thrombosis (DVT), which is a blood clot in his extremities, is seen by his diabetes educator for education. He is taking glipizide and insulin for his diabetes and warfarin, a blood thinner, for the DVT. He has heard that some complementary therapies may be useful for diabetes, and he has heard that he may even be able to discontinue insulin. Products that he has heard are useful include gymnema sylvestre, fenugreek, ginseng, and chromium.

Questions for Discussion
1 Which of the complementary therapies for diabetes that he has heard about may have an effect in lowering blood glucose?
2 What side effects could be produced by these agents?
3 Can any of them interact with his sulfonylurea? With his warfarin?

Discussion

1 All of the complementary therapies that he has heard about (gymnema, fenugreek, chromium, and ginseng) may have an effect in lowering blood glucose.

2 A side effect that may be produced by all of these agents is hypoglycemia.

3 There is the potential for additive hypoglycemia since he is taking both a sulfonylurea and insulin. Fenugreek also may produce allergic reactions and adverse gastrointestinal effects. Chromium may produce adverse renal effects and dermatologic reactions, and it may adversely affect mood. Ginseng may cause edema, increased blood pressure, and anxiety. Another concern is that both fenugreek and ginseng may interact with warfarin.

4 The patient may consider that if complementary therapies are to be used, the patient should closely monitor their effect on blood glucose and A1C levels and inform his healthcare provider so the patient may be monitored. Consider that the complementary therapy may have no impact whatsoever on blood glucose or A1C levels.

Learning Assessment: Case Study 2

A postmenopausal woman with diabetes who has retinopathy and peripheral neuropathy asks her diabetes educator about using complementary therapies to treat these complications of diabetes. In addition to diabetes, she has hypertension, hyperlipidemia, intermittent claudication, and depression. She is taking Glucovance (a combination of metformin plus glyburide), Lipitor (a statin used to treat hyperlipidemia), Norvasc (a calcium-channel blocker used to treat hypertension), Prempro (hormone replacement therapy), and Zoloft® (a serotonin-specific reuptake inhibitor [SSRI] antidepressant).

Questions for Discussion

1 What complementary therapies are thought to be useful for treating diabetes complications?
2 Are there any complementary therapies that may be useful to treat her other conditions?
3 What potential drug interactions may occur if the patient uses complementary therapies?

Discussion

1 Agents that may be useful for diabetes complications are alpha-lipoic acid, gamma linolenic acid, and bilberry.

2 Possible agents that may have some possible benefit to her other conditions are garlic for hypertension and hyperlipidemia, gingko for the intermittent claudication, and St John's wort for depression.

3 Potential drug interactions may occur with use of complementary therapies, such as additive hypoglycemia between her Glucovance and gymnema, fenugreek, momordica, ginseng, chromium, and several other botanical products. Ginseng may attenuate the beneficial effects of her antihypertensive and produce additive estrogenic effects with her hormone replacement therapy. St John's wort may produce serotonin syndrome in combination with the SSRI. Finally, St John's wort may lower blood levels of her antihypertensive medications, and she may experience an increase in blood pressure. If St John's wort is used and then stopped, consider that the dose of the antihypertensive may have to be adjusted. Specifically, if St John's wort is used, the dose of the antihypertensive may have to be increased; if stopped, the antihypertensive dose may then have to be decreased.

References

1 Marwick C. Alterations are ahead at the OAM. JAMA. 1998;280:1553-1554.

2 Eisenberg DM, Kessler RC, Foster C, Norlock FE, Calkins DR, Delbanco TL. Unconventional medicine in the United States: prevalence, costs, and patterns of use. N Engl J Med. 1993;328:246-252.

3 Miller LG, Hume A, Mehra Harris IM, Jackson EA, Kanmaz TJ, Cauffield JS, et al. White paper on herbal products. Pharmacotherapy. 2000;20:877-891.

4 Eisenberg DM, Davis RB, Ettner SL, Appel S, Wilkey S, Van Rompay, et al. Trends in alternative medicine use in the United States, 1990-1997: results of a follow-up national survey. JAMA. 1998;280:1569-1575.

5 Kaufman DW, Kelly JP, Rosenberg L, Anderson TE, Mitchell AA. Recent patterns of medication use in the ambulatory adult population of the United States. JAMA. 2002;287:337-344.

6 Gill GV, Redmond S, Garratt F, Paisey R. Diabetes and alternative medicine: cause for concern. Diabet Med. 1994;11:210-213.

7 Egede LE, Ye X, Zeng D, Silverstein MD. The prevalence and pattern of complementary and alternative medicine use in individuals with diabetes. Diabetes Care. 2002;25:324-329.

8 Leese GP, Gill GV, Houghton GM. Prevalence of complementary medicine usage within a diabetes clinic. Pract Diabetes Int. 1997;14:207-208.

9 Ryan EA, Pick ME, Marceau C. Use of alternative medicines in diabetes mellitus. Diabet Med. 2001;218:242-245.

10 Yeh GY, Eisenberg DM, Davis RB, Phillips RS. Use of complementary and alternative medicine among persons with diabetes mellitus: results of a national survey. Am J Public Health. 2002;92:1648-1652.

11 Kim C, Kwok YS. Navajo use of native healers. Arch Intern Med 1998;158:2245-2249.

12 Noel PH, Pugh JA, Larme AC, Marsh G. The use of traditional plant medicines for non-insulin dependent diabetes mellitus in South Texas. Phytother Res. 1997;11:512-517.

13 Mull DS, Nguyen N, Mull JD. Vietnamese diabetic patients and their physicians: what ethnography can teach us. West J Med. 2001;175:307-311.

14 Astin JA. Why patients use alternative medicine—results of a national study. JAMA. 1998;279:1548-1553.

15 Elder NC, Gillcrist A, Minz R. Use of alternative health care by family practice patients. Arch Fam Med. 1997;6:181-184.

16 Anderson DL, Shane-McWhorter L, Crouch B, Andersen SJ. Alternative medication use in rheumatology and geriatric patients. Pharmacotherapy. 2000;8:958-966.

17 Shaw D, Leon C, Koley S, Murray V. Traditional remedies and food supplements: a 5-year toxicological study (1991-1995). Drug Safety. 1997;17:342-356.

18 Boullata JI, Nace AM. Safety issues with herbal medicine. Pharmacotherapy. 2000;20:257-269.

19 Miller LG. Herbal medicinals: selected clinical considerations focusing on known or potential drug-herb interactions. Arch Intern Med. 1998;158:220-222.

20 Fugh-Berman A. Herb-drug interactions. Lancet. 2000;355:134-138.

21 Keen RW, Deacon AC, Delves HT, Moreton JA, Frost PG. Indian herbal remedies for diabetes as a cause of lead poisoning. Postgrad Med J. 1994;70:113-114.

22 Beigel Y, Ostfeld I, Schoenfeld N. Clinical problem-solving: a leading question. N Engl J Med. 1998;339:827-830.

23 Bonati A. How and why should we standardize phytopharmaceutical drugs for clinical validation? J Ethnopharmacol. 1991;32:195-197.

24 Grant KL. Patient education and herbal dietary supplements. Am J Health Syst Pharm. 2000;57:1997-2003.

25 Nortier JL, Muniz Martinez MC, Schmeiser HH, et al. Urothelial carcinoma associated with the use of a chinese herb (Aristolochia fangchi). N Engl J Med. 2000;342:1686-1692.

26 US Food and Drug Administration. Regulation on statements made for dietary supplements concerning the effect of the product on the structure or function of the body. Fed Register. 2000;65:1000-1050.

27 Blumenthal M. Industry alert: plantain adulterated with digitalis. Herbal Gram. 1997;350:1598-1599.

28 US Food and Drug Administration. Dietary supplement strategy (ten year plan). Center for Food Safety and Applied Nutrition. Washington, DC. January 2000. Available at: http://www.cfsan.fda.gov/~dms/ds-strat.html. Accessed March 2001.

29 USP dietary supplement verification program overview. US Pharmacopeia. Available at: http://www.USP-DSVP.Org). Accessed June 14, 2003.

30 NSF dietary supplements certification program. NSF International. Ann Arbor, Mich. Available at: http://www.nsf.org.) Accessed June 14, 2003.

31 ConsumerLab.com. White Plains, NY. Available at: http://www.consumerlab.com.

32 Peterson A. New seals of approval certify unregulated herbs, vitamins. The Wall Street Journal. July 10, 2002.

33 What's in this stuff? Consumer Reports. March 1999.

34 Sarubin A. The Health Professional's Guide to Popular Dietary Supplements. Chicago: American Dietetic Association; 2000.

35 Blumenthal M, Busse WR, Goldberg A, et al, eds. The Complete German Commission E Monographs: Therapeutic Guide to Herbal Medicines. Klein S, trans. Boston: American Botanical Council; 1998.

36 The Review of Natural Products by Facts and Comparisons. St Louis, Mo: Wolters Kluwer Co; 1999.

37 Jellin JM, Gregory PJ, Batz F, Hitchens K, et al. Pharmacist's Letter/Prescribers Letter Natural Medicines Comprehensive Database 5th ed. Stockton, Ca: Therapeutic Research Faculty; 2003.

38 Kapoor LD. Handbook of Ayurvedic Medicinal Plants. Boca Raton, Fla: CRC Press; 1990:200-201.

39 Shanmugasundaram ER, Panneerselvam C, Samudram P, Shanmugasundaram ERB. Enzyme changes and glucose utilization in diabetic rabbits: the effect of gymnema sylvestre. J Ethnopharmacol. 1983;7:205-234.

40 Persaud SJ, Al-Majed H, Raman A, Jones PM. Gymnema sylvestre stimulates insulin release in vitro by increased membrane permeability. J Endocrinol. 1999;163:207-212.

41 Shanmugasundaram ERB, Gopinath KL, Radha Shanmugasundaram KR, Rajendran VM. Possible regeneration of the islets of langerhans in streptozotocin-diabetic rats given gymnema sylvestre leaf extracts. J Ethnopharmacol. 1990;30:265-279.

42 Shanmugasundaram ERB, Rajeswari G, Baskaran K, et al. Use of gymnema sylvestre leaf extract in the control of blood glucose in insulin-dependent diabetes mellitus. J Ethnopharmacol. 1990;30:281-294.

43 Baskaran K, Kizar B, Ahamath K, Radma Shanmugasundaram K, Shanmugasundaram ERB. Antidiabetic effect of a leaf extract from gymnema sylvestre in non-insulin-dependent diabetes mellitus patients. J Ethnopharmacol. 1990;30:295-306.

44 Madar Z. Fenugreek (trigonella foenum-graceum) as a means of reducing postprandial glucose levels in diabetic rats. Nutr Rep Int. 1984;29:1267-1273.

45 Raghuram TC, Sharma R, Sivakumar D, Sahay BK. Effect of fenugreek seeds on intravenous glucose disposition in non-insulin dependent diabetic patients. Phytotherapy Res. 1994;8:83-86.

46 Patil SP, Niphadkar PV, Bapat MM. Allergy to fenugreek (trigonella foenum graecum). Ann Allergy Asthma Immunol. 1997; 78:297-300.

47 Lambert JP, Cormier A. Potential interaction between warfarin and boldo-fenugreek. Pharmacotherapy. 2001;21:509-512.

48 Sharma RD, Raghuram TC, Sudhakar Rao N. Effect of fenugreek seeds on blood glucose and serum lipids in type 1 diabetes. Eur J Clin Nutr. 1990;44:301-306.

49 Madar Z, Abel R, Samish S, Arad J. Glucose-lowering effect of fenugreek in non-insulin dependent diabetics. Eur J Clin Nutr. 1988;42:51-54.

50 Sharma RD, Sarkar A, Hazra DK, et al. Use of fenugreek seed powder in the management of non-insulin-dependent diabetes mellitus. Nutr Res. 1996;16:1331-1339.

51 Gupta A, Gupta R, Lal B. Effect of Trigonella foenum-graecum (fenugreek) seeds on glycaemic control and insulin resistance in type 2 diabetes mellitus: a double blind placebo controlled study. J Assoc Physicians India. 2001;49:1057-1061.

52 Ali K, Khan AK, Mamum MI, Mosihuzzaman M, Nahar N, Nur-e-Alam M, Rokeya B. Studies on hypoglycaemic effects of fruit pulp, seed, and whole plant of momordica charantia on normal and diabetic model rats. Planta Med. 1993;56:408-412.

53 Aslam M, Stockley IH. Interaction between curry ingredient (karela) and drug (chlorpropamide). Lancet. 1979;i:607.

54 Ahmad N, Hassan MR, Halder H, Bennoor KS. Effect of momordica charantia (karolla) extracts on fasting and postprandial serum glucose levels in NIDDM patients. Bangladesh Med Res Counc Bull. 1999;25:11-13.

55 Khanna P, Jain SC, Panagariya A, Dixit VP. Hypoglycemic activity of polypeptide-p from a plant source. J Nat Prod. 1981;44:648-655.

56 Akhtar MS. Trial of momordica charantia linn (karela) powder in patients with maturity-onset diabetes. J Pak Med Assoc. 1982;32:106-107.

57 Srivastava Y, Venkatakrishna-Bhatt H, Verma Y, Venkaiah K. Antidiabetic and adaptogenic properties of Momordica charantia extract: an experimental and clinical evaluation. Phytother Res. 1993;7:285-289.

58 Raman A, Houston P. Herbal products—ginseng. Pharm J. 1995;255:150-152.

59 Vogler BK, Pittler MH, Ernst E. The efficacy of ginseng, a systematic review of randomized clinical trials. Eur J Clin Pharmacol. 1999;55:567-575.

60 Vuksan V, Sievenpiper JL, Koo VY, et al. American ginseng (Panax quinquefolius L) reduces postprandial glycemia in nondiabetic subjects and subjects with type 2 diabetes mellitus. Arch Intern Med. 2000;160:1009-1013.

61 Siegel RK. Ginseng abuse syndrome: problems with the panacea. JAMA. 1979;241:1614-1615.

62 Cui J, Garle M, Eneroth P, Bjorkhem I. What do commercial ginseng preparations contain [letter]? Lancet. 1994;344:134.

63 Harkey MR, Henderson GL, Gershwin ME, Stern JS, Hackman RM. Variability in commercial ginseng products: an analysis of 25 preparations. Am J Clin Nutr. 2001;73:1101-1106.

64 Sotaniemi EA, Haapakoski E, Rautio A. Ginseng therapy in non-insulin dependent diabetic patients. Diabetes Care. 1995;18:1373-1375.

65 Vuksan V, Stavro MP, Sievenpiper JL, et al. Similar postprandial glycemic reductions with escalation of dose and administration time of American ginseng in type 2 diabetes. Diabetes Care. 2000;23:1221-1226.

66 Hong B, Ji YH, Hong JH, Nam KY, Ahn TY. A double-blind crossover study evaluating the efficacy of korean red ginseng in patients with erectile dysfunction: a preliminary report. J Urol. 2002;168:2070-2073.

67 Ibanez-Camacho R, Roman-Ramos R. Hypoglycemic effect of opuntia cactus. Arch Invest Med. 1979;10:223-230.

68 Frati-Munari AC, Gordillo BE, Altaminrano P, Ariza CR. Hypoglycemic effect of opuntia streptacantha lemaire in NIDDM. Diabetes Care. 1988;11:63-66.

69 Frati AC, Gordillo BE, Altamirano P, Ariza CR, Cortes-Franco R, Chavez-Negrete A. Acute hypoglycemic effect of opuntia streptacantha lemaire in NIDDM [letter]. Diabetes Care. 1990;13:455-456.

70 Ghannam N. The antidiabetic activity of aloes: preliminary clinical and experimental observations. Horm Res. 1986;24:288-294.

71 Muth ER, Laurent JM, Jasper P. The effect of bilberry nutritional supplementation on night visual acuity and contrast sensitivity. Alternative Med Rev. 2000;5:164-173.

72 Pepping J. Alternative therapies—milk thistle: silybum marianum. Am J Health Syst Pharm. 1999;56:1195-1197.

73 Velussi M, Cernigoi AM, De Monte A, Dapas F, Caffau C, Zilli M. Long-term (12 months) treatment with an anti-oxidant drug (silymarin) is effective on hyperinsulinemia, exogenous insulin need and malondialdehyde levels in cirrhotic diabetic patients. J Hepatol. 1997;26:871-879.

74 Flora K, Hahn M, Rosen H, Benner K. Milk thistle (silybum marianum) for the therapy of liver disease. Am J Gastroenterol. 1998;93:139-143.

75 Ravina A, Slezak L, Mirsky N, Bryden NA, Anderson RA. Reversal of corticosteroid-induced diabetes mellitus with supplemental chromium. Diabet Med. 1999;16:164-167.

76 Food and Nutrition Board. Institute of Medicine. Dietary Reference Intakes for Vitamin A, Vitamin K, Arsenic, Boron, Chromium, Copper, Iodine, Iron, Manganese, Molybdenum, Nickel, Silicon, Vanadium, and Zinc. Washington, DC: National Academy Press; 2001.

77 Anderson R, Polansky M, Bryden N, Canary J. Supplemental chromium effects on glucose, insulin, glucagon, and urinary chromium losses in subjects consuming controlled low-chromium diets. Am J Clin Nutr. 1991;54:909-916.

78 Anderson RA, Cheng N, Bryden NA, et al. Elevated intakes of supplemental chromium improves glucose and insulin variables in individuals with type 2 diabetes. Diabetes. 1997;46:1786-1791.

79 Cefalu WT, Bell-Farrow AD, Stegner J, et al. Effect of chromium picolinate on insulin sensitivity in vivo. J Trace Elem Exp Med. 1999;12:71-83.

80 Jovanovic L, Gutierrez M, Peterson CM. Chromium supplementation for women with gestational diabetes mellitus. J Trace Elem Exp Med. 1999;12:91-107.

81 Abraham AS, Brooks BA, Eylath U. The effects of chromium supplementation on serum glucose and lipids in patients with and without non-insulin-dependent diabetes. Metabolism. 1992;41:768-771.

82 Uusitupa MJ, Mykkanen L, Siitonen O, et al. Chromium supplementation in impaired glucose tolerance of elderly: effects on blood glucose, plasma insulin, C-peptide and lipid levels. Br J Nutr. 1992;68:209-216.

83 Althuis MD, Jordan NE, Ludington EA, Wittes JT. Glucose and insulin responses to dietary chromium supplements: a meta analysis. Am J Clin Nutr. 2002;76:148-155.

84 Fawcett JP, Farquhar SJ, Walker RJ, Thou T, Lowe G, Goulding A. The effect of oral vanadyl sulfate on body composition and performance in weight-training athletes. Int J Sport Nutr. 1996;6:382-390.

85 Fantus IG, Tsiani E. Multifunctional actions of vanadium compounds on insulin signaling pathways: evidence for preferential enhancement of metabolic versus mitogenic effects. Mol Cell Biochem. 1998;182:109-119.

86 Cohen N, Halberstam M, Shlimovich P, Chang CJ, Shamoon H, Rossetti L. Oral vanadyl sulfate improves hepatic and peripheral insulin sensitivity in patients with non-insulin-dependent diabetes mellitus. J Clin Invest. 1995;95:2501-2509.

87 Domingo JL, Gomez M, Liobet JM, Corbella J, Keen CL. Oral vanadium administration to streptozotocin-diabetic rats has marked negative side effects which are independent of the form of vanadium used. Toxicology. 1991;66:279-287.

88 Boden G, Chen X, Ruiz J, van Rossum GDV, Turco S. Effects of vanadyl sulfate on carbohydrate and lipid metabolism in patients with non-insulin dependent diabetes mellitus. Metabolism. 1996;45:1130-1135.

89 Goldfine AB, Simonson DC, Folli F, Patti ME, Kahn CR. Metabolic effects of sodium metavanadate in humans with insulin-dependent and non-insulin-dependent diabetes mellitus: in vivo and in vitro studies. J Clin Endrocrinol Metab. 1995;80:3311-3320.

90 Pepping J. Alternative therapies—Coenzyme Q10. Am J Health Syst Pharm. 1999;56:519-521.

91 McCarty MF. Can correction of suboptimal coenzyme Q status improve beta-cell function in type II diabetes? Med Hypotheses. 1999;52:397-400.

92 Shigeta Y, Izumi K, Abe H. Effect of coenzyme Q7 treatment on blood sugar and ketone bodies of diabetics. J Vitaminol. 1966;12:293-298.

93 Henriksen JE, Andersen CB, Hother-Nielsen O, et al. Impact of ubiquinone (coenzyme Q10) treatment on glycaemic control, insulin requirement and well-being in patients with type 1 diabetes mellitus. Diabetic Med. 1999;16:312-318.

94 Elliott RB, Pilcher CC, Fergusson DM, et al. A population-based strategy to prevent insulin-dependent diabetes using nicotinamide. J Pediatr Endocrinol Metab. 1996;501-509.

95 Pozilli P, Browne PD, Kolb H, and the Nicotinamide Trialists. Meta-analysis of nicotinamide treatment in patients with recent-onset IDDM. Diabetes Care. 1996;19:1357-1363.

96 Polo V, Saibene A, Pontiroli AE. Nicotinamide improves insulin secretion and metabolic control in lean type 2 diabetic patients with secondary failure to sulphonylureas. Acta Diabetol. 1998;35:61-64.

97 Head KA. Type 1 diabetes: prevention of the disease and its complications. Alternative Med Rev. 1997;2:256-281.

98 Schatz DA, Bingley PA: Update on major trials for the prevention of type 1 diabetes mellitus: the American Diabetes Prevention Trial (DPT-1) and the European Nicotinamide Diabetes Intervention Trial (ENDIT). J Pediatr Endocrinol Metab. 2001;14(suppl 1):619-622.

99 Nichols TW. Alpha-lipoic acid: Biological effects and clinical implications. Alternative Med Rev. 1997;2:177-183.

100 Evans JL, Goldfine ID. Alpha-lipoic acid: a multi-functional antioxidant that improves insulin sensitivity in patients with type 2 diabetes. Diabetes Technol Ther. 2000;2:401-413.

101 Packer L. Antioxidant properties of lipoic acid and its therapeutic effects in prevention of diabetes complications and cataracts. Ann NY Acad Sci. 1994; 738:257-264.

102 Giugliano D, Ceriello A, Paolisso G. Oxidative stress and diabetic vascular complications. Diabetes Care. 1996;19: 257-267.

103 Ziegler D, Hanefeld M, Ruhnau K-J, et al, and the ALADIN Study Group. Treatment of symptomatic diabetic peripheral neuropathy with the anti-oxidant alpha-lipoic acid. A 3-week multicentre randomized controlled trial (ALADIN Study I). Diabetologia. 1995;38:1425-1433.

104 Reljanovic M, Reichel G, Rett K, et al, and the ALADIN II Study Group. Treatment of diabetic polyneuropathy with the antioxidant thioctic acid (alpha-lipoic acid): a two year multicenter randomized double-blind placebo controlled trial (ALADIN II). Alpha Lipoic Acid in Diabetic Neuropathy. Free Radic Biol Med. 1999;31:171-179.

105 Ziegler D, Hanefeld M, Ruhnau K-J, et al, and the ALADIN III Study Group. Treatment of symptomatic diabetic polyneuropathy with the antioxidant alpha-lipoic acid. A 7-month multicenter randomized controlled trial (ALADIN III Study). Diabetes Care. 1999;22:1296-1301.

106 Ziegler D, Reljanovic M, Mehnert H, Gries FA. Alpha-lipoic acid in the treatment of diabetic polyneuropathy in Germany: current evidence from clinical trials. Exp Clin Endocrinol Diabetes. 1999;107:421-430.

107 Jamal GA, Carmichael H. The effect of gamma-linolenic acid on human diabetic peripheral neuropathy: a double-blind placebo-controlled trial. Diabetic Med. 1990;7:319-323.

108 Keen H, Payan J, Allawi J, et al. Treatment of diabetic neuropathy with gamma-linolenic acid. The Gamma-Linolenic Acid Multicenter Trial Group. Diabetes Care. 1993;16:8-15.

109 Kleijnen J, Knipschild P. Ginkgo biloba. Lancet. 1992;340:1136-1139.

110 Pittler MH, Ernst E. Ginkgo biloba extract for the treatment of intermittent claudication: a meta analysis of randomized trials. Am J Med. 2000;108:276-281.

111 Cohen AJ, Bartlik B. Ginkgo biloba for antidepressant-induced sexual dysfunction. J Sex Marital Ther. 1998;24:139-143.

112 Shon M, Sikora R. Ginkgo biloba extract in the therapy of erectile dysfunction. J Sex Educ Ther. 1991;17:53-61.

113 LeBars PL, Katz MM, Berman N, Itil TM, Freedman AM, Schatzberg AF. A placebo-controlled, double-blind, randomized trial of an extract of gingko biloba for dementia. North American Egb Study Group. JAMA. 1997;278:1327-1332.

114 Kudolo GB. The effect of 3-month ingestion of Gingko biloba extract (Egb 761) on pancreatic beta-cell function in response to glucose loading in individuals with non-insulin-dependent diabetes mellitus. J Clin Pharmacol 2001;41:600-611.

115 Granger AS. Gingko biloba precipitating epileptic seizures. Age Ageing. 2001;30: 523-525.

116 Galluzzi S, Zanetti O, Binetti G, Trabucchi M, Frisoni GB. Coma in a patient with Alzheimer's disease taking low dose trazodone and gingko biloba. J Neurol Neurosurg Psychiatry. 2000;68:679-680.

117 Castleman M. The Healing Herbs. Emmaus, Penn: Rodale Press; 1991.

118 Pareddy SR, Rosenberg JM. Does garlic have useful medicinal purposes? Hosp Pharm Rep. 1993;8:27.

119 Rose KD, Croissant PD, Parliament CF, Levin MB. Spontaneous spinal epidural hematoma with associated platelet dysfunction from excessive garlic ingestion: a case report. Neurosurgery. 1990;2:880-882.

120 German K, Kumar U, Blackford HN. Garlic and the risk of TURP bleeding [letter]. Br J Urol. 1995;76:518.

121 Burnham BE. Garlic as a possible risk for postoperative bleeding [letter]. Plast Reconstr Surg. 1995;95:213.

122 Stevinson C, Pittler MH, Ernst E. Garlic for treating hypercholesterolemia, a meta-analysis of randomized clinical trials. Ann Intern Med. 2000;133:420-429.

123 Silagy CA, Neil HA. A meta-analysis of the effect of garlic on blood pressure. J Hypertens. 1994;12:463-468.

124 Ackermann RT, Mulrow CD, Ramirez G, Gardner CD, Morbidoni L, Lawrence VA. Garlic shows promise for improving some cardiovascular risk factors. Arch Intern Med. 2001;161:813-814.

125 Gulick RM, McAuliffe V, Holden-Wiltse J, et al. Phase I studies of hypericin, the active compound in St John's wort, as an antiretroviral agent in HIV-infected adults. Ann Intern Med. 1999;130:510-514.

126 Beckman SE, Sommi RW, Switzer J. Consumer use of St John's wort. A survey on effectiveness, safety, and tolerability. Pharmacotherapy. 2000;20:568-574.

127 Ferko N, Levine MA. Evaluation of the association between St John's wort and elevated thyroid-stimulating hormone. Pharmacotherapy. 2001;21:1574-1578.

128 Hauben M. The association of St John's wort with elevated thyroid-stimulating hormone. Pharmacotherapy. 2002;22:673-675.

129 Lantz MS, Buchalter DO, Giambanco V. St John's wort and antidepressant drug interactions in the elderly. J Geriatr Psychiatry Neurol. 1999;12:7-10.

130 Linde K, Mulrow CD. St John's wort for depression. Cochrane Rev [computer software]. In: The Cochrane Library. Oxford: Update software; 2000.

131 Woelk H. Comparison of St John's wort and imipramine for treating depression: randomized controlled trial. BMJ. 2000;321:536-539.

132 Shrader E. Equivalence of St John's wort (ZE117) and fluoxetine: a randomized, controlled study in mild-moderate depression. Int Clin Psychopharmacol. 2000;15:61-68.

133 Brenner R, Azbel V, Madhusoodanan S, Pawlowska M. Comparison of an extract of hypericum (LI 160) and sertraline in the treatment of depression: a double-blind, randomized pilot study. Clin Ther. 2000;22:411-419.

134 Selton RC, Keller MB, Gelenberg A, et al. Effectiveness of St John's wort in major depression; a randomized control trial. JAMA. 2001;285:1978-1986.

135 Hypericum Depression Trial Study Group. Effect of Hypericum perforatum (St John's wort) in major depressive disorder: a randomized controlled trial. JAMA. 2002;287:1807-1814.

136 Yeh GY, Eisenberg DM, Kaptchuk TJ, Phillips RS. Systematic review of herbs and dietary supplements for glycemic control in diabetes. Diabetes Care. 2003;26:1277-1294.

137 US Preventive Services Task Force. Guide to Clinical Preventive Services: An Assessment of the Effectiveness of 169 Interventions. Baltimore, MD: Williams and Wilkins, 1989.

138 American Diabetes Association. Standards of medical care for patients with diabetes mellitus (position statement). Diabetes Care. 2002;25(suppl 1):S33-S49.

139 American Diabetes Association. Unproven therapies (position statement). Diabetes Care. 2003;26:S142.

Suggested Readings and Web Sites

Bisset NG, ed. A Handbook for Practice on a Scientific Basis. Boca Raton, Fla: Medpharm Scientific Publications CRC; 1996.

Dietary Supplement Strategy (Ten Year Plan), Letter From the Director. Washington, DC: US Food and Drug Administration Center for Food and Safety and Applied Nutrition; January 2000. Available on the Internet at: http://www.cfsan.fda.gov/~dms/ds-strat.html. Accessed January 2003.

Food and Nutrition Board. Institute of Medicine. Dietary Reference Intakes. Washington, DC: National Academies Press; 2002. Available on the Internet at: http//www.nap.edu. Accessed May 2003.

FDA public health advisory: Risk of drug interactions with St John's Wort and Indinavir and other drugs. Washington, DC: US Food and Drug Administration Center for Drug Evaluation and Research; February 10, 2000. Available on the Internet at www.fda.gov/cder/drug/advisory/stjwort.htm. Accessed June 14, 2003.

FDA talk paper: FDA finalizes rules for claims on dietary supplements. Rockville, Md: US Food and Drug Administration Center for Food Safety and Applied Nutrition. January 5, 2000. Available on the Internet at: http://vm.cfsan.fda.gov/~lrd/tpdsclm.html. Accessed January 2003.

Food and Nutrition Information Center. US Department of Agriculture Agricultural Research Service, National Agricultural Library. Available on the Internet at: http://www.nal.usda.gov/fnic. Accessed May 2003.

Gruenwald S, Brenoller T, Jaenicke L, eds. PDR for Herbal Medicine. Montvale, NJ: Medical Economics Co; 1999.

International Bibliographic Information on Dietary Supplements (IBIDS) Database. National Institutes of Health Office of Dietary Supplements. Available on the Internet at: http://ods.od.nih.gov/databases/ibids.html. Accessed January 2003.

Leung AY, Foster S. Encyclopedia of Common Natural Ingredients Used in Foods, Drugs, and Cosmetics. 2nd ed. New York: John Wiley & Sons; 1995.

National Council Against Health Fraud. Available on the Internet at: http://www.ncahf.org. Accessed January 2003.

National Institutes of Health National Center for Complementary and Alternative Medicine (NCCAM). Available on the Internet at: http://www.nccam.nih.gov. Accessed January 2003.

Newall CA, Anderson LA, Phillipson JD. Herbal Medicines: A Guide for Health-Care Professionals. London: Pharmaceutical Press; 1996.

Tips for the Savvy Supplement User; Available on the Internet at http://www.cfsan.fda.gov/~dms/ds-savvy.html

Tyler VE. Herbs of choice. In: The Therapeutic Use of Phytomedicinals. Binghamton, NY: Pharmaceuticals Products Press; 1994.

United States Pharmacopeia (USP). Available on the Internet at: http://www.usp.org. Accessed January 2003.

Yeh GY, Eisenberg DM, Kaptchuk TJ, Phillips RS. Systematic review of herbs and dietary supplements for glycemic control in diabetes. Diabetes Care. 2003; 26:1277-1294.

Learning Assessment: Post-Test Questions

Biological Complementary Therapies in Diabetes   **7**

1 Legislation that determines that complementary therapies may be sold as dietary supplements is called:
  A The FDA 10-year plan
  B Dietary Supplement Health and Education Act (DSHEA)
  C Complementary and Alternative Medicine ruling
  D There is no official legislation

2 The most likely mechanism of action of gymnema is:
  A Inhibition of glucose absorption
  B Beta cell stimulation and/or increase in insulin release
  C Increase in cell permeability to insulin
  D All of the above

3 Which of the following is a cofactor in the Krebs cycle?
  A Alpha-lipoic acid
  B Vanadium sulfate
  C Chromium
  D Nicotinamide

4 Which of the following agents may be used to treat complications of diabetes?
  A Alpha-lipoic acid
  B Gamma linolenic acid
  C Gingko biloba
  D All of the above

5 Which of the following complementary therapies have antiplatelet activity?
  A Garlic
  B Gingko biloba
  C Fenugreek
  D Vanadium
  E All of the above
  F None of the above

6 Which of the following is thought to lower serum concentrations of other drugs?
  A St John's wort
  B Nicotinamide
  C Alpha-lipoic acid
  D Vanadium sulfate

7 Which of the following are derived from botanicals?
  A Alpha-lipoic acid
  B Vanadium sulfate
  C Nicotinamide
  D All of the above
  E None of the above

8 Which of the following have more than one form that is used medicinally?
  A Aloe
  B Bilberry
  C Nicotinamide
  D All of the above
  E A and B only

9 Which of the following could potentially cause nephrotoxicity?
  A Alpha-lipoic acid
  B Nicotinamide
  C Vanadium sulfate
  D Chromium

10 What are some practical tips that may be provided to patients with diabetes who want to use complementary therapies?
  A Always evaluate the effect of these therapies on blood glucose
  B Tell your healthcare provider what complementary therapies you are using
  C Tell your healthcare provider about any problems you may be having with the complementary therapies
  D All of the above

See next page for answer key.

Post-Test Answer Key

Biological Complementary Therapies in Diabetes   **7**

1	B	**6**	A
2	D	**7**	E
3	A	**8**	D
4	D	**9**	D
5	E	**10**	D

A Core Curriculum for Diabetes Education

Research

A Core Curriculum for Diabetes Education
Diabetes in the Life Cycle and Research

The Importance of Research

8

James A. Fain, PhD, RN, BC-ADM, FAAN
University of Massachusetts Worcester
Graduate School of Nursing
Worcester, Massachusetts

Introduction

1 Diabetes educators practicing in all care settings (ie, acute-care facility, community agency, inpatient/outpatient setting, education centers, private practice) are expected to provide quality care and education that reflects the translation of scientific evidence and professional consensus into practice.

2 Diabetes educators have the responsibility and opportunity for assuming an active role in scientifically based practice by
  A Having sufficient knowledge of the research process in order to determine what constitutes valid conclusions and recommendations of a given study.
  B Developing the skills of reading and evaluating research reports to determine the accuracy and applicability of study findings.
  C Participating in research opportunities.

3 Diabetes educators can employ the process of scientific method to enrich and evaluate their everyday practice.

4 This chapter provides an overview of the importance of research and outcome measures to daily clinical care. Application of the research process with discussion of approaches to research and the role of the research consumer are presented.

Objectives

Upon completion of this chapter, the learner will be able to
1 Explain the importance of research for diabetes educators.
2 Distinguish between a quantitative and qualitative approach to research.
3 Define different types of research studies.
4 List the 5 general phases of the research process.
5 Identify the basic elements of a research report.
6 Distinguish between experimental and nonexperimental research.
7 Describe the importance of identifying and measuring diabetes outcomes.
8 Explain strategies for participating in research opportunities.

The Importance of Research

1 The challenges confronting the healthcare system today have made it necessary for healthcare providers to strive to enhance the quality and value of health care while reducing costs. Diabetes educators must validate their practice by using evidence-based guidelines and by documenting outcomes.

2 When diabetes educators use research findings as their foundation for clinical decision making in providing the "best care" possible, the outcome is evidence-based practice.

3 *Evidence-based practice* is defined as the conscientious, explicit, and judicious use of current best evidence in making decisions about the care of an individualized patient.[1]

4 *Evidence-based health care* happens when clinicians make healthcare decisions for a population or group of patients using research evidence.

5 The development of a discipline such as diabetes education is marked by the knowledge that is useful in solving problems encountered in practice.
   A By actually conducting research studies or understanding and translating the research results of other investigators, diabetes educators contribute to the knowledge base that serves as a reference for the practice of diabetes care and education.
   B Evidence-based health care cannot occur unless healthcare providers are skilled in reading, critiquing, and synthesizing research findings. Diabetes educators must focus on improving their understanding of the research process and developing skills to evaluate published research reports.

Definition of Research

1 *Research* is defined as a systematic process in which the scientific method is employed to answer questions. The goal of research is to explain, predict, and/or control phenomena.[2]

2 Research often is considered synonymous with problem-solving. While the intent of research is the generation of new knowledge for broad application to inform or guide practice, problem-solving seeks to satisfy or reach resolution of a given, specific situation.

3 Research employs the rigorous process of scientific method for generating new knowledge.
   A Application of the scientific method moves in an orderly and systematic fashion, imposing conditions (*control*) on the research situation so that biases are minimized and validity maximized. Evidence is collected in the research process via a method that can be readily reviewed or replicated by others.[2]
   B The following research tasks are part of the scientific method:
   • Selecting and defining a problem
   • Formulating research questions and/or hypotheses
   • Collecting data
   • Analyzing data
   • Reporting results

Quantitative and Qualitative Research Methods

1 Two major approaches to scientific inquiry are quantitative and qualitative research methods.

2 *Quantitative research* is defined as a systematic, formal process that involves the quantitative methods to explore factors of interest. Quantitative research seeks to describe, identify, explain, or predict relationships. Quantitative methods are used and categorized by the level of control applied (whether something occurred by chance). Depending on the method used, the research can describe variables, examine relationships, or predict outcomes. The strength of a quantitative study lies in the ability to offer findings that suggest maximum control (ie, results did not happen by chance) or findings that are valid and applicable to other similar groups.[2]

A There are different types of quantitative research. Table 8.1 defines the types of quantitative research. However, study designs often overlap.

B Key research terms are listed in Table 8.2.

C Data collected in quantitative studies are translated into numbers with use of statistical analysis to convey not only the effect of the study (ie, 80% of low-income individuals with diabetes living in the Northeast describe themselves as having little or no tangible social support), but whether or not the results occurred by chance. The phrase, "The group who received social support training were more likely to demonstrate improved A1C levels compared to the group who did not receive social support training ($P = .03$)" means that as a researcher you are willing to accept 3 times out of 100 the possibility that the difference in A1C levels occurred by chance alone.

D An example of a quantitative approach to research[3] is displayed in Figure 8.1 The purpose of the study in the example was to provide baseline information on the perceptions, use, and knowledge of A1C values among home healthcare nurses and patients. Data was collected from telephone interviews (patients) and written questionnaires (nurses). Medical records reviews were analyzed using descriptive methods. Data collected included gender, age, race, educational level, household type, and duration of diabetes and was quantified and presented using summary statistics (ie, frequencies and percentages).

E Quantitative studies are further categorized by the design used that implies the level of control.

F The *randomized controlled trial* (RCT) is the most rigorous approach to research. The RCT is a prospective study comparing the effect of an intervention against a control. In an RCT, the researcher randomly assigns subjects to an intervention (experimental group) and control group. The most important features of this design include randomization of groups along with use of a control group for comparison.[2]

G In making decisions about care and treatment of patients, it is important for clinicians to critically appraise the various grades of evidence in addressing clinical questions. Strongest levels of evidence are associated with RCTs.[1]

3 *Qualitative research* also uses a systematic approach to identify those variables or aspects of a person's experience and/or meaning of some specific phenomenon. Examples include the experience of 'becoming diabetic,' the experience of learning diabetes self-management, or the phenomenon of fear of hypoglycemia.

A Qualitative methods incorporate the subject's own words and narrative summaries of observable behavior to express data, rather than using numbers. Questions that lend themselves to qualitative inquiry are generally broad and seek to understand why particular phenomena occur. Collecting qualitative data often leads to development and design of a quantitative research project.

B A description of a qualitative approach to research[4] is shown in Figure 8.2. The purpose of this qualitative approach was to explore the concept of fatalism in relation to diabetes self-management behavior in African Americans with type 2 diabetes. Data were collected from focus group interviews with 39 participants. Seven focus groups were conducted; sessions were tape recorded, transcribed, and analyzed to identify themes related to fatalism and diabetes self-management.

Table 8.1. Types of Quantitative Research Studies

Intervention or Controlled Research – Study subjects (whether human or animal) are selected according to relevant characteristics, and then randomly assigned to either an experimental or control group. The experimental group is generally manipulated based on the study question, so the study question can be answered.

- *Basic Research* – Generates data by investigating biochemical substances or biological processes. Basic research may be conducted *in vitro* (such as in test tubes), or with animals.
- *Clinical Trials* – Attempts to determine whether the findings of basic research are applicable to humans, or to confirm the results of epidemiological research. *Double-Blind Placebo-Controlled Studies* are considered the "gold standard" of clinical research studies. They provide dependable findings that are free of bias introduced by the subject or the researcher. Unfortunately, it is almost never possible to blind educational studies.

Observational Research – Examines specific factors in defined groups of subjects in order to investigate relationships between those factors and aspects of health or illness. As these are observational studies, there is no manipulation of either study group.

Epidemiological Research – The study of the distribution and determinants of diseases or other health outcomes in human populations; is often observational, but may also be experimental (a manipulation to answer the study question is done). Observational studies look at free-living subjects that are usually much larger than groups in clinical trials. There are 3 main types of observational studies:

- *Cross-Sectional Study* – Measures the status of an individual with respect to the presence or absence of both exposure (eg, to dietary factors, physical activity levels, or actual exposure to disease-causing agent) and disease at the same time. It is like a "snapshot."
- *Case-Control Study* – One group of people with a certain disease or set of characteristics is compared to a suitable group without that disease or those characteristics (control). The 2 groups are evaluated by comparing past exposure to some identifiable risk factor.
- *Cohort Study* – Large groups of people are followed over a long period of time in an attempt to identify possible causes and/or preventives associated with certain predetermined biological endpoints. There are 2 types of cohort studies: prospective and retrospective.

    Prospective Study – Epidemiological research that follows a group of people over a period of time to observe the potential effects of diet, behavior and other factors on health or the incidence of disease. In general, considered a more valid research design than retrospective research.

    Retrospective Study – Research that relies on recall of past data or on previously recorded information. Often, this type of research is considered to have limitations, due to the fact that the number of variables cannot be controlled and because memory is not infallible.

Meta-Analysis – A quantitative technique in which the results of many individual studies are pooled to yield overall conclusions. To conduct a meta-analysis, a systematic review of research, generally published, relative to the topic is undertaken.

Outcomes Research – Type of research used by the health industry which provides information on the results of a specific procedure or therapy: the subject (clinical safety and efficacy); educational, clinical, or behavioral measures; the subject's physical functioning and lifestyle; economic considerations such as savings/prolonged life and avoiding costly complications.

Population-Based Interventions – This study is a cross between an epidemiological study and a clinical trial in which a large number of free-living subjects are given either a treatment or a placebo. They are then observed to see what outcomes occur.

Table 8.2. Definitions of Key Research Terms

Bias – Problems in study design that can lead to effects that are not related to the variables being studied.

Blind, Single or Double – In a single-blind study, the subjects do not know whether they are receiving an experimental treatment or a placebo. In a double-blind study, neither the researchers nor the participants are aware of which subjects receive the treatment until after the study is completed.

Confounding Variable or Confounding Factor – A "hidden" variable that may cause an association, which the researcher attributes to other variables.

Control Group – The group of subjects in a study to whom a comparison is made in order to determine whether an observation or treatment has an effect. In an experimental study, it is the group that does not receive a treatment. Subjects are as similar as possible to those in the test group.

Correlation – An association, or when one phenomenon is found to be accompanied by another. A correlation does not prove cause and effect. Correlation may also be defined statistically.

Experimental Group – The group of subjects in an experimental study that receives an active treatment.

Generalizability – The extent to which the results of a study are able to be applied to the general population.

Incidence – The number of new cases of a disease during a given period of time in a defined population.

Placebo – "Fake" treatment that seems identical to the real treatment. Placebo treatments are used to eliminate bias that may arise from the expectations that a treatment should produce an effect.

Prevalence – The number of existing cases of a disease in a defined population at a specified time.

Randomization or Random Assignment – A process of assigning subjects to experimental or control groups in which the subjects have an equal chance of being assigned to each group. Utilized to control for known, unknown, and difficult-to-control-for variables.

Random Sampling – A method by which subjects are selected to participate in a study in which all individuals in a population have an equal chance of being chosen. Helps ensure the generalizability of the study results.

Reliability – Whether a test or instrument used to collect data, such as a questionnaire, gives the same results if repeated on the same person at different times. A reliable test gives reproducible results.

Research Design – How a study is set up to collect information or data. For valid results, the design must be appropriate to answer the question or hypothesis being studied.

Residual Confounding – The effect that remains after one has attempted to statistically control for variables that cannot be measured perfectly. A particularly important concept in epidemiological studies because knowledge of human biology is still developing. Unknown variables may exist that could significantly change conclusions made on the basis of epidemiological research.

Risk – A term encompassing a variety of measures of the probability of an outcome. It is usually used in reference to unfavorable outcomes such as illness or death. It is important to distinguish between absolute and relative risk.

Risk Factor – Anything statistically shown to have a relationship with the incidence of a disease. Although risk factors usually imply a contributory (ie, casual) influence, they do not necessarily infer cause and effect. Actual cause and effect can only be determined by an intervention study.

Statistical Power – A mathematical quantity that indicates the probability a study has of obtaining a statistically significant effect. A power of 80 percent, or 0.8, indicates that the study—if conducted repeatedly—would produce a statistically significant effect 80 percent of the time. On the other hand, a power of only 0.1 means there would be a 90 percent chance that the research missed the effect—if one exists at all.

Statistical Significance – The statistical probability, or chance, that the observed outcome would have occurred if, in reality, the outcome was merely due to chance. A *P* value of less than 5 percent (*P*<.05) means the result would occur less than 5 percent of the time if there were no effect, and it is generally to be considered evidence of a true treatment effect or a true relationship.

Validity – The extent to which a study or study instrument measures what it is intended to measure. Refers to accuracy or truthfulness in regard to a study's conclusion.

Variable – Any characteristic that may vary in study subjects, such as gender, age, body weight, diet, behavior, attitude, or other attribute. In an experiment, the treatment is called the *independent variable*; it is the factor being investigated. The variable that is influenced by the treatment is the *dependent variable*; it may change as a result of the effect of the independent variable.

Figure 8.1. Example of a Quantitative Approach to Research

A convenience sample (44 patients, 26 nurses) from a Medicare-certified home care agency was surveyed using an investigator-developed demographic and knowledge questionnaire. Patients' medical records also were examined to obtain demographic (eg, age and gender) and treatment-related information, including type of antidiabetic medication(s), classification of type of diabetes, and presence of a documented A1C value. Nurses' perceptions of their practice patterns were measured; however, these responses were not matched to specific patient records, documented care, or laboratory values.

Source: Excerpted from Setter, Corbett, Campbell, Cook, Gates.[3]

4 Regardless of the research methods used, researchers have the responsibility of conducting a study with rigor and skill. *Rigor* is defined as the striving for excellence in research using discipline, scrupulous adherence to detail, and strict accuracy.

Figure 8.2. Example of a Qualitative Approach to Research

Seven focus groups were conducted between March and June of 2001. Thirty-nine study participants were invited to participate in the study. Each participant received a $25 honorarium for attending the 2-hour focus group. The principle investigator or an experienced focus group facilitator moderated all sessions. Facilitators were of the same ethnicity and gender as participants. An interview guide was used to facilitate discussion across groups. Audiotapes of each focus group session were transcribed and entered into a word processing program.

Source: Excerpted from Egede and Bonadonna.[4]

▲ *Multimethod research* blends both quantitative and qualitative methods to collect data.[2] Some research findings can be strengthened by including a multimethod type of research approach. For example, a study could apply a quantitative approach to examine the effect of social support on patient education and diabetes self-management by measuring knowledge, type of social support, and diabetes self-management before and after an educational program. A qualitative component could explore what daily self-management is like for subjects who have social support and those who do not have social support.

The Research Process

1 The intent of the research process is to describe the general thinking of researchers. Although many different research models exist, the research process consists of standard elements; the order may vary and the steps may overlap in different research situations. The 5 general phases of the research process are presented in Figure 8.3.

2 The research process is circular. When conducting a study, researchers may need to rethink and reconceptualize a problem several times. For example, researchers continually review the literature to keep up with the most current information and refer to previous research reports to get ideas for sampling, operational definitions, and research designs. In addition, research is circular in that research leads to further research, and the process starts over again.

How to Read and Critique a Research Report

1 As consumers of research, diabetes educators need to develop the ability to understand and apply research findings to their practices. Becoming familiar with research terminology along with critically reviewing research reports allows the diabetes educator to translate findings into practice if practical.

2 Research reports are divided into sections with headings and subheadings. Examples of headings may include an abstract, introduction, research questions and/or hypotheses, methods, results, and discussion of conclusions.[2]

Figure 8.3. Phases of the Research Process

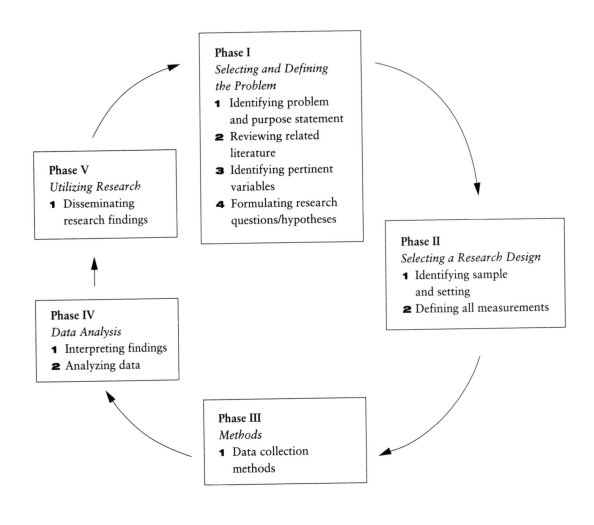

A The *abstract* is located at the beginning of a research report and provides a brief, concise summary of the study. The abstract provides an overview and is helpful in understanding if the study design and methods were appropriate to the concluded study findings. Many journals use a structured abstract form, limiting the number of words to approximately 100.

 • An example of an abstract[5] is presented in Figure 8.4. The abstract is written in a structured format (ie, purpose, methods, results, and conclusions) to help readers determine whether the research is appropriate for their needs and if the complete article is something they may want to read.

Figure 8.4. Example of a Typical Structured Abstract

Purpose

The purpose of this study was to compare the efficacy of outpatient versus inpatient programs on medical, cognitive, behavioral, and psychosocial outcomes.

Methods

Using 3 large, tertiary medical centers in the United States, the sample of 32 children newly diagnosed with diabetes and their parents were recruited. Children and parents who received outpatient education were compared with those who received inpatient education. The following outcome variables were compared: (1) rates of hospital readmissions and/or emergency room visits for either severe hypoglycemia or ketoacidosis, (2) knowledge, (3) sharing of responsibilities, (4) adherence, (5) family functioning, (6) coping, and (7) quality of life.

Results

In general, no statistically significant differences were found between the groups. A trend was noted in the outpatient group with regard to improved use of emergency precautions on the adherence measure, roles on the family functioning measure, maintaining family integration on the parental coping measure, and disposition on the children's coping instrument.

Conclusions

Findings support the safety and efficacy of the outpatient program method.

Source: Excerpted from Siminerio, Charron-Prochownik, Banion, Schreiner.[5]

B The *introduction* of a research article contains 3 parts: a problem statement, a review of related literature, and a purpose statement.
  - The *problem statement* provides direction for the research study and is typically stated at the beginning of a research article. The problem statement provides justification for the research by citing background information about the problem to support the need for conducting the proposed study.[2] The discussion of previous research can be as brief as 1 or 2 sentences or as long as several pages.
  - *Literature reviews* involve identifying and analyzing relevant publications that contain information related to the proposed research problem. Literature reviews are conducted to uncover what is already known about the topic and problem, to determine consistencies and gaps in knowledge about the problem, to describe strengths and weaknesses of designs and methods of inquiry, and to generate useful research questions and/or hypotheses.[2] A review of literature can be as brief as 3 or 4 sentences or as long as 2 or 3 pages. Comprehensive reviews of the literature are usually not found in most research reports due to space limitations, but may be published separately as a literature or technical review study.
  - The *purpose statement* is a single statement that identifies why the problem is being studied, specifies the overall goal and intent of the research, and clarifies the knowledge to be gained.[2]

- The statement presented in Figure 8.5 provides the reader with a clear understanding of the problem being studied and why it is important.[5] The literature review is concise and reflects the relevant background that is necessary to support the rationale for the study. The literature review ends with a purpose statement that delineates the population (newly diagnosed children with type 1 diabetes) and outcome measures (medical, cognitive, behavioral, and psychosocial measures) to be evaluated.

Figure 8.5. Example of a Problem Statement With a Purpose Statement

Problem Statement:

The management of type 1 diabetes is a complex lifelong process that requires a great deal of self-management. The tasks required to achieve good metabolic control are taking injections, testing blood glucose levels, and monitoring food intake and exercise. The fundamental prerequisite for diabetes self-management is patient education that is considered to be the cornerstone of diabetes management. In this time of health care reform, the question of where education should occur is being revisited. Traditionally, children have been hospitalized for constant supervision, education, metabolic stabilization, and initiation of insulin. Although hospitalization allows for intense support and medical supervision, it presents several problems. First, hospitalization is a traumative experience for children. Second, achieving metabolic control during hospitalizations can be difficult. Meals, activities, and schedule are different in the hospital than in the home. Adjusting insulin doses within a relatively controlled hospital environment is not comparable to the child's home life. Making the transition can be difficult. An alternative to hospitalizing newly diagnosed children with diabetes is providing outpatient education. Comparative studies have been performed; however, these studies have been limited to retrospective reports and chart reviews, and focus on medical outcomes and costs. The purpose of this study is to compare the efficacy of outpatient versus inpatient programs on medical, cognitive, behavioral, and psychosocial outcomes.

Source: Excerpted from Siminerio, Charron-Prochownik, Banion, Schreiner.[5]

---

c Hypotheses and/or research questions are formulated after the literature review has been completed. Before stating hypotheses and/or research questions, the researcher needs to identify variables that are pertinent to the study.
- A *hypothesis* is defined as a statement that explains or predicts the relationship or differences between 2 or more variables in terms of expected results or outcomes of a study.[2] Hypotheses provide direction for the research design and the collection, analysis, and interpretation of data. When the purpose of a study is to explain the nature and strength of relationships among variables, hypotheses are used.
- Researchers do not set out to prove a hypothesis but rather to collect data that either support or refute the hypothesis.

- The variables that are identified in hypotheses are operationally defined. An operational definition specifies how the variables will be measured in terms of the instruments and/or scales to be used.[2]
- The *dependent variable*, or outcome, represents the area of interest under study and reflects the effect of or the response to the independent variable. Dependent variables are sometimes thought of as the results of conducting a study or the outcome measure. Dependent variables are sometimes referred to as criterion or outcome variables.
- The *independent variable* is perceived as contributing to or preceding a particular outcome. It is sometimes referred to as the variable that is manipulated by the researcher, and its effect on the dependent variable is observed. Depending on the research approach, the independent variable may be classified as an experimental, treatment, intervention, or predictor variable.
- The following statement is an example of hypothesis: *Individuals with type 2 diabetes who receive instruction on an individual basis will exhibit better glycemic control (measured by A1C tests) than those individuals who receive instruction in a group setting.* The dependent variable associated with the hypothesis is glycemic control (measured by A1C tests). Individual versus group setting is the independent variable for the hypothesis.
- Research studies do not always contain hypotheses but may instead be organized around research questions. A *research question* is defined as a concise, interrogative statement that is written in the present tense and includes 1 or more variables.[2]
- Research questions focus on describing the variable(s), examining relationships among variables, and determining differences between 2 or more groups regarding the selected variable(s).
- Examples of specific research questions are displayed in Figure 8.6. In this study, 221 members of the American Association of Diabetes Educators (AADE) listed in the 1995 membership directory in the state of Georgia completed the Diabetes Educator Responsibilities Questionnaire (DERQ).[6] In the first research question, educators were asked to rate how frequently they carried out certain responsibilities associated with their position using a 5-point Likert scale (1 = Never, 2 = Rarely, 3 = Sometimes, 4 = Frequently, 5 = Always). In the second research question, responses from diabetes educators in Georgia were compared to diabetes educators in New York City. Finally, in the third research question, diabetes educators were again asked to rate the frequency with which they employed certain behavioral strategies in their practice using a 5-point Likert scale.

D The methods section of a research report contains information about how a study is conducted. This section is the most important part of the research report and needs to be written clearly and concisely. The first part of the methods section is the study design.

- The *research design* is defined as a set of guidelines by which a researcher obtains answers to the research question(s). The research design provides a methodological direction and specifies procedures such as site selection, sampling techniques, selection of instruments, and data analysis.
- A wide variety of study designs are used in research, including quantitative and qualitative approaches (see Table 8.3). Quantitative research designs are classified as experimental or nonexperimental.

- *Experimental research* refers to studies in which the researcher manipulates and controls 1 or more variables and observes the effect(s) on another variable.[2]
- Experimental designs are sometimes referred to as intervention studies whereby a particular method or treatment is expected to influence 1 or more outcomes. Such studies enable researchers to assess the effectiveness of various teaching methods, curriculum models, and other variables at influencing the characteristics of individuals or groups.

Figure 8.6. Example of Research Questions

The purpose of this study was to identify and describe the scope of practice of diabetes educators in the state of Georgia. This study was a replication of a research investigation originally published in 1992 by Cypress and colleagues. Information obtained from this study could be used to develop future practice guidelines and health promotion activities of diabetes educators in the state of Georgia and elsewhere in the United States. The following research questions were proposed for this study:

1 What are the primary responsibilities of diabetes educators in the state of Georgia?

2 How do the responsibilities of diabetes educators in Georgia (1996) compare with those of diabetes educators in New York City (1991)?

3 Are behavioral strategies being used by diabetes educators in Georgia to help people with diabetes make lifestyle modifications?

Source: Excerpted from Kaufman, All, Davis.[6]

- *Quasi-experimental designs* refer to a modified experimental approach. Researchers may use a quasi-experimental design and still be able to manipulate the independent variable (experimental condition) and exercise some control over the study. However, random assignment of subjects to control or experimental groups is not feasible using quasi-experimental designs.
- *Nonexperimental research* refers to studies in which the researcher examines variables in natural environments and does not include researcher-imposed treatments.[2] Nonexperimental research is classified as descriptive and/or correlational.
- *Descriptive research* provides information about the characteristics of a particular individual, event, or group for the purpose of discovering new information, describing what exists, and determining the frequency with which something occurs.[2]
- *Correlational research* provides a description of the relationship between 2 or more variables and the nature of that relationship (eg, positive or negative).[2] Descriptive correlational research attempts to describe what exists and identify several interrelationships. Variables are not manipulated, and the setting is not controlled. Analysis of data often leads to forming hypotheses that can be tested experimentally.

Table 8.3. Types of Quantitative and Qualitative Approaches to Research

1 Quantitative Approach to Research
 A Experimental Research
  • Experimental designs (eg, randomized clinical trials)
  • Quasi-experimental designs
 B Nonexperimental Research
  • Descriptive designs
  • Correlational designs
  • Longitudinal designs
  • Time-series designs

2 Qualitative Approach to Research
 A Phenomenological research
 B Ethnographic research
 C Grounded theory research

E Details of the methods section are presented in the following subsections: subjects/setting, data collection procedures, data collection instruments, and specific statistical procedures for analyzing data.
  • Discussion of subjects (study sample) includes the criteria for selecting subjects to participate in the study, sample size, sample characteristics, and setting. Research reports also include a sentence documenting that subjects have read and signed an informed consent form and that the study was approved by an institutional review board (IRB) for the protection of human subjects' rights.
  • The methods section should contain all necessary information so that another researcher can replicate the study. For example, educational interventions should be described in detail.
  • The example in Figure 8.7 illustrates criteria for study eligibility along with a rationale for why only women participated in the study.[7] A statement about approval from an Office of Regulatory Compliance is mentioned along with how subjects were invited to participate in the study. Informed consent forms must also be signed by study participants. Data collection procedures are described so that the reader can follow the procedural flow of the study. These procedures include a detailed explanation of what subjects were asked to do, who collected the data, and how often measurements were taken. Data collection instruments (surveys, scales) identify the variables that are measured.
F The results section of a research report provides a description of the findings from the study based on statistical analysis of the data. The results of a study are organized according to the research purpose or objectives and the hypotheses and/or research questions.
G The discussion section of a research report combines and gives meaning to information from the other sections and includes major findings, limitations of the study, conclusions drawn from the findings, and implications/recommendations for further research.

Figure 8.7. Example of a Methods Section With Inclusion Criteria

Women between the age of 40 and 60 years and diagnosed with NIDDM (type 2 diabetes) at least 12 months prior to the initiation of the study were recruited from a rural community. Age was restricted to 40 to 60 years because NIDDM is usually diagnosed after the age of 40 years and the label-reading habits of older women (>65 years) differ from those of younger women. Women were the focus of this study because they were frequent label readers as well as primary food shoppers. A uniform group of women in terms of diagnosis and use of nutrition labels was desired. Participants were recruited through advertisements in newspapers and public service announcements on television. The study was described as a general consumer research study rather than a nutrition study to minimize social desirability effects. All methods were approved by the Office for Regulatory Compliance at a major university. Three procedures were followed for data collection: (1) a telephone screening interview to determine subject eligibility; (2) written questionnaire about location and frequency of grocery shopping, diabetes education, and demographic characteristics mailed to participants to be completed at home; and (3) participation in either a focus group or an in-depth interview. Both the data collection and data analysis of the focus groups and in-depth interviews are further described.

Source: Excerpted from Miller, Probart, Achterberg.[7]

Diabetes Outcomes

1 The issue of outcomes of care have achieved national prominence, and measures of these outcomes have become a requirement for determining the quality of performance of providing health care within a clinic or organization. In some instances, these reports form the basis for funding or allocation of resources. The Center for Medicare & Medicaid Services (CMS), the Agency for Health Care Research and Quality (AHRQ), and accrediting bodies such as the Joint Commission on Accreditation of Health Care Organizations (JCAHO) and National Center for Quality Assurance (NCQA) use organizational reports of outcomes to determine resource allocation and standards. In the past few years, these and other agencies have joined with the American Diabetes Association (ADA) advisory groups to determine diabetes outcomes for which health-care programs/organizations should be held accountable.

2 An outcome is another term for 'endpoint.' For health care, the endpoints of interest are health status, costs, and satisfaction.[1,8] In chronic disease conditions, the endpoint itself is not always directly measurable within a short period of time. For example, the health status change of reducing end-stage renal disease may be the desired outcome, but the measure will be how many patients with diabetes in a particular practice are screened and treated early for proteinuria.

3 Outcomes are often determined by 'indicators' of care. For example, an A1C level is a clinical indicator, as are blood pressure and microalbuminuria, whereas a patient's activity of monitoring blood glucose 4 times a day would be an indicator of diabetes self-management.

4 The National Standards of Diabetes Self-Management Education (DSME)[9] have recently been revised to define quality diabetes education that can be implemented in diverse settings to facilitate improvement in healthcare outcomes. Measures of diabetes self-management lead to improved health status, patient satisfaction, and contained costs of care, especially the kinds of self-management education/support that diabetes educators engage in.

5 The American Association of Diabetes Educators (AADE) has developed the *National Diabetes Education Outcomes Systems* (NDEOS). The purpose of the NDEOS is to provide the diabetes care and education team with a complete system to gather, track, and aggregate outcome measures unique to diabetes education and to support the integration of diabetes education into clinical care.
  A *Outcome measures* associated with diabetes education programs include medical, behavioral, and psychosocial factors.[10]
  - *Medical factors* are identified in the patient's medical history (eg, present health status, health resource utilization, risk factors).
  - *Behavioral factors* focus on goals and intentions that mediate the program effect on self-care (eg, blood glucose, monitoring, medications, eating habits, exercise, prevention/management of complications, knowledge). The most common technique for measuring self-care is patient self-report (or parent reports in the case of young children and caregiver reports in the case of the elderly).
  - *Psychosocial factors* evaluate social support systems (eg, family, peer, health professional) and health beliefs and attitudes. In addition, barriers to learning and socioeconomic factors are addressed.

6 Just as it is important to consider the kinds of outcomes sought as the result of a program or care intervention, it is also important to make certain that what is used to measure that outcome is, indeed, a reliable and valid measure of the outcome.
  A *Reliability* of a measure is the consistency with which an instrument, questionnaire, scale, or test provides accurate information.[2] Validity is the degree to which an instrument, questionnaire, scale, or test measures what it is supposed to measure.[2] As an example, an oral glucose tolerance test (OGTT) is not a reliable test for diagnosing diabetes because so many things can affect the test results. However, the OGTT is a valid measure of blood glucose levels because it does measure what it is supposed to (blood glucose levels following a dose of oral glucose). Another example could be that of an educator who wants to measure whether a person's health beliefs have an effect on the level of glycemic control. The researcher asks the patient to fill out a questionnaire on diabetes knowledge that has been reported to be reliable. The questionnaire provides a reliable measure of the individual's diabetes knowledge, but it will not be a valid measure of health beliefs.
  B Another consideration to keep in mind is how data are collected in a research study (that is, the process a researcher follows). Using the last example, suppose the questionnaire was a valid and reliable measure of health beliefs, but the questionnaire

was administered with the patient's immediate family members present. The patient may 'adjust' his or her answers towards what he/she thinks the family wants to hear and not disclose true feelings about health beliefs.

Research and the Diabetes Educator

1 The role of the researcher is defined on a continuum by the degree of active or passive participation in the research process. At one end of the continuum are diabetes educators who are consumers of research while at the other end are those who are principal investigators (PIs) of large research studies.

2 The role of the research consumer includes the ability to read and evaluate research reports. Diabetes educators are increasingly expected to maintain, at minimum, this level of involvement in research. Developing skills to critically read and understand research takes time, knowledge of the research process, and repeated practice.

3 Diabetes educators who are PIs are those who conduct research and are responsible for designing, implementing, and evaluating a study. Diabetes educators who are members of a research team collaborate on the development of an idea and actually participate in the design, production, and final reporting of a study.

4 Participation in research activities can occur at all levels. Several research-related activities in which diabetes educators may participate are listed in Table 8.4.

Table 8.4. Research-Related Activities

1 Participating in a journal club that involves regular meetings among educators to discuss research articles

2 Attending research presentations at professional meetings and conferences

3 Evaluating published research for possible use in the practice setting

4 Assisting in collecting research information (eg, distributing questionnaires to patients/clients or observing/recording behaviors)

5 Collaborating in the development of an idea for a research project

6 Joining an institutional review board where ethical aspects of a proposed study are discussed

7 Serving on committees or task forces of professional organizations

8 Developing clinical guidelines

9 Publishing review papers

10 Serving as a journal manuscript reviewer

11 Serving as principal investigator (PI) or coprincipal investigator (Co-PI) of a study

Key Educational Considerations

1 Diabetes educators are responsible for assuming an active role in developing a body of knowledge that serves as a reference for the science and art of diabetes education and care. As research consumers, diabetes educators need to develop the skills of reading and critiquing published research reports.

2 Quantitative and qualitative approaches to research refer to an organizing framework that contains a set of assumptions or values that relates to the purpose of the study. Different types of research are used depending on the question being asked and the study design.

3 The 5 general phases of the research process are
- Selecting and defining the problem
- Selecting a research design
- Collecting data
- Analyzing data
- Using research findings

4 Published research reports are divided into several sections and usually include the following:
- Abstract
- Introduction
- Research question/hypotheses
- Methods
- Results
- Discussion of conclusions

5 The problem statement (usually located within the introduction) presents the topic to be studied along with a description of the background and rationale for its significance.

6 A literature review involves identifying, obtaining, and analyzing literature that is related to the research problem.

7 The purpose statement is expressed as a single statement or research question that specifies the overall goal of the study.

8 Hypotheses provide direction to the study and determine research methodologies and type of data to be collected. Hypotheses state clearly and concisely the expected relationship between 2 or more variables.

9 Research questions are cited in published research reports when prior knowledge about a particular phenomenon is limited and the researcher seeks to identify and/or describe that phenomenon (exploratory or descriptive studies).

10 Independent variables are used to explain or predict a result or outcome. These are sometimes referred to as experimental or treatment variables.

11 Dependent variables reflect the effects of or responses to the independent variables and sometimes are referred to as outcome variables.

12 Research designs are classified as experimental versus nonexperimental.

13 Several organizations have come together to evaluate the quality of care delivered to individuals with diabetes. Health outcomes include measurements of glycemic control, lipid levels, blood pressure, urinary protein, and frequency of self-monitoring of blood glucose. Patient-centered outcomes include patient satisfaction, well-being, and quality of life.

14 Evaluation of diabetes education programs includes assessment of medical factors (health status, health resources), behavioral factors (diabetes knowledge and skills, health behaviors and goals), and psychosocial factors (social support systems, health beliefs, and attitudes).

Self-Review Questions

1 What is the value of research for diabetes educators?

2 What are several research-related activities in which diabetes educators can participate?

3 What is the difference between a quantitative and qualitative approach to research?

4 What types of information are usually found in an abstract associated with a published research report?

5 What is the difference between a problem statement and purpose statement?

6 Why is it important for a researcher to review literature pertinent to the research topic before planning a study?

7 What is the purpose of a hypothesis?

8 What is the definition of the terms independent variable and dependent variable?

9 What is the difference between true experiments and quasi-experiments? In what ways are true experiments better than quasi-experiments? In what ways are quasi-experiments better than true experiments?

10 As consumers of research, diabetes educators must be able to read, critique, understand, and apply findings to practice. What strategies would you apply to read, critique, and understand published research reports?

References

1 Sackett DL. Evidence-based medicine: what it is and what it isn't. BMJ. 1996;312:71-72.

2 Fain JA. Reading, Understanding, and Applying Nursing Research: A Text and Workbook. Philadelphia, Pa: FA Davis Company; 2002.

3 Setter SM, Corbett CF, Campbell RK, Cook, D, Gates BJ. A survey of the perceptions, knowledge, and use of A1C values by home care patients and nurses. Diabetes Educ. 2003; 29:144-152.

4 Egede LE, Bonadonne RJ. Diabetes self-management in African Americans: An exploration of the role of fatalism. Diabetes Educ. 2003;29:105-115.

5 Siminerio LM, Charron-Prochownik D, Banion C, Schreiner B. Comparing outpatient and inpatient diabetes education for newly diagnosed pediatric patients. Diabetes Educ. 1999;25:895-906.

6 Kaufman MW, All AC, Davis H. The scope of practice of diabetes educators in the state of Georgia. Diabetes Educ. 1999; 25;56-64.

7 Miller CK, Probart CK, Achterberg CL. Knowledge and misconceptions about the food label among women with non-insulin-dependent diabetes. Diabetes Educ. 1997;23:425-432.

8 White EB, Sanderson-Austin J. Outcomes measurement: measuring success. Group Practice J. 2000;49:32-34.

9 Mensing C, Boucher J, Cypress M, et al. National standards for diabetes self-management education. Diabetes Care. 2003;26(suppl 1):S149-S156.

10 Peyrot M. Evaluation of patient education programs: how to do it and how to use it. Diabetes Spectrum. 1996;9:86-93.

Suggested Readings

American Association of Diabetes Educators. Diabetes Educational and Behavioral Research Summit. Diabetes Educ. 1999;25(suppl 1).

American Diabetes Association. Report of the Task Force on the Delivery of Diabetes Self-Management Education and Medical Nutrition Therapy. Diabetes Spectrum. 1999;12: 44-47.

Beauchamp TC, Childress JF. Principles of Biomedical Ethics. 4th ed. New York: Oxford University Press; 1994.

Denzin N, Lincoln Y. Handbook of Qualitative Designs. Thousand Oaks, Calif: Sage Publications; 1994.

Funk SG, Champagne MT, Wiese RA, Tornquist EM. Barriers to using research findings in practice. The clinician's perspective. Appl Nurs Res. 1991;4:90-95.

Glasgow RE. Outcomes of and for diabetes education research. Diabetes Educ. 1999;25(suppl 1):74-88.

Locke LF, Spirdusco WW, Silverman SJ. Proposals That Work. 3rd ed. Newbury Park, Calif: Sage Publications; 1995.

Marrero DG, Peyrot M, Garfield S. Promoting behavior research in diabetes. Diabetes Care. 2001;24:1-2.

Peyrot MF. Theory in behavioral diabetes research. Diabetes Care. 2001;24:1703-1705.

Wheeler ML, Wylie-Rosett J, Pichert JW. Diabetes education research. Diabetes Care. 2001;24:421-422.

Wylie-Rosett J, Wheeler M, Krueger K, Halford B. Opportunities for research-oriented dietitians. J Am Diet Assoc. 1990;90:1531-1534.

Learning Assessment: Post-Test Questions

The Importance of Research

8

1 The scientific method incorporates the procedures used by researchers in the pursuit of new knowledge. The first step of the scientific method is:

A Developing a theoretical framework

B Reviewing the related literature

C Formulating a research problem and purpose

D Formulating research objectives, questions, and hypotheses

2 A research approach to acquire knowledge that describes life experiences is classified as:

A Quantitative

B Qualitative

C Experimental

D Quasi-experimental

3 Multimethod research refers to the process of:

A Reaching agreement among members of a research team

B Collecting data using more than 1 research approach

C Abstracting themes into theoretical constructs

D Examining problems to gain knowledge about improving health care

4 Research uses a systematic approach to explain or predict phenomena. The research process itself may best be characterized as a:

A Random manner of assigning people to various groups to prove a hypothesis

B Set of steps carried out in prescribed order as part of the research design

C Set of regulations which must always be followed in the implementation phase

D Flexible and circular planning and decision-making process

5 A problem statement includes all of the following except:

A Justification for the study

B Population

C Statement of need

D Design

6 Abstracts of research reports include information about all of the following except:

A Purpose and importance of study

B Description of methods

C Overall project costs

D Highlights of data analysis

Consider the following hypothesis in answering questions 7 and 8:
"Patients with type 2 diabetes who receive instruction on an individual basis will be more compliant than those who receive instruction in a group setting."

7 What is the dependent variable in the hypothesis above?

A Type 2 diabetes mellitus

B Individual versus group setting

C Type of instruction undergone

D Patient compliance

8 What is the independent variable?

A Type 2 diabetes mellitus

B Individual versus group setting

C Content of instruction undergone

D Patient compliance

9 Where in the research report would you expect to find the following statement: *"The study was conducted within the Grady Health Systems, a public health-care facility serving 2 urban counties in Atlanta."*

A Introduction

B Methods

C Results

D Conclusions

10 Where in the research report would you expect to find the following statement: *"The purpose of this study was to examine the relationship between care-giving burden and social support in spouses of individuals with type 1 diabetes."*

A Introduction

B Methods

C Results

D Conclusions

11 In choosing a quasi-experimental design over a true experimental design, the researcher realizes that the study would involve less:
A Bias
B Control
C Rigor
D Significance

12 A correlational study identifies:
A Relationships among variables
B Causal link between an independent variable and an outcome
C Difference between an independent and dependent variable
D The effect of 1 variable on another

13 Choosing a validated instrument as an outcome measure provides:
A Confidence in the results
B Reliable results regardless of when the instrument is administered
C A biased sampling of the target population
D Qualitative research data

14 The purpose of an operational definition is to:
A Assign numerical values to investigational variables
B Specify how variables will be explained and measured
C Stipulate expected relationship between the variables
D Designate the overall plan which drives the research

See next page for answer key.

Post-Test Answer Key

The Importance of Research

8

1	C	**8**	B
2	B	**9**	B
3	B	**10**	A
4	D	**11**	B
5	D	**12**	A
6	C	**13**	A
7	D	**14**	B

A Core Curriculum for Diabetes Education
Diabetes in the Life Cycle and Research

Index

Copyright Permission

a CORE Curriculum for Diabetes Education, 5th Edition
American Association of Diabetes Educators

Contact: AADE, 800/338-3633; fax 312/424-2427

The information contained in a CORE Curriculum for Diabetes Education, 5th Edition, is based on the collective experience of the diabetes educators who assisted in its production. Reasonable steps have been taken to make it as accurate as possible based on published evidence as of June 2003. But the Association cannot warrant the safety or efficacy of any product or procedure described in a CORE Curriculum for Diabetes Education, 5th Edition, for application in specific cases. Individuals are advised to consult an appropriate healthcare professional before undertaking any diet or exercise program or taking any medication referred to in a CORE Curriculum for Diabetes Education, 5th Edition. Healthcare professionals must use their own professional judgment, experience, and training in applying the information contained herein. The American Association of Diabetes Educators and its officers, directors, employees, agents, and members assume no liability whatsoever for any personal or other injury, loss, or damages that may result from use of a CORE Curriculum for Diabetes Education, 5th Edition.

TO WHOM IT MAY CONCERN:
Permission is hereby granted from the American Association of Diabetes Educators under the following terms:

ISSN/ISBN #1-881876-15-2

Book Title: _____

Chapter Title: _____

Page Numbers: _____

Permission Granted To: _____

Permission is granted for one-time use only and for educational purposes only.

Complete credit line should appear on all reproductions as follows:
"Reprinted with permission from A Core Curriculum for Diabetes Education, copyright _____, the American Association of Diabetes Educators."

_____   _____
AADE PUBLISHER   DATE